T0275705

NEURAL NETWORKS AND PSYCHOPATHOLOGY

Connectionist models in practice and research

Research on connectionist models is one of the most exciting areas in cognitive science, and neural network models of psychopathology have immediate theoretical and empirical appeal. This volume aims to bring clinicians and computer modellers into closer contact, recognizing that clinical science often lacks an adequate theoretical framework for integrating neurobiological and psychological data, while neural networks, which have been tremendously successful in modelling a range of important psychological phenomena, have focused less on models of psychopathology.

The contributors to this pioneering book review theoretical, historical and clinical issues, including the contribution of neural network models to diagnosis, pharmacotherapy and psychotherapy. Models are presented for a range of disorders, including schizophrenia, obsessive–compulsive disorder, dissociative phenomena, autism and Alzheimer's disease.

This book will appeal to a broad audience. On the one hand, it will be read with interest by psychiatrists, psychologists and other clinicians and researchers in psychopathology. On the other, it will appeal to those working in cognitive science and artificial intelligence, and particularly those interested in neural network or connectionist models.

DAN J. STEIN is Director of the MRC Research Unit on Anxiety and Stress Disorders in the Department of Psychiatry, University of Stellenbosch, South Africa.

JACQUES LUDIK is Senior Lecturer in the Department of Computer Science, University of Stellenbosch, South Africa.

NEURAL NETWORKS AND PSYCHOPATHOLOGY

Connectionist models in practice and research

DAN J. STEIN

Department of Psychiatry
University of Stellenbosch

JACQUES LUDIK

Department of Computer Science
University of Stellenbosch

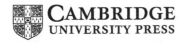

CAMBRIDGE
UNIVERSITY PRESS

CAMBRIDGE UNIVERSITY PRESS
Cambridge, New York, Melbourne, Madrid, Cape Town, Singapore, São Paulo

Cambridge University Press
The Edinburgh Building, Cambridge CB2 2RU, UK

Published in the United States of America by Cambridge University Press, New York

www.cambridge.org
Information on this title: www.cambridge.org/9780521571630

First published 1998
This digitally printed first paperback version 2007

A catalogue record for this publication is available from the British Library

Library of Congress Cataloguing in Publication data

Neural networks and psychopathology : connectionist models in practice
and research/ [edited by] Dan J. Stein, Jacques Ludik.
    p. cm.
Includes index.
ISBN 0 521 57163 4 (hardback)
1. Psychology, Pathological–Computer simulation.   2. Neural
networks (Neurobiology).   3. Cognitive psychology.   4. Neural
networks (Computer science).   I. Stein, Dan J.   II. Ludik, Jacques,
1960–
    [DNLM: 1. Mental Disorders–physiopathology.   2. Neural Networks
(Computer)   3. Mental Disorders–diagnosis.   4. Mental Disorders–
therapy.   5. Psychopathology–methods.   WM 140 N494 1998]
RC455.2.D38N48   1998
616.89–dc21
DNLM/DLC
for Library of Congress 98-5826 CIP

ISBN-13 978-0-521-57163-0 hardback
ISBN-10 0-521-57163-4 hardback

ISBN-13 978-0-521-03606-1 paperback
ISBN-10 0-521-03606-2 paperback

For our families, with thanks for their support.
D.J.S.
J.L.

Contents

Contributors

German E. Berrios
Department of Psychiatry, University of Cambridge, Addenbrooke's Hospital, Cambridge CB2 2QQ, UK

Franz Caspar
Institute of Psychology, University of Bern, Muesmattstrasse 45, 3000 Bern 9, and Psychiatric Hospital Sanatorium Kilchberg, Switzerland

Eric Y. H. Chen
Department of Psychiatry, University of Hong Kong, Hong Kong

Ira L. Cohen
Division of Behavioral Assessment and Research, Institute for Basic Research in Developmental Disabilities, 1050 Forest Hill Road, Staten Island, NY 10314-6399, USA

David V. Forrest
New York State Psychiatric Institute, 722 W. 168th Street, New York, NY 10032, USA

Michael E. Hasselmo
Department of Psychology, Harvard University, 33 Kirkland Street, Cambridge, MA 02138, USA

David Hestenes
Arizona State University, Tempe, AZ 85287, USA

Dan Lloyd
Department of Philosophy, Trinity College, 300 Summit Street, Hartford, CT 06106, USA

Jacques Ludik
Department of Computer Science, University of Stellenbosch, PO Box 19063, Tygerberg 7505, South Africa

S. B. G. Park
*University Department of Psychiatry, Duncan Macmillan House,
Porchester Road, Nottingham NG3 6AA, UK*

John H. Poole
*San Francisco Veterans Administration Medical Center – 116C, 4150
Clement Street, San Francisco, CA 94121, USA*

Manfred Spitzer
*Universitätsklinikum Ulm, Abteilung Psychiatrie 111, Leimgrubenweg 12–
14, 89075 Ulm, Germany*

Dan J. Stein
*Department of Psychiatry, University of Stellenbosch, PO Box 19063,
Tygerberg 7505, South Africa*

Sophia Vinogradov
*San Francisco Veterans Administration Medical Center – 116C, 4150
Clement Street, San Francisco, CA 94121, USA*

Gene V. Wallenstein
*Department of Psychology, Harvard University, 33 Kirkland Street,
Cambridge, MA 02138, USA*

Jason Willis-Shore
*San Francisco Veterans Administration Medical Center – 116C, 4150
Clement Street, San Francisco, CA 94121, USA*

Preface

This volume of essays on neural networks and psychopathology is aimed at an unusually diverse audience. On the one hand, we hope that the volume will be read by psychiatrists, psychologists, and other clinicians and researchers interested in psychopathology and its treatment. On the other hand, we hope that it will be read by those who work in the fields of cognitive science and artificial intelligence, and particularly those interested in neural network or connectionist models.

We believe that it is timely for clinicians and computational modellers to be in closer contact. While recent decades have seen dramatic advances in pharmacological and psychological treatments of psychiatric disorders, clinical science often lacks an adequate theoretical framework for integrating neurobiological and psychological data. Conversely, while neural networks have been tremendously successful in modelling a range of important psychological phenomena and in analysing data from a wide range of other sciences, less work has focused on connectionist models of psychopathology.

Neural network models of psychopathology have immediate theoretical and empirical appeal. They are theoretically interesting because they seem to incorporate neurobiological and psychological data in a seamless model of the way in which representational processes emerge from assemblies of neuron-like processing elements. They are empirically useful because they have been able to allow rigorous and elegant simulations of such uniquely human phenomena as pattern recognition, categorization, and learning; simulations that have in turn led to new insights into the phenomena under study.

In aiming at a diverse audience, contributors to this volume have had to tread a fine line between ensuring that their chapters are not only relevant to clinical practice and research, but also tackle basic questions about how the brain–mind works and about how best this can be operationalized using computational models. Any such pioneering attempt to straddle two such different camps runs the risk of drawing criticism from some clinicians who find that computational models are too removed from clinical experience, or from some cognitivists who find clinical phenomena abstruse.

However, we believe that our contributors have succeeded remarkably in reaching out to all members of the intended audience. An introductory chapter by Stein and Ludik introduces the concept of neural networks and considers some of the potentials and pitfalls of using connectionist models to investigate psychopathology. In a second background chapter, Spitzer provides important historical context, outlining the long use of neural networks in clinical theory. For example, in his abandoned 'Project for a scientific psychology', Freud drew on the neuroscience of his day to develop an approach that is in many ways reminiscent of current connectionism.

Other contributions in Part one of the volume show how neural network models may have value in several different arenas of clinical practice and research. These range from diagnosis (Chen and Berrios) to pharmacotherapy (Park) and psychotherapy (Caspar). Hestenes concludes this part of the volume with an overview of the implications of neural network theory for approaching the neurobiology of clinical disorders.

In the second part of the volume, contributors develop models of a range of different clinical disorders. These include examples from the psychotic, anxiety, dissociative, and cognitive psychiatric disorders. Specifically, models are provided for schizophrenia (Chen and Berrios; Vinogradov and colleagues), obsessive–compulsive disorder (Ludik and Stein), dissociative phenomena (Lloyd), autism (Cohen), and Alzheimer's disease (Wallenstein and Hasselmo).

Finally, Forrest, who has long been working at the interface of neural networks and psychiatry, provides an epilogue and a vision for the future.

We hope that this brief outline of the volume sufficiently whets the appetite of both clinicians and connectionists to pursue the exciting interchange between these fields more fully. Ultimately, we look forward to the development of a strong field of cognitive clinical science, in which computational models inform clinical practice and research, and in which clinical data provide an important impetus for work in connectionism.

It is left only for us to add a few brief words of thanks. First, to each of the contributors for their generous participation in this volume. Second, to our publisher director, Dr Richard Barling, who provided sound advice throughout the project. Third, to the many colleagues who have supported our work, particularly Professor Robin Emsley, Head of the Department of Psychiatry at the University of Stellenbosch. And finally, to our wives and families, who have always been supportive and encouraging of our academic lives.

Dan J. Stein
Jacques Ludik

Part one

General concepts

1

Neural networks and psychopathology: an introduction

DAN J. STEIN and JACQUES LUDIK

The recent shift in psychiatry from a predominantly psychodynamic model towards a neurobiological paradigm has led to important advances in our understanding and management of many mental disorders. At the same time, this shift has been characterized as a move from a brainless psychiatry to a mindless one (Lipowski, 1989). Certainly, the continued existence of different psychiatric schools with widely divergent approaches to psychopathology and its treatment suggests that psychiatry continues to lack an adequate theoretical underpinning.

During the same time that psychiatry has undergone a paradigm shift, academic psychology has also experienced a revolution – the so-called cognitive revolution against behaviorism (Gardner, 1985). Cognitive science, a multidisciplinary arena encompassing cognitive psychology, artificial intelligence, neuroscience, linguistics, anthropology, and philosophy, and based on computational models of the mind, is now a predominant approach. Not surprisingly, clinicians have asked whether the constructs and methods of cognitive science are also applicable to psychopathology.

Indeed, a promising dialogue between clinical and cognitive science has emerged (Stein and Young, 1992). Both cognitive–behavioral therapists and psychodynamic researchers have increasingly drawn on cognitivist work in their theoretical and empirical studies of psychopathology and psychotherapy. Schema theory, for example, has been applied to a range of clinical phenomena (Stein, 1992). Such cognitivist work is often immediately attractive to the clinician insofar as it incorporates a range of theoretical disciplines and insofar as it is based on hard empirical studies.

One of the most important developments in modern cognitive science has been connectionism, the field concerned with neural network models (Rumelhart et al., 1986a). Whereas early work in cognitive science

3

emphasized 'top-down' symbolic architectures and the manipulation of mental representations, connectionism has focused on 'bottom-up' models that specify the interactions of simple processing units. In contrast to the serial processing of traditional symbolic models, in neural networks information processing occurs simultaneously in all units (parallel distributed processing). Increasingly, neural networks are being applied in the clinical arena, again offering the clinician a set of constructs and methods that seem sophisticated and robust (Hoffman, 1987; Park and Young, 1994).

This book provides a forum for the presentation of pioneering work at the intersection of clinical science and connectionism. This introductory chapter details some of the defining features of the connectionist paradigm, and considers some of the advantages and possible limitations of this approach for clinical science.

Features of neural networks

Connectionist models focus on sets of processing units (idealized neurons) and their interactions. Some of the earliest connectionist work was done by Donald Hebb (1949) in his speculations about the basis of neuronal functioning. He put forward the idea of cell assemblies, and proposed that simultaneous activation of two cells resulted in strengthening of their connection (Hebb's rule). Other theorists helped develop sophisticated mathematical theories to describe such neuronal networks (Grossberg, 1980; McCulloch and Pitts, 1943; Rosenblatt, 1962; Selfridge and Neisser, 1960), and the development of modern computers allowed ready implementation of detailed connectionist models.

Any particular neural network model can be described in terms of its specific processing units, the way these are put together, and the way in which they learn (Hanson and Burr, 1990). Like neurons, each unit has inputs (dendrites) from other units, and outputs (axons) to other units. Each input has a particular weight (synapse), which can be positive (excitatory) or negative (inhibitory). Whether or not a unit is activated is determined by this net input and by its current activation.

The topology of a neural network is the way in which units are joined to one another. In a totally connected network, such as the Hopfield network (Hopfield, 1982, 1984), all units are connected to one another (Fig. 1.1). In a feedforward unit, information flows in only one direction, from input units to output units. In multilayer networks, there are also hidden units between input and output units (Fig. 1.2).

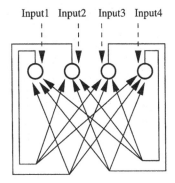

Fig. 1.1 A Hopfield neural network in which all units are connected to one another.

Learning takes place in networks via modification of synaptic weights. Neural networks, for example, can be trained to associate particular input patterns with particular output patterns. During training, input patterns are presented and synaptic weights are changed according to a learning rule. In a multilayer network, error can be measured across the output units and then compensatory changes can be made at each level of the network (back-propagation).

How are memories stored in a network? Many networks can be conceptualized as constraint networks in which each unit represents a hypothesis (i.e., a feature of the input), and in which each connection represents constraints among the hypotheses (Rumelhart et al., 1986b). A variation of Hebb's rule, for example, states that if features A and B often co-exist, then the connection between the two will be positive. On the other hand, when the two features exclude one another, then the connection will be negative. When the network runs, it settles into a locally optimal state in which as many as possible of the constraints are satisfied.

The information processing of a network from state to state can be conceptualized in terms of movement over a goodness-of-fit landscape (Rumelhart et al., 1986b). The system processes input by shifting from state to state until it reaches a state of maximal constraint satisfaction, that is, it climbs upward until it reaches a goodness maximum. A landscape can be described in terms of the set of maxima which the system can find, the size of the region that feeds into each maximum, and the height

Dan J. Stein and Jacques Ludik

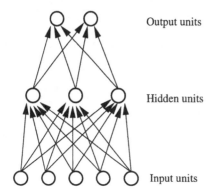

Output units

Hidden units

Input units

Fig. 1.2 A multilayer neural network in which hidden units intervene between input and output unit.

of the maximum itself (Fig. 1.3). The positions of the system correspond to the possible interpretations, the peaks in the space correspond to the best interpretations, the extent of the foothills surrounding a particular peak determines the likelihood of finding the peak, and the height of the peak corresponds to the degree that the constraints of the network are actually met (Rumelhart et al., 1986b).

Schemas versus neural networks

Characterizing neural networks in terms of a goodness-of-fit landscape has immediate intuitive appeal. This characterization allows neural networks to be compared with schemas – cognitivist constructs that are, as noted earlier, increasingly familiar to clinicians. A schema is a prototypical abstraction that develops from past experience and that guides the organization of new information (Thorndyke and Hayes-Roth, 1979; Stein, 1992). Schemas allow rapid processing of information, but also result in typical biases (Winfrey and Goldfried, 1986).

Similarly, a particular neural network, prompted by a given set of data, rapidly moves toward a previously acquired landscape. This allows rapid information processing, but, again, may result in certain distortions (Rumelhart et al., 1986b). This view of schemas is perhaps more fluid than the conventional one; for example, schemas can be defined as inflexible (narrow peaks in the goodness-of-fit landscape) or more flexible (with

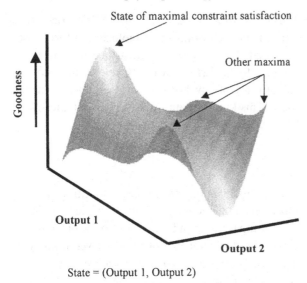

State = (Output 1, Output 2)

Fig. 1.3 The goodness-of-fit landscape for a neural network as function of the activation of two output units. A state is represented here by an (output 1, output 2) pair. For every state of the network, the pattern of inputs and connection weights determines a value of the goodness-of-fit function. The network processes its input by moving upward from state to state until it reaches a state of maximum goodness.

broad plateaus allowing for movement in the region of the maximum) (Rumelhart et al., 1986b).

Consider, for example, a woman who has been abused in childhood. She may develop a mistrust schema according to which others are not easily to be trusted. She is consequently liable to bias her interpretation of reality in particular ways, perhaps drawing false generalizations about authority figures or viewing neutral situations as unsafe. Both schemas and neural networks provide a way of explaining how such biases are 'built in', without having to rely on explicit cognitive rules.

Rumelhart et al. (1986b) conclude that the relationship between neural network models and schema models is largely a matter of a different degree of analysis. Whereas schema models are predominantly 'top-down' in their approach, neural network models work from the 'bottom-up'. An advantage of the neural network approach is its ability to demonstrate in fine detail how cognitive phenomena emerge from interactions of simple elements of the system.

Similarly, in the clinical situation, the neural network approach may allow a better understanding of the microstructure of schemas. While schemas have allowed an integration of different kinds of theories, they have been less successful at incorporating neurobiological information than some would have hoped. For example, while a theory of mistrust schemas does exist (Young, 1990), this is not easily able to incorporate such clinical data as the efficacy of psychotropic medication in patients with personality disorders. This kind of data might be better understood if the cognitivist model used was a bottom-up one.

The grounding problem

Why should neural network modelers pay attention to clinical science? It may be argued that clinical phenomena are particularly challenging insofar as they necessarily encompass a broad range of levels of analysis. Thus, it may be argued that such phenomena demand a level of analysis that extracts the maximum potential from cognitive science.

There remains, for example, a basic problem in cognitive science that may be characterized (following Harnad, 1990) as the symbol-grounding problem. This concerns how the meanings of the symbols in a system can be grounded so that they have meaning independently of an external interpreter. This problem may lie at the heart of a number of important debates in cognitive science.

Consider, for example, Searle's (1980) well-known argument against symbolic models of the mind. Searle notes that while a Turing computer could conceivably implement a range of rules necessary for translating Chinese symbols into English ones, it cannot be argued that this computer understands Chinese. For example, while it might be possible for a person to memorize all the syntactical rules employed by such a program, this would not necessarily mean that the person had a grasp of the semantic meanings of Chinese.

Similarly, a range of so-called situated cognitivists argue against conventional symbolic cognition (Norman, 1993). Symbolic cognitivists hold that cognitive processing essentially involves the manipulation of symbols, and that the task of cognitive science is to provide formalized descriptions of these transformations. Situational cognitivists hold that cognitive processes necessarily take place within a particular interactive social context, and that the task of cognitive science is to understand how cognitive processes are situated in experience.

A clinical example may be useful here. Consider once again the mistrustful patient. In a pioneering project in early artificial intelligence, Colby (1981) developed a computer program, PARRY, which simulated paranoid thought processes. The program relied on a symbolic architecture, and incorporated a number of rules that governed the manipulation of symbols. For example, one rule stated that when self-esteem score decreased, level of suspicion would be increased. PARRY was highly successful insofar as experienced clinicians interacting with it were sometimes unable to tell whether they were dealing with a computer or with a person (the Turing Test).

From Searle's perspective, however, the claim that PARRY is in fact paranoid should not be taken seriously. PARRY is a computer program that implements syntactic rules, but that lacks semantic understanding and intentionality. Similarly, from the perspective of a situated cognitivist, although it might be conceded that PARRY devotes attention to the interpersonal context of paranoid behavior, its focus on the manipulation of symbols means that it ultimately fails to come to terms fully with this phenomenon.

Indeed, from a clinical viewpoint, although PARRY was a pioneering contribution to the intersection between clinical and cognitive science, and although it provided an interesting hypothesis for and test of the cognitive processes underlying paranoia, its success was only partial. In particular, PARRY ignored many aspects of the clinical phenomenon of paranoid thinking, including data on the neurobiology of psychosis. Ultimately, PARRY was unable to explain the underlying mechanisms upon which its rules were based.

Harnad (1989) has proposed a variant of the Turing Test, the Total Turing Test (TTT), in order to help solve the symbol-grounding problem. In addition to simulation of pen-pal (symbolic) interactions, passing the TTT demands simulation of 'robotic capacity' – all of our sensorimotor capacity to discriminate, recognize, identify, manipulate, and describe the world we live in. Harnad argues that a system is grounded only when it has the symbolic and robotic capacity to pass the TTT in a coherent way, that is when its symbolic capacity is grounded in its robotic capacity rather than being mediated by an outside interpretation projected onto it.

To return to the Chinese room, the question is no longer whether the Turing Test candidate really understands Chinese or can merely be interpreted as if he or she were understanding it, but rather whether the TTT candidate (a robot with optical transducers) really sees the Chinese letters and really writes the English version down or whether it is merely interpretable as if it were doing this. If Searle now attempted to implement the

TTT candidate without seeing or writing (as he attempted to implement the TT candidate without understanding), this would be impossible.

Insofar as real transduction is essential to TTT capacity, a TTT candidate would satisfy the demands of a situated cognitivist. This candidate would not simply be manipulating symbols, but would in fact demonstrate cognitive processes that were situated in experience. Such cognitive processes could no longer be said to be independent of their physical instantiations (as symbolic cognitivists are so fond of averring).

Similarly, from a clinical viewpoint, modeling sensory transduction is indeed necessary if psychopathological phenomena such as paranoia are to be fully understood. Cognitive clinical science needs to take cognizance of the growing emphasis by cognitivists on the embodiment of cognition (Lakoff, 1987), both in the sense of being embodied within the physicality of the brain and in the sense of being embodied within particular social situations. Given the increased understanding of the neurobiology underlying psychopathology, models that incorporate this kind of understanding may well be possible.

Consider, for instance, a pioneering example of work at the intersection of connectionism and the clinic, the research of Jonathan Cohen and David Servan-Schreiber (1992) on schizophrenia. In their model of this disorder they model how changes in neurotransmitter function (dopamine gain) result in dysfunction on neuropsychological testing. The model therefore moves toward providing a seamless integration of the neurobiology and psychology of this complex disorder. Although the model only attempts to cover limited aspects of schizophrenia and could not pass the TTT, it does not simply involve syntactic rule transformation, and it provides a preliminary account of how psychopathological processes in schizophrenia are in fact embodied.

Some difficulties

Different kinds of neural network models may be applicable to different arenas within psychiatry. For example, there is currently work on neural network approaches to diagnosis (see Chapter 3), neural network modeling of psychopharmacological data (see Chapter 4), and neural network modeling of psychotherapeutic processes (See Chapter 5) and psychodynamic phenomena (see Chapter 10). Nevertheless, much work follows the pioneering lines taken by Hoffman (1987) and Cohen and Servan-Schreiber (1992), in which 'lesions' to neural network models are made in the hope of simulating psychopathological data.

It may be argued that there remains an important disjunction between phenomena as they are witnessed by the clinician (e.g., schizophrenic delusions) and the kind of inputs and outputs that are processed by neural networks (e.g., numerical patterns, results on a neuropsychological test). Psychiatric research methodologies such as functional brain imaging are currently allowing insights into the concrete mechanisms that underlie specific clinical phenomena (e.g., basal ganglia activation in obsessions and compulsions); in contrast, neural networks are experience distant.

This distance between clinical experience and neural network analysis may also account for the worrying fact that particular neural networks are used by various authors to account for a range of different psychopathological phenomena. For example, Cohen and Servan-Schreiber's network for schizophrenia has also been used to account for other kinds of phenomena including obsessive–compulsive disorder (OCD). Certainly, a single neurotransmitter system may in fact be involved in several different psychiatric disorders. However, the use of a single neural network to explain diverse clinical phenomena also appears to suggest that it can explain everything.

To some extent, however, a similar issue arises in schema theory. Is there anything about minds that schema theory does not explain? Given that schemas and neural networks seem to incorporate general rules of cognition, their application to any clinical phenomena will perhaps always result in at least a partial ring of truth. The trick for future researchers will be to specify the details of these applications with increasing depth, so that specific differences in the neural networks/schemas of different clinical phenomena become increasingly clear.

So much for the issue of phenomenology. What are the objections that a strict neurobiological approach may have for neural network theory? It seems clear that many processes in the brain do operate according to the principles of parallel distributed processing. Nevertheless, neural network models of clinical phenomena typically fail to incorporate many of the fine details of neurobiological knowledge, and they may even directly contradict the findings of modern neuroscience. For example, the fact that units typically have both inhibitory and excitatory connections is at odds with neurobiological data that most neurons are either inhibitory or excitatory.

However, this criticism fails to take adequate account of the level of analysis that neural network models hope to achieve. While computational models of neurophysiological and neuropathological processes are often extremely relevant to psychiatry, neural networks that aim to model clinical phenomena often aim at a higher level of analysis. Certainly, they may aim to incorporate neurobiological data (e.g., Cohen and Servan-Schreiber (1992) attempt to integrate basic findings on dopamine), but this may ultimately be with the goal of understanding relevant cognitive processes (such as neuropsychological dysfunction in schizophrenia).

Nevertheless, it is true that by focusing on higher level processes, neural networks of psychopathology may lose detail. Neural network modelers of neurophysiological processes may find more clinically oriented neural networks too sketchy and vague. In the future, as our understanding of the neurobiology of psychiatric disorders grows, an attempt will need to be made to incorporate ever-more detailed neuro-physiologically based models into our connectionist work on clinical phenomena.

Work on the interface of two disparate disciplines is always open to attack by both fields. Neural network theorists may find the psychiatric phenomena of interest to clinicians overly nebulous, while clinicians may find the mathematics of neural network models somewhat esoteric. We hope that by providing concrete examples of interesting work at this intersection, we will be able to foster its growth and to temper this kind of criticism. Certainly, we hope that this volume will provide an impetus to both clinicians and cognitivitists to explore the potentially fertile intersection between these fields more fully.

Acknowledgment

Dr Stein is supported by a grant from the South African Medical Research Council.

References

Cohen, J.D. & Servan-Schreiber, D. (1992). Context, cortex, and dopamine: a connectionist approach to behavior and biology in schizophrenia. *Psychological Review*, **99**, 45–77.

Colby, K.M. (1981). Modeling a paranoid mind. *Behavioral Brain Science*, **4**, 515–60.

Gardner, H. (1985). *The Mind's New Science: A History of the Cognitive Revolution*. New York: Basic Books.

Grossberg, S. (1980). How does the brain build a cognitive code? *Psychological Review*, **87**, 1–51.

Hanson, S.J. & Burr, D.J. (1990). What connectionist models learn: learning and representation in connectionist networks. *Behavioral Brain Science*, **13**, 471–518.

Harnad, S. (1989). Minds, machines, and Searle. *Journal of Theoretical and Experimental Artificial Intelligence*, **1**, 5–25.

Harnad, S. (1990). The symbol grounding problem. *Physica*, **42**, 335–46.

Hebb, D.O. (1949). *The Organization of Behavior*. New York: Wiley.

Hoffman, R.E. (1987). Computer simulations of neural information processing and the schizophrenia–mania dichotomy. *Archives of General Psychiatry*, **44**, 178–88.

Hopfield, J.J. (1982). Neural networks and physical systems with emergent collective computational abilities. *Proceedings of the National Academy of Science*, **79**, 2554–8.

Hopfield, J.J. (1984). Collective processing and neural states. In *Modeling and Analysis in Biomedicine*, ed. C. Nicolini, pp. 369–89. New York: Elsevier Science.

Lakoff, G. (1987). *Women, Fire, and Dangerous Things: What Categories Reveal about the Mind*. Chicago: University of Chicago Press.

Lipowski, Z.J. (1989). Psychiatry: Mindless or brainless, both or neither. *Canadian Journal of Psychiatry*, **34**, 249–54.

McCulloch, W.S. & Pitts, W. (1943). A logical calculus of ideas immanent in nervous system activity. *Bulletin of Mathematical Physics*, **5**, 15–133.

Norman, D.A. (1993). Cognition in the head and in the world: An introduction to the special issue on situated action. *Cognitive Science*, **17**, 1–6.

Park, S.B.G. & Young, A.H. (1994). Connectionism and psychiatry: a brief review. *Philosophy, Psychiatry & Psychology*, **1**, 51–8.

Rosenblatt, F. (1962). *Principles of Neurodynamics*. New York: Spartan.

Rumelhart, D.E., Hinton, G.E. & The PDP Research Group (1986a). *Parallel Distributed Processing: Explorations in the Microstructure of Cognition*. Cambridge, MA: MIT Press.

Rumelhart, D.E., Smolensky, P., McClelland, J.L. & Hinton, G.E. (1986b). Schemata and sequential thought processes in PDP models. In *Parallel Distributed Processing: Explorations in the Microstructure of Cognition*, Vol. 2, ed. J.L. McClelland & D.E. Rumelhart, pp. 5–57. Cambridge, MA: MIT Press.

Searle, J.R. (1980). Minds, brains and programs. *Behavioral Brain Science*, **3**, 417–24.

Selfridge, O.G. & Neisser, U. (1960). Pattern recognition by machine. *Scientific American*, **203**, 60–8.

Stein, D.J. (1992). Schemas in the cognitive and clinical sciences: an integrative construct. *Journal of Psychotherapy Integration*, **2**, 45–63.

Stein, D.J. & Young, J.E. (1992). *Cognitive Science and Clinical Disorders*. San Diego: Academic Press.

Thorndyke, P.W. & Hayes-Roth, B. (1979). The use of schemata in the acquisition and transference of knowledge. *Cognitive Psychology*, **11**, 82–106.

Winfrey, L.P.L. & Goldfried, M.R. (1986). Information processing and the human change process. In *Information Processing Approaches to Clinical Psychology*, ed. R.E. Ingram, pp. 241–58. New York: Academic Press.

Young, J.E. (1990). *Cognitive Therapy for Personality Disorders: A Schema-focused Approach*. Sarasota: Professional Resource Exchange.

2

The history of neural network research in psychopathology

MANFRED SPITZER

Introduction

The use of neural networks for the study of psychopathological phenomena is not new, but rather has a rich historical tradition. One striking feature of this tradition is that from the very inception of the idea of the neuron, psychiatrists have used the notion of networks and their pathology to account for psychopathological phenomena. Moreover, many advances in neural network research were either made by psychiatrists or were put forward in relation to psychopathology. In other words, neural network studies of psychopathological phenomena are by no means a 'late add on' to the mainstream of neural network research, but have always been at the heart of the matter. Neural networks were drawn by Freud and Exner to explain disorders of cognition, affect and consciousness. Carl Wernicke (1906) coined the term 'Sejunktion' to denote the functional decoupling of cortical areas, which he suggested was the cause of psychotic symptoms such as hallucinations and delusions. Emil Kraepelin (1892) and his group of experimentally oriented psychiatrists reasoned about associative networks and psychosis. Not least, Eugen Bleuler (1911/1950) – inspired by the experimental work carried out by his resident Carl-Gustav Jung (1906/1979) – saw the disruption of these networks as the hallmark of schizophrenia.

Various developments in many fields have contributed to the present surge of neural network research. The historical material discussed in this chapter is organized by time and by topic.

Present-day connectionism takes it for granted that there are neurons, summing up action potentials coming via the connections among them, the synapses. These fundamental ideas, however, have their history, and are the starting point of this chapter. Some of these ideas, in turn, may be history in the near future, which is where the discussion ends.

From sponges to networks of neurons

The idea of a neural network is crucially dependent upon the idea of the neuron, which was not 'discovered' in a single act but rather was the result of a scientific battle that lasted for almost 100 years (cf. Breidbach, 1993; Dierig, 1993; Finger, 1994). In the 1830s, several authors (Christian Gottfried Ehrenberg, Jan Evangelista Purkyné, Gabriel Gustav Valentin) described 'ganglia-globules' (Ganglienkugeln) in various neural tissues, including the central nervous system. These globules were found to be enmeshed within a dense 'felt' of fibres, and the question of the exact nature of globules and fibres arose. A few years later, the globules were identified as ganglia cells within the framework of the newly developed general cell theory of tissue and pathology by Rudolf Virchow. In 1844, Robert Remak published the first drawings of ganglia cells, which clearly showed vermiform projections containing fibres, and in a paper published by Otto Friedrich Karl Deiters in 1865 (two years after his death), axons and dendrites were distinguished for the first time.

Paralleling the increasing anatomical detail, functional aspects of neuronal tissue were also worked out. In 1846, Rudolf Wagner proposed the first reflex arc of a sensory fibre to the spinal cord to motor neurons. Studies of degenerating fibres after experimental nerve injuries clarified that fibres were dependent upon cell bodies. These observations led Wilhelm His, in 1886, to postulate that any nerve fibre comes from a single cell: the neuron was born but did not yet have a name. Five years after its birth, the nerve cell was baptized 'neuron' in a highly influential paper written by the German anatomist Heinrich Wilhelm Gottfried Waldeyer, and published in the *Deutsche Medizinische Wochenschrift*, a weekly medical journal, in October 1891.

In an ironic twist of history, the man who made the most crucial discovery in the field was also the one who drew the decisively wrong conclusions from his ensuing observations. The Italian physician Camilo Golgi had been trying to stain the meninges. By accident, he thereby discovered that silver stains have the peculiar feature of making only one in about 100 neurons visible, offering unprecedented detail. Golgi used the technique to describe nervous tissue in detail, concluding that fibres grow into each other and thereby form direct connections.

It was the Spanish neuroanatomist Santiago Ramón y Cahal who noticed that neurons do not, as Golgi maintained, form a sponge-like seamless structure, a syncytium, but rather are discrete entities. Ramón y Cahal noticed that there were gaps between the ends of nerve fibres –

slightly thickened, button-like structures – and the adjacent cells. Both
Golgi and Ramón y Cahal received the Nobel Prize in 1906, but even at
that time they were still engaged in fierce debates. Golgi just could not
accept the notion developed by his Spanish colleague. In particular, he
did not accept that there were gaps between neurons, which already had
been christened 'Synapse' in 1897 by Sir Charles Scott Sherrington.

From associated ideas to associated neurons

The concept of the neuron was highly successful. Within a few years after
its inception and naming, it conquered the imagination of scientists and
physicians. Consider the writings of Sigmund Freud and Sigmund Exner,
prime examples in point.

Exner was a physiologist and in 1894 published a monograph, entitled
Project for Physiological Explanations of Mental Phenomena, which contains an impressive number of drawings of neural networks, meant to
bring about various mental phenomena (Figs. 2.1 and 2.2). Freud worked

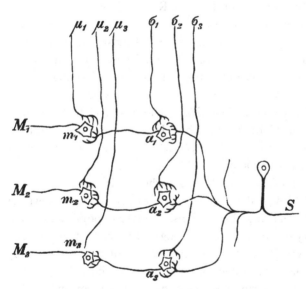

Fig. 2.1 Neural network drawn by Sigmund Exner (1894, p. 164). The schema is
supposed to account for the effect of selective attention on choice reaction time
experiments. Sensory input (S) is flowing in from the right to sensory cells (a_1, a_2
and a_3) and relayed to motor output cells (m_1, m_2 and m_3) on the left. The
processing of specific inputs can be primed, according to Exner, by additional
input from higher centres (Exner refers to them as the 'organ of consciousness')
either to the sensory input layer or to the motor output layer (cells μ and σ).

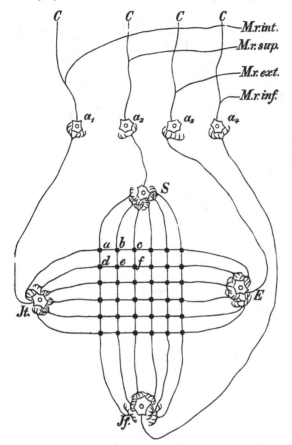

Fig. 2.2 Neural network by Exner (1894, p. 193), which was meant to explain visual motion detection. The dot-like connections in the lower half of the drawing closely ressemble modern recurrent networks as described by Hopfield in 1982.

as a neurologist in private practice and had a background in neuroanatomy from his work at the University of Vienna. In 1895, he was trying very hard to incorporate the latest neuroscience research findings into a treatise on psychological functions. He sent the chapters of the book in the form of letters to his friend Wilhelm Fliess, and these were later published as *Project for a Scientific Psychology*. In this book Freud produced drawings of networks of neurons carrying out specific functions (Fig. 2.3). The entire idea was later abandoned, possibly because Freud felt that there was not enough neuroscientific evidence for such a neurocognitive theory. Freud therefore rewrote his entire theory using purely psychological terms.

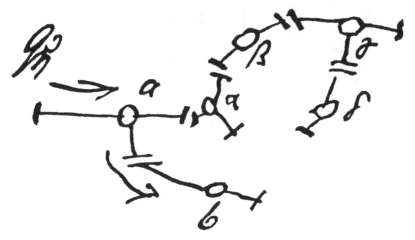

Fig. 2.3 Neural network drawn by Sigmund Freud in 1895. The arrow on the left marks incoming energy, which is rerouted within the network to a side-chain of associated neurons. Freud links these neurophysiological concepts with the associations of ideas that can sidetrack to unusual contents.

As has been pointed out by a number of authors, *The Interpretation of Dreams*, Freud's first major work on the foundations of psychoanalysis, is in many respects a neurocognitive model in the disguise of psychological theory (Pribram & Gill, 1976; Hobson and McCarley, 1977; Sulloway, 1984).

The concept of neurons associated with each other to form larger networks was also highly successful. One of the reasons for this success was that the idea fell on the highly fertile and receptive ground of *association psychology*, the major scientific paradigm within the newly established science of psychology during the last two decades of the 1800s. On the shoulders of associationist ideas which had been around for centuries, the technique of word associations had just been introduced in 1879 by Francis Galton, who had already come very close to the concept of the unconscious as we know it from the writings of Freud (Spitzer, 1992). It is likely that Freud knew Galton's work on associations, although he did not mention Galton in this respect and claims to have developed the method of free associations by 'following a dark presentiment' (Jones, 1978; p. 293). The similarities between Galton and Freud are, at any rate, striking.

Regarding the very young discipline of academic psychology, Wilhelm Wundt founded the world's first psychological laboratory in Leipzig,

Germany, in 1879. In this laboratory a great deal of research on associations was either performed or stimulated. Emil Kraepelin worked in Wundt's laboratory, and was not only highly influenced by the empirical spirit of Wundt (Spitzer and Mundt, 1994), but also was able to use some of the methods developed in Wundt's laboratory for purposes of experimental psycho*patho*logy. It is beyond the scope of this chapter even to summarize the enormous work on the associations of normal people done by psychiatrists in the two decades before and after 1900 (Spitzer, 1992). To mention just a few examples: Kraepelin studied the effects of drugs on word associations, and his disciple, Gustav Aschaffenburg, pursued research on the effects of fatigue. Carl-Gustav Jung performed similar experimental studies, and applied the dual task method to research on attentional effects on word associations.

As mentioned above, with the advent of physiology and neuroanatomy, the term 'association' gained a new 'biological' meaning: Not ideas, but rather brain parts – neurons – were thought to be associated, i.e. connected in a specific way. As the then leading American psychologist William James put it, '. . . so far as association stands for a *cause*, it is between *processes in the brain* . . .' (James, 1892/1984; p. 225 – italics in original). James avoided any reference to ideas but mentions the *brain*. However, it is important to note that the flow of *ideas* was the very subject of his discussion. In his review of the actual laws of associations, however, James nonetheless used mentalistic terms. It is therefore obvious that his explicit 'reductive' approach was merely a programme and not a finding. The law of contiguity, for example, was introduced as follows:

. . . objects once experienced together tend to become associated in the imagination, so that when any one of them is thought of, the others are likely to be thought of also . . . the most natural way to account for it [the law] is to conceive it as a result of the laws of habit in the nervous system; in other words, it is to ascribe it to a physiological cause.
(James, 1890/1983; p. 529)

As can be seen, a mentalistic description of the association law is given first, and then a physiological cause is stipulated. Along the same lines, the arguments in Exner's and Freud's *Projects* were constructed. Similarly, Carl Wernicke (1906) wrote his famous textbook of psychiatry, arguing that hallucinations and delusions were the result of the severing of connections between association areas of the human cortex ('sejunction'). These approaches remained speculative, as no one had developed a theoretical understanding of how associations of neurons were related to associations of ideas. This is probably the main reason why association psychology, in spite of the many bright minds working on it and the many papers published, was abandoned by the second decade of the 1900s. In fact, it took the idea of neural networks to bridge the very gap between the associated neuron and the associated idea, a gap that became evident 100 years ago.

From energy to information

The problem of linking the association of concepts to the association of nerve cells has been a major motivational force for the development of neuroscience in the twentieth century. Exner, Freud, and James, as we have already seen, could merely stipulate such links.

The first attempt to bridge mind and matter on a neuronal basis was made by McCulloch and Pitts (1943/1988). Quite strikingly, the particular assumptions about the functioning of neurons that were made by these authors in their famous paper, 'A logical calculus of the ideas immanent in nervous activity', later turned out to be wrong. However, McCulloch and Pitts were able to show that neurons could be conceived of as computing devices capable of performing propositional logic. In this view, neurons were no longer capacitors storing energy, with cables attached to them conducting energy. Instead, they were switches that corresponded to logical propositions, and fibres were links between those switches. A neural network was therefore no longer a device for handling energy, but became a device for handling information. The importance of this conceptual change cannot be overestimated.

It was clear to McCulloch and Pitts that this view had to have profound consequences for any attempt to understand how the mind works, including malfunction. In the very paper in which the idea of the neuron as information-processing device was proposed, the authors commented on psychopathological phenomena. Referring to 'tinnitus paraesthesias, hallucinations, delusions, confusions and disorientations' (p. 25), they claim that their account of the functioning of neuronal assemblies allows for a physiological account of psychopathology: 'Certainly for the psychiatrist, it is more to the point that in such systems "Mind" no longer "goes more ghostly than a ghost." Instead, diseased mentality can be understood without loss of scope or rigor, in the scientific terms of neurophysiology' (McCulloch & Pitts, 1943/1988, p. 25).

From Hebbian learning to long-term potentiation

William James clearly saw the necessity for change in mental associations and he speculated on brain processes that might account for it. Given that the word 'neuron' had not yet arrived from across the Atlantic Ocean, he wrote about 'points' within the cortex and their connections:

The amount of activity at any given point in the brain-cortex is the sum of the tendencies of all other points to discharge into it, such tendencies being proportionate (1) to the number of times the excitement of each other point may have accompanied that of the point in question; (2) to the intensity of such excitements; and (3) to the absence of any rival point functionally disconnected with the first point, into which the discharges might be diverted.
(James 1892/1984; p. 226)

James obviously foresaw an organizing principle of neural networks even before he knew about neurons. If we replace 'point' with 'neuron,' we get the idea that the activity of a neuron is equal to the sum of its weighted input. James even formulated a learning rule:

When two elementary brain processes have been active together or in immediate succession, one of them, on re-occurring, tends to propagate its excitement into the other.
(James, 1892/1984; p. 226)

Half a century later, the Canadian physician and psychologist Donald Hebb (1949/1988) built not only upon these ideas, but also upon the growing body of physiological knowledge. In 1949, he published a highly influential book entitled *The Organization of Behavior*, in which he speculated upon the workings of cell assemblies and proposed a mechanism by means of which associations of neurons could actually be influenced through experience. He clearly saw that neurons in brains need such a mechanism if learning is to be possible. Hebb outlined the operating principles of the 'association' of single nerve cells, the synapse, and developed a scheme of how such associations could be influenced by 'meaningful' associations, i.e. something to be learnt:

When an axon of cell A is near enough to excite a cell B and repeatedly or persistently takes part in firing it, some growth process or metabolic change takes place in one or both cells such that A's efficiency, as one of the cells firing B, is increased.
(Hebb, 1949/1988; S. 50)

Only seven years later, the first successful computer simulation of synaptic change in neural networks was reported (Rochester et al., 1956/1988), which implemented a slightly modified version of Hebb's idea. Neurons and connections were simulated, and patterns of coordinated activity appeared in the simulated 'cells' after learning had occurred. The mechanisms of such synaptic changes in biological cells were unknown at that time, however. Progress in this area was stimulated by the psychiatrist Eric Kandel, who used a very simple organism, the sea snail *Aplysia californica*, to show how learning and synaptic modification occur in parallel (for a review see Kandel, 1991). Once the connection between learning and synaptic change was clearly established, the mechanism of synaptic modification in more complex brains became the subject of intense study. In the early 1970s, experimental work on the hippocampus of rats first demonstrated the plasticity of synaptic connections caused by artificial neural excitation. The phenomenon was called long-term potentiation (LTP) and has since been the subject of intensive neurobiological research (Baudry and Davis, 1997). More recently, long-term depression (LTD) has been studied extensively and is now seen as the mirror image of LTP. Neither LTP nor LTD is restricted to the site where it was first discovered, the hippocampus and the cerebellum, but instead both have been shown to be much more widespread in the brain. Hence, these mechanisms of synaptic change are good candidates for the mechanisms needed to implement learning and memory in biological neural networks.

From computers and concepts to computer simulations

The history of neural network research, in a strict sense, began with the concepts just outlined and took off with the first neurocomputer, the *Mark I Perceptron*, developed by Frank Rosenblatt and coworkers at the Massachusetts Institute of Technology in 1957 and 1958 (Rosenblatt, 1958/1988). In the late 1950s and 1960s, neural network flourished during what is sometimes called the first blossom of neural network research (Zell, 1994). It was brought to a rather sudden end by the publication of a book entitled *Perceptrons* (Minsky and Papert, 1969), in which the authors pointed out several serious limitations of the networks then in use. As these limitations were widely believed to apply to neural networks in general and not just to the specific type the perceptron, neural network research was thought to be a 'dead end' and funding stopped almost completely.

The ensuing 12 to 15 years are now sometimes referred to as the quiet, or 'dark age' of neural network research, although several highly important papers were published (Anderson and Rosenfeld, 1988). In particular,

Stephen Grossberg (1980) published a number of innovative papers during this period.

The early phase of neural network research was done at a time when the conventional computer, as we all know it at present, was conceived. These digital computers not only served as tools for computing in research, but also were soon taken as models for any 'thinking machine,' including the brain. Named after the person whose brainchild it was, the von Neumann machine was the model for all computers. Most of the computers of the present day still work like the machines designed 40 years ago. It is important to discuss the main general features of these machines briefly, since neural networks, biological and simulated, are very different. These differences have driven neural networks to some extent, since it became increasingly obvious that computers are very much *unlike* brains.

In a conventional digital computer, information is processed serially, i.e. a central processing unit (CPU) handles a single 'chunk' of information at a time. To compensate for this limitation, such processing happens very quickly. Compared to the switching devices on silicon computer chips, neurons are terribly slow: for example, the computer used to type this chapter contains memory chips with a switching speed of less than a tenth of a microsecond (< 0.0000001 s), whereas neurons take a few milliseconds (> 0.001 s) to respond to input, i.e. to switch. If we take reaction time data from the experiments reported above and below as examples, i.e. reaction times as low as 500 ms, we can conclude that the neural algorithm which performs, for example, lexical decisions cannot consist of more than about a hundred consecutive steps (Rumelhart, 1989; p. 135). However, everyone who has some experience with computer programming knows that a 100-step program is far too limited to accomplish even quite simple tasks.

This directly implies that most psychological tasks cannot be performed by neurons working in the same manner as a personal computer. It is quite obvious that the rather slow neurons must work massively in parallel to perform the many computations necessary for even simple word-recognition or face-recognition experiments.

In addition to the argument from considerations of speed, a similar argument in favour of a parallel design for the associations-handling device called 'brain' can be made from considerations of precision. In a classic monograph, *The Computer and the Brain*, John von Neumann (1958) pointed out that the level of precision that can be accomplished by neurons is several orders of magnitude less than the level of precision that computers can achieve. This implies that long programs relying on many steps cannot possibly be handled by such systems because an error occurring within one such step will be easily propagated and multiplied in subsequent steps.

Computers may fail completely upon a single faulty connection. Brains, in striking contrast, show a more graceful degradation of function when neurons die. In fact, it is sometimes striking that patients with very little brain tissue left by a disease process are discovered by chance, i.e. these patients show very little, if any, cognitive impairment notwithstanding major brain defects.

For these reasons, although many psychological theories of the 1950s and 1960s took the computer as a metaphor for the mind, the idea that computers are very different from biological information-processing systems was gradually accepted by psychologists. However, it was not until the 1980s that the idea of neural networks, simulated by using conventional computers in a different way, became the new paradigm for research in cognitive neuroscience. In these networks, idealized neurons, i.e. computing devices, are supposed to be in a certain state of activity (represented by a number), and are connected to other neurons with connections of varying strength (also represented by a number). Hence the name connectionism for the entire approach to the architecture of ideal systems neurons. Because in these systems neurons work in parallel, and because the work is done in different locations (rather than in only a single CPU), the term parallel distributed processing (PDP) has been used to characterize these models. As David Rumelhart, a major proponent of the connectionist approach, has put it:

> The basic strategy of the connectionist approach is to take as its fundamental processing unit something close to an abstract neuron. We imagine that computation is carried out through simple interactions among such processing units. Essentially the idea is that these processing elements communicate by sending numbers along the lines that connect the processing elements. . . The operations in our models then can best be characterized as 'neurally inspired.' . . . all the knowledge is in the connections. From conventional programmable computers we are used to thinking of knowledge as being stored in the state of certain units in the system. . . This is a profound difference between our approach and other more conventional approaches, for it means that almost all knowledge is implicit in the structure of the device that carries out the task rather than explicit in the states of the units themselves.
> (Rumelhart, 1989; pp. 135–6)

At present, neural network models and simulations of cognitive functions are commonplace in psychology and neuroscience. The models vary a great deal in biological plausibility, complexity, specificity, and explanatory power. Further, they have been used in order to capture features of such different functions as language, attention, memory, and cognitive development. In the next sections, examples from psycho*pathol*ogy will be discussed.

From psychopathology to network dysfunction

There is hardly a psychopathological symptom or disorder for which no network models exist. This is surprising, since the field is only about ten years old. In 1987, the Yale psychiatrist Ralph Hoffman published the first major paper on neural network models of psychopathology. While he has refined his models in subsequent papers (Hoffman et al., 1995), his early work was a landmark in that it laid out how simulations and psychopathology could be linked.

Hoffman trained recurrent networks to store input patterns. In these networks every neuron is connected to every other neuron except itself. These connections make the network behave such that upon the presentation of an input it will settle into a certain state, which can be interpreted as the stored memory trace. Such recurrent networks have a certain capacity.

The way in which recurrent networks perform can be characterized by saying that upon the presentation of a given input, the pattern of activation of the neurons in the network converges to a specific output state, a stable activation pattern of the neurons in the network called attractors. If the sequence of states upon activation by an input is closely scrutinized, one observes that the pattern of activation changes such that it becomes increasingly like the stable state that most closely resembles the input pattern. The network converges to the attractor that is closest to the input pattern. All possible states of the network can be metaphorically likened to a landscape of energy, where the attractors form valleys between mountains of non-stable network states.

According to the simulations performed by Hoffman, information overload of the networks leads to network behaviour that can be likened to hallucinations in schizophrenic patients, in that the spontaneous activation of some stored patterns occurs. Hoffman describes how if real biological neural networks are diminished in size and for storage capacity by some pathological process, they can no longer handle the experiences of the person. Eventually, information overload will lead to the deformation of the landscape, described by Hoffman as follows:

Memory overload . . . causes distortions of energy contours of the system so that
gestalts no longer have a one-to-one correspondence with distinct, well delineated
energy minima.
(Hoffman, 1987; p. 180)

In addition to the deformation of the structure of the network, new
attractors are formed, which Hoffman called 'parasitic'. Such parasitic
attractors are produced by the amalgamation of many normal attractors,
whereby particularly stable attractors, i.e. 'deep valleys' in the energy
landscape, are produced. These deep valleys are therefore the end state
of the system starting out from a large number of positions. In this way,
these parasitic attractors are reached with almost any input to the system.
According to Hoffman, these attractors are the basis of voices and other
major symptoms of schizophrenia:

These parasitic states are the information processing equivalents of 'black holes in
space' and can markedly disrupt the integrity of neural network functioning by
inducing 'alien forces' that distort and control the flow of mentation. If a similar
reorganization of the schizophrenic's memory capabilities has taken place, it
would not be at all surprising for him to report one or more schneiderian symptoms, namely, that he no longer has control of his thoughts, or that his mind is
possessed by alien forces.
(Hoffman, 1987; p. 180)

Hoffman and coworkers (1995) have proposed other, more detailed
models of schizophrenic hallucinations that encompass the specific
effects of neuronal loss in the frontal lobes and the effects of dopamine.
Nonetheless, the model just discussed led to the development of an
entire new field, which may be called neurocomputational psychopathology.

From network dysfunction to neuropathology

In this section, the ideas of Michael Hasselmo, from Harvard University,
on network function are taken as an example of how detailed models of
computer-simulated neural networks can be used to understand patterns
of neuropathology.

Hasselmo starts with the fact that in neural network simulations the
learning phases have often to be distinguished from the retrieval phase.
During learning, the spreading of activation through the network must be
prevented to some degree, otherwise synaptic activation and change
would spread like an avalanche through the entire network. Hasselmo
was able to show that whenever overlapping patterns have to be learned –

which is what happens in biological systems – such runaway synaptic modification, as he called the phenomenon, occurs. The end result of the process is that every input pattern activates all output neurons. This is equivalent to a network that has not learned anything, since learning always implies discrimination. A network that leads to the activation of all output neurons in response to an input is computationally useless.

In most computer-simulated network models, runaway synaptic modification is prevented by inhibiting the spread of activation within the network during learning, since such spread interferes with learning, as we have just seen. Only during the process of retrieval (i.e. whenever the network carries out what it has previously learned) does the spread of activation through it become essential. This change in the spread of activation within computer simulations of networks can be implied in various ways by mathematical procedures. The question, however, is how runaway synaptic modification is prevented in biological systems such as the human brain.

To repeat the problem, during learning, the network must be sensitive to activation from outside, but the spread of activation via internal connections must also be suppressed, whereas during recall, activation must be able to spread through the network via internal connections. Within this framework, recent neurobiological findings on the role of *acetylcholine* in the dynamics of cortical activation are of special importance. For a long time, acetylcholine has been related to processes of learning and memory. The substance is produced by a small number of neurons that are clustered together in the nucleus basalis Meynert. From there, acetylcholine is spread out through almost the entire brain via tiny fibres that proceed to the cortex.

Experiments in slices of the entorhinal cortex have demonstrated that acetylcholine selectively suppresses excitatory synaptic connections between neurons of the same cortical region. In contrast, signals from other cortical areas can pass through synapses unimpaired. Thus, acetylcholine has the very function needed in neuronal networks to prevent runaway synaptic modification such that learning of new and overlapping patterns can occur. In order to do its work, acetylcholine must be liberated during learning but not during retrieval. This in turn presupposes the existence of a fast-acting mechanism that evaluates and detects the novelty of an incoming stimulus pattern and sends the result of this evaluation to the nucleus basalis Meynert. The existence of such a mechanism in the brain is conceivable and has in fact been assumed for other reasons as well, even though there is no detailed view on it so far (Hasselmo, 1994; p. 22).

For many years it has been known that in Alzheimer's disease the amount of acetylcholine in the brain is decreased. However, before Hasselmo's model it was not clear how the lack of this substance has an effect on learning. Within the framework of Hasselmo's model, however, a prediction can be made about what happens if acetylcholine is lacking in the brain. The model explains why in Alzheimer's disease the learning of new information is affected severely at an early stage. Furthermore, it is known that overly active neurons using the transmitter glutamate may be damaged by their own excessive activity. This phenomenon is referred to as excitotoxicity and is well described for glutamatergic neurons. For years, such excitotoxicity has been implicated in the neuronal loss observed in Alzheimer's disease. The functional role of acetylcholine in the prevention of runaway synaptic modification explains how the lack of the substances can lead to excitotoxicity and neuronal loss.

If acetylcholine is decreased or lacking, the number of associations that form within neural networks increases. This causes the increased activation of neurons within the network upon the presence of any input. In short, acetylcholine puts the brakes on cortical excitation during encoding, and if this is malfunctioning, cortical excitation increases. Hence, any new learning causes changes in desired as well as in undesired synaptic connections, which not only interferes with learning, but also leads to the increased activation of glutamatergic neurons. As just mentioned, this activity can be toxic for the neurons themselves.

Hasselmo's model predicts the spatial pattern of neuropathology observed in the brains of deceased patients with Alzheimer's disease. Such pathology should occur in those brain areas that are highly involved in associative learning, such as the hippocampus. The typical pathological changes of Alzheimer's disease, most importantly the Alzheimer tangles, become visible earliest and most frequently in the hippocampus. Even within the hippocampus, the Alzheimer-related pathology occurs in regions that are known to have the most easily modifiable synaptic connections (notably those in which the process of LTP was first discovered). Hasselmo (1994; see also Chapter 12) discusses a number of further neuropathological changes that can be explained easily within his model, which, like other neural network models, can put together a number of otherwise inexplicable or unrelated characteristics of the disorder.

From integration to coincidence detection?

Most present-day network theories assume that information is coded in the frequency of the action potential and that the neuron is a device that integrates incoming signals, thereby extracting the information. Since the speed of synaptic transmission is limited to at most 1 kHz, and since it takes a few transmissions to detect the mean frequency of the signal – which is the variable that supposedly carries the information – there is a principal speed limit for any neural information processing of this type. In other words, neural processes cannot work, let alone be accurate, at the sub-millisecond level. However, this is exactly what has been observed in some instances.

A prominent case in point is the auditory system of the barn owl. When flying in the dark, the owl is able to detect the horizontal angle of an incoming acoustic signal by measuring the difference in the time of arrival of the signal at the two ears. Given the speed of sound in air (300 m/s) and the distance between the ears (6 cm), this difference is 0.2 ms. It is detected by a cleverly arranged set of neurons that pass the impulses from the left and the right ear towards one another and detect where they arrive. A difference in time is thereby translated into a point on a spatial map. This example shows that neurons within this system are capable of detecting the coincidence of two incoming spikes and thereby process information much more quickly and efficiently than by using a frequency code.

As this example shows that neurons can, in principle, be more efficient than the standard model assumes, the question is whether such efficiency is actually used in the most sophisticated of all neuronal systems, i.e. the human cortex. One argument in favour of such a view draws upon evolutionary considerations. It stipulates that, given neurons have been shown to be capable of using highly efficient time codes, it does not make sense to assume that they do so only in special cases, such as in the auditory system of the owl and some other species. In brief, 'why waste all the hardware with such inefficient coding?', as John Hopfield put it on the occasion of a conference devoted to this topic.[1] While this argument is appealing, it has been questioned by Shadlen and Newsome (1994, 1995). A second argument in favour of precise time coding within the cortex, put forward by Softky and Koch (1993), relies upon a careful analysis of the temporal sequence of spikes in cortical neurons, and runs as follows. Cortical neurons integrate hundreds, if not thousands, of highly variable signals, and their firing rate therefore represents the mean of these signals. As the fluctuation of the means of a fluctuating variable is a function of the number of events taken to calculate the mean, it can be demonstrated that the statistical properties of such means are different from what is observed, in that statistically these means should be quite uniform (because of the large sample size) but in fact they are not (as highly fluctuating activity is the rule in cortical neurons). The argument concludes that the signal integration model of neuronal coding does not explain the observed firing patterns of cortical neurons. Hence, more precise time coding may be at work (Softky, 1995).

The debate as to whether cortical neurons are integrators or coincidence detectors is far from resolved (Koch, 1997; Thomson, 1997). It is advanced enough, however, to draw some conclusions for neural network models of psychological and psychopathological phenomena. First, if neurons use some form of time code, the principal assumptions of most present-day network models are wrong. This does not imply, however, that the discoveries made by the models must necessarily be dismissed. As James McClelland once put it on the occasion of a conference on neural networks and pathology (Reggia, Ruppin and Berndt, 1997),[2] 'all models may be wrong, but some of the principles I discovered may be right'. After all, we know that present-day network models are simplifications of biological neurons, and in fact have to be, like all good models. As far as these models capture some essential feature of reality, provide parsimonious accounts of otherwise unrelated or incomprehensible sets of data, and generate new hypotheses that can be put to empirical tests, they are useful tools for cognitive neuroscience research, including the field of psychopathology.

Kohonen-networks (self-organizing feature maps) may be a case in point. They rely on the neuron as integrator assumption and allow the study of map formation on the basis of input regularities. Since we know that the cortex is a map-formation device, and we know that temporal information can be used to drive map reorganization, we may use Kohonen-networks or variants of them to discover principles governing the organization and reorganization of cortical representations, as long as we are aware of the model's limitations.

Neural networks are no longer just a curiosity in the field of psychopathology. These neurocomputational accounts of psychobiological phenomena represent the sorely needed bridge between psychopathological and neurobiological models of disorders and no doubt have already provided important theoretical insights. In conjunction with clinical attentiveness and the available neurobiological tools, neural networks will be part of the psychiatry of the near future.

Summary

A little more than 100 years ago, the neuron was found to be the functional unit of the central nervous system. Shortly thereafter, a number of people interested in physiology, including Freud and Exner, conceived of the flow of energy through 'networks' of neurons, and speculative neurophysiological ideas were used to explain psychopathological phenomena. About 50 years later, McCullough and Pitts were the first to posit the neuron as a device that carries and processes information, rather than energy, which set the stage for preliminary models and ideas regarding psychopathological applications. In fact, McCullough and Pitts themselves explicitly placed the conundrums of psychopathology, such as hallucinations and delusions, within the scope of neural network research. The first surge of interest in neural networks during the 1950s and 1960s had little, if any, impact on psychopathology, a fact possibly caused by the states of both fields during this period. After the renaissance of neural network research, beginning in the 1980s, and after the classic paper by Ralph Hoffman in 1987, an increasing number of network models of forms for psychopathology have been proposed. Psychopathology is not a late 'add on' to neural network research, nor is network research just a curiosity in psychopathology. Instead, neurocomputational models represent the sorely needed bridge between neuropathology and psychopathology.

Endnotes

1 The Role and Control of Random Events in Biological Systems: workshop held in Sigtuna, Sweden, September 4–9, 1995.
2 Neural Modelling of Cognitive and Brain Disorders: workshop held at the University of Maryland, USA, June 8–10, 1995.

References

Anderson, J.A. & Rosenfeld, E. (eds) (1988). *Neurocomputing. Foundation of Research*. Cambridge, MA: MIT Press.
Baudry, M. & Davis, J.L. (1997). *Long-term Potentiation*, Vol. 3, Cambridge, MA: MIT Press.

Bleuler, E. (1911/1950). *Dementia Praecox or the Group of Schizophrenias*, translated by J. Ziskin & N.D. Lewis. New York: International Universities Press.

Breidbach, O. (1993). Nervenzellen oder Nervennetze? Zur Entstehung des Neuronenkonzepts. In *Das Gehirn – Organ der Seele?*, ed. E. Florey & O. Breidbach, pp. 81–126. Berlin: Akademie-Verlag.

Dierig, S. (1993). Rudolf Virchow und das Nervensystem. Zur Bergründung der zellulären Neurobiologie. In *Das Gehirn – Organ der Seele?*, ed. E. Florey & D. Breidbach, pp. 55–89. Berlin: Akademie-Verlag.

Exner, S. (1894). *Entwurf zu einer physiologischen Erklärung der psychischen Erscheinungen*. Leipzug, Wien: Deuticke.

Finger, S. (1994). *Origins of Neuroscience. A History of Explorations into Brain Functions*. Oxford: Oxford University Press.

Freud, S. (1895/1978). Project for a scientific psychology. *The Standard Edition of the Complete Psychological Works of Sigmund Freud*, Vol. 1, pp. 283–397. London: Hogarth Press.

Grossberg, S. (1980). How does the brain build a cognitive code? *Psychological Review*, **87**: 1–51.

Hasselmo, M.E. (1994). Runaway synaptic modification in models of cortex: implications for Alzheimer's disease. *Neural Networks*, **7**(1), 13–40.

Hebb, D.O. (1949/1988). The organization of behavior (1949). Quoted from *Neurocomputing. Foundations of Research*, ed. J.A. Anderson & E. Rosenfeld, pp. 45–56. Cambridge, MA: MIT Press.

Hobson, J.A. & McCarley, R.W. (1977). The brain as a dream state generator. *American Journal of Psychiatry*, **134**, 1335–48.

Hoffman, R.E. (1987). Computer simulations of neural information processing and the schizophrenia–mania dichotomy. *Archives of General Psychiatry*, **44**, 178–85.

Hoffman, R.E., Rapaport, J., Ameli, R., McGlashan, T.H., Harcherik, D. & Servan-Schreiber, D. (1995). The pathophysiology of hallucinated 'voices' and associated speech perception impairments in psychotic patients. *Journal of Cognitive Neuroscience*, **7**, 479–96.

James, W. (1890/1983). *Principles of Psychology*. Cambridge, MA: Harvard University Press.

James, W. (1892/1984). *Psychology: Briefer Course*. Cambridge, MA: Harvard University Press.

Jones, E. (1978). *The Life and Work of Sigmund Freud*.

Jung, C.G. (1906/1979). *Experimentelle Untersuchungen über Assoziationen Gesunder*. Gesammelte Werke 2 (Experimentelle Untersuchungen), pp. 15–213. Olten, Freiburg: Walter.

Kandel, E.R. (1991). Cellular mechanisms of learning and the biological basis of individuality. In *Principles of Neuroscience*, 3rd edn, ed. E.R. Kandel, J.H. Schwarz & T.M. Jessell, pp. 1009–31. Amsterdam: Elsevier Science.

Koch, C. (1997). Computation and the single neuron. *Nature*, **385**, 207–10.

Kraepelin, E. (1892). Über die Beeinflussung einfacher psychischer Vorgänge durch einige Arzneimittel. Jena: G. Fischer.

McCulloch, W.S. & Pitts, W. (1943/1988). A logical calculus of the ideas immanent in nervous activity. In *Neurocomputing. Foundations of Research*, ed. J.A. Anderson, & E. Rosenfeld, pp. 18–27. Cambridge, MA: MIT Press.

Minsky, M. & Papert, S. (1969). *Perceptrons*. Cambridge, MA: MIT Press.

Pribram, K.H. & Gill, M.M. (1976). *Freud's Project Re-assessed.* New York: Basic Books.

Reggia, J., Ruppin, E. & Berndt, R. (eds.) (1997). *Neural Modeling of Brain and Cognitive Disorders.* Singapore: World Scientific Press.

Rochester, N., Holland, J.H., Haibt, L.H. & Duda, W.L. (1956/1988). Tests on a cell assembly theory of the action of the brain, using a large digital computer. In *Neurocomputing. Foundations of Research*, ed. J.A. Anderson & E. Rosenfeld, pp. 68–79. Cambridge, MA: MIT Press.

Rosenblatt, F. (1958/1988). The perceptron: a probabilistic model for information storage and organization in the brain. In *Neurocomputing. Foundations of Research*, ed. J.A. Anderson & E. Rosenfeld, pp. 92–114. Cambridge, MA: MIT Press.

Rumelhart, D.E. (1989). The architecture of mind: a connectionist approach. In *Foundations of Cognitive Science*, ed. M.I. Posner, pp. 133–59. Cambridge, MA: MIT Press.

Shadlen, M.N. & Newsome, W.T. (1994). Noise, neural codes and cortical organization. *Current Opinion in Neurobiology*, 4, 569–79.

Shallen, M.N. & Newsome, W.T. (1995). Is there a signal in the noise? *Current Opinion in Neurobiology*, 5, 248–50.

Softky, W.R. (1995). Simple codes versus efficient codes. *Current Opinion in Neurobiology*, 5, 239–47.

Softky, W.R. & Koch, C. (1993). The highly irregular firing of cortical cells is inconsistent with temporal integration of random EPSPs. *Journal of Neuroscience*, 13, 334–59.

Spitzer, M. (1992). Word-associations in experimental psychiatry: a historical perspective. In *Phenomenology, Language and Schizophrenia*, ed. M. Spitzer, F.A. Uehlein, M.A. Schwartz & C. Mundt, pp. 160–96. New York: Springer.

Spitzer, M. & Mundt, C. (1994). Interchanges between philosophy and psychiatry: the continental tradition. *Current Opinion in Psychiatry*, 7, 417–22.

Sulloway, F.I. (1984). *Freud, Biologist of the Mind.* New York: Basic Books.

Thomson, A.M. (1997). More than just frequency detectors. *Science*, 275, 179–80.

von Neumann, J. (1958). *The Computer and the Brain.* New Haven: Yale University Press.

Wernicke, C. (1906). *Grundriß der Psychiatrie in klinischen Vorlesungen*, 2nd edn. Leipzig: Deuticke.

Zell, A. (1994). *Simulation neuronaler Netze.* Bonn: Addison-Wesley.

3

Neural network models in psychiatric diagnosis and symptom recognition

ERIC Y. H. CHEN and
GERMAN E. BERRIOS

Matters historical

Psychiatric diagnosis has been conceptualized as either a 'one-off' ('recognition') type of cognitive act or as a 'recursive (constructional) process'. History teaches us that scientists choose their models not on the basis of some 'crucial empirical test' (such tests do not exist at this level of abstraction) but on the more humdrum (but rarely owned up to) dictate of fashion. For example, during the eighteenth century, when the so-called 'ontological' notions of disease (as it was then based on the *more botanico* tradition) (Berg, 1956; López-Piñero, 1983), reigned supreme, there was little problem in accepting the view that the diagnosis (recognition) of disease happened at one fell (cognitive) swoop. This was because the Platonic (ontological) assumption lurking behind such a notion amply justified the belief that disease was 'fully bounded and out there' and, furthermore, that inklings of its existence had been planted at birth (like everything else) in the mind of the diagnostician. The *a priori* privileging of some features of a disease (the successful strategy that Linné had already tried on plants), and the view that such features actually 'signified' the disease, was just one version of the ontological approach. Indeed, a century earlier, a similar view had governed the study of linguistics (Aarsleff, 1982). That it was fashion and *Zeitgeist* that sustained the popularity of the ontological view is illustrated by the fact that a rival approach put forward at the time by Adanson was given short shrift (Stevens, 1984). Adanson's claim that all features have the same weight *ab initio*, and that *a priori* privileging is unwarranted, only came to fruition as 'numerical taxonomy' more than 150 years later (Vernon 1988)!

During the nineteenth century, new notions of disease quietly appeared, and the most popular (in terms of the physiology of the period) was one that postulated a continuity between the 'normal and the pathological' (Canguilhem, 1975). The need to identify thresholds encouraged physicians to develop descriptive routines and biological markers, which since those days have been assumed to have enough discriminant power to determine the cut-off where normality 'ends' and disease 'begins' (Faber, 1923; Riese, 1953). The arrival during the twentieth century of probabilistic concepts (Gigerenzer et al., 1989) soon showed that such cut-offs were relative and shifting notions and that new strategies were required for the definition and recognition of disease. For example, the notion of 'caseness' is a late product of such conceptual change (Ragin and Becker, 1992). The adoption first of factor analysis and then of discriminant and cluster analysis seemed to offer an opportunity to define boundaries as regions of rarity. Failure to identify such regions between the various psychoses led, in some cases, to premature pessimism (Kendell, 1975). Most researchers, however, have soldiered on (Mezzich and Solomon, 1980; Guimón, Mezzich and Berrios, 1988). In this regard, resorting to neural networks is but the latest strategy (as were Bayesian routines in the 1960s) (e.g. Hall, 1967) to map the chiaroscuro between normality and disease.

During the 1980s, nosological fashion encouraged a return to the old Weberian idea of 'ideal types' (e.g. Schwartz and Wiggins, 1986; 1987), and led to calls for a 'scientific psychiatric nosology' (Kendler, 1990) and interesting conceptual developments (Sadler, Wiggins and Schwartz, 1994). Although the future remains obscure, it can be predicted that the relentless progress of genetics will cause once again a major shift in nosological theory, and that something like a new ontological model of disease will develop, this time divested of its old metaphysical elements (strong at the time it was abandoned by Bichat – see Haigh, 1984) but dependent upon complex mathematical models (e.g. Neale and Cardon, 1992).

It is against this historical context that the current use of neural networks in psychiatry must be understood. It is, indeed, tempting to feel that, by considering medical diagnosis as a typical pattern recognition task (e.g. Ripley, 1996; p. 1), we have at long last come upon the right solution. This is not necessarily so, although as always occurs with new techniques, neural networks will end up modifying our thinking about psychiatric disease, and about diagnostic clinical algorithms. This means that, in the current climate, there may be no alternative to characterizing medical diagnosis as a complex, multidimensional, and recursive process.

When trying to make sense of the mental symptoms and signs presented by a patient, the psychiatrist can be said to have embarked on 'pattern recognition' and 'decision-making' routines. Surprisingly, few of these processes are well defined and understood, particularly from the point of view of the new cognitive psychology. (By this is meant what, for example, Newell (1990) and Baars (1986) have described in their work.) One reason may be the lack of models comprehensive enough to handle the complexity of the diagnostic process. Another, that there is still a tendency to resort to 'operational definitions' (Bridgman, 1927) without realizing that this conceptual trick is based on obsolete assumptions about science and the mind. It is thus the case that the new models should not only have face validity, and be able to generate empirical questions, but also show conceptual reasonableness.

Using the brain itself, rather than computers, to create analogues for its functioning and that of the 'mind', is a clever idea, and one that has proven surprisingly fruitful. As oft-repeated in this book, neural networks (neurocomputational models) are conceived of as sets of processing units so richly connected that their reciprocal interactions may generate complex patterns of activity (Rumelhart and McClelland, 1986). This property (and others to be mentioned below) make such models attractive with regard to modelling the processes of disease diagnosis and symptom recognition, and also to creating models to explain some of the symptoms and diseases themselves. Because there has been, in general, far more work on disease diagnosis, this chapter emphasizes the new problem of symptom recognition (on which, after all, disease diagnosis is based). Some of the conceptual issues besetting current views on the diagnosis or 'recognition' of mental symptoms are identified first, and then some solutions are offered.

Conceptual issues

Psychiatric diagnosis and symptom recognition

The term 'psychiatric diagnosis' is ambiguous, and its meaning varies according to the theoretical perspective of its practitioner; for example, it means something different to a psychoanalyst and to a biological psychiatrist. A good understanding of psychiatric diagnosis, therefore, will need to take into account its descriptive, semantic and therapeutic dimensions. If so, it could be concluded that computers (and those who have forgotten what psychiatric diagnosis is about) may not be able to implement it, because psychiatric diagnosis involves more than cognition. This wide view of psychiatric diagnosis, popular in the good psychodynamic days of American psychiatry – before, that is, DSM-III (APA, 1980) –

has suddenly become an embarrassment, particularly to those who want to conceive it as a cognitive act.

But the disambiguation of psychiatric diagnosis also depends upon sound conceptualizing. Like all medical acts, it includes, as hinted above, attitudinal components such as cognition, emotion, and volition, and is embedded in a 'pragmatics' context. When complete, psychiatric diagnosis is also a 'speech act', i.e. the mark of successful communication, the beginning of a relationship between two human beings around the promise of 'help without harm'. It would seem, therefore, that psychiatric diagnosis, as understood by neural network modellists, is a far cry from this. The issue is whether it is possible to abstract the intellectual component of psychiatric diagnosis from its Gestaltic context and still claim that one is dealing with it.

This chapter sticks to its brief and assumes that psychiatric diagnosis (also) involves the cognitive (intellectual) identification of certain clinical features as presented by a given patient in a given context. Such identification becomes a psychiatric diagnosis when it is carried out according to certain public guidelines. Such guidelines include techniques to fit exemplars into classes, a taxonomic theory, and professional warrants to legitimize the cognitive act (i.e. both in folk psychology terms and in law, a psychiatric diagnosis issued by a layman will be considered as 'less valid' than one issued by a mental health professional). In this context, 'class' refers to 'disease', a concept whose usage, extension, intension, epistemological basis, and general meaning vary a great deal in medicine. For example, whilst diseases with known genetics are regaining what could be called an ontological basis, those that still depend upon descriptions alone (such as some in psychiatry) are dependent upon 'criteria', mental set, and cognition. Auditing the conceptual efficiency of these types of disease shows marked differences. In the case of diseases defined in terms of genes or known histopathology, the measurement of sensitivity and specificity can be set against 'gold standards' and 'prototypes'. In the absence of the latter, psychiatric diagnosis becomes a bootstrapping operation primarily defined in terms of 'clusters' of features (Katz, Cole and Barton, 1965), and in which the clustering rules depend both on 'nature' and social authority. The lack of a biological invariant tends to cause amongst psychiatrists yearnings for 'reliability'. This and no other is the explanation for recent attempts to operationalize diagnostic criteria (e.g. DSM-IV, APA, 1994). Because the 'operations' in terms of which the clinical entities in question are 'defined' are mostly intuitive and blurred cognitive acts (very different from the measurement and experimental operations that Bridgman had intended), this approach tends to trivialize psychiatric diagnosis and neglect its connection with the republic of objects (i.e. its validity). It is assumed in this chapter that both reliability and validity are equally important.

The diagnosis of mental symptoms (symptom recognition) has, on the other hand, received less attention in the literature. For some reason, it has been assumed that psychiatric diagnosis is more problematic and that mental symptoms are easy to recognize (Berrios and Chen, 1993; see below).

Parallel processing and algorithmic approaches

Conventional artificial intelligence (AI) models for decision making involve the use of algorithmic trees in which 'complex' decisions (e.g. diagnostic processes) are broken down into component branches and nodes (e.g. identification of individual symptoms) (Berrios and Chen, 1993). In such trees, individual loci represent the status of the decisional process at a moment in time, as it progresses in discrete steps. One well-known problem with such algorithms is deciding on whether there is a 'natural' ordinal sequence for decisions or whether an 'arbitrary' hierarchy should be imposed. In a parallel processing system, on the other hand, this problem is obviated because each and every individual decision contributes towards the overall decisional process, i.e. all decisions are taken into account at each step of the process. (Crucial to this process is a fool-proof mechanism to save information, namely that no individual decision is allowed to override the processing of other decisions.) Equally important is the fact that 'horizontal' interactions between different component decisions are also possible. The ensuing system, therefore, imposes very few *a priori* constraints. Likewise, components are related 'structurally', i.e. in terms of reciprocal connections whose strength is modifiable in response to empirical data.

Symptom recognition in psychiatry

Mental symptoms can be defined as verbal and non-verbal expressions of aberrant subjective experiences, and play a central role in all official systems for psychiatric diagnosis. Their elicitation and recognition, however, are limited in a number of ways, and research into this field has just started. Mental symptoms are usually 'reported' by the patient in a speech act whose medium is assumed to be ordinary (folk) language.

Depending upon fashion and taste, the lexicons built into the latter have been considered as 'rich and creative' (and hence up to the task of describing complex emotional and subjective states) or as 'rudimentary, rigid, vicarious, and second-hand' (and hence as inappropriate for such descriptions).

Current diagnostic practice focuses on the mapping of preconceived units of behaviour by 'symptoms', and these by 'diagnosis'. Some systems have formalized this action by the generation of certain operationalized criteria. If this approach was to be followed rigidly, then models for diagnosis would be well represented by decision charts, flow diagrams and algorithms rather than by computational models. The shortcomings of rigid, algorithmic approaches, however, have already been indicated (Berrios and Chen, 1993). A crucial problem here is that the serial nature of decision charts impedes the revision of early decisions in the light of late ones (see below).

Neurocomputational models have been applied to many clinical situations (Cho and Reggia, 1993) including psychiatry (Davis et al., 1993; Modai et al., 1993). In general, neural networks have been used as pattern-recognition devices susceptible to training by means of empirical diagnostic data (i.e. to map symptoms and diagnoses). Given a set of adequately operationalized symptoms, these programmes can be implemented by means of a variety of neural network architectures. Approaches that make use *simpliciter* of the pattern-recognition capacity of neural networks will not be dealt with further in this chapter.

Some problems at the descriptive level

As always, things are more complicated at the stage of data collecting. Patients rarely 'volunteer' full reports of their mental symptoms: most of the time, symptom description and recognition result from an overt or covert negotiation between patient and interviewer. Hence, it is disingenuous to see it as consisting of a simple and uncontaminated transfer of 'phenomenological' information. Mental symptoms result from 'descriptive contracts' whereby 'basic experiences' ('primordial soups') are formatted in terms of personal, cultural and clinical codes (Marková and Berrios, 1995a), the latter being provided by the technical language of psychopathology. (For discussion of the formation and history of the such codes, see Berrios, 1996.)

It is conventionally claimed that mental symptoms are 'private to the patients experiencing them', and hence 'unverifiable' in the sense of not being susceptible to public measurement by instruments calibrated against objects in the physical world. Whereas most psychiatrists will agree with the general drift of this claim, it is important to ask what 'private' means in this context, what aspects or components of the mental symptom are to be considered 'private' in this sense, and what empirical and scientific implications are to be drawn from this claim. The view that, as compared with our knowledge of public things at large (where we seem to share in a common epistemological enterprise), our knowledge of our own mind and its contents is characterized by a special authority, has a long pedigree, and goes beyond Descartes to Plotinus (Plotinus, 1966; pp. 1, 4, 10) and his definition of consciousness as a private sanctuary. This is not the place to discuss the pros and cons of this view (Saunders and Henze, 1967; Jones, 1971; Bailey, 1979). Suffice it to say that the issue here is not so much whether such private access should make one doubt the existence of mental states, or their susceptibility to scientific treatment. The issue is what the meaning and force of 'special authority' are. Does it mean 'infallibility' (i.e. that one cannot be wrong about describing one's mental states) or 'incorrigibility' (i.e. that one can be wrong but cannot be corrected by others) or simply 'self-intimation' (i.e. not only that they are directly and transparently available to us but that our descriptions are neither infallible nor incorrigible)?

But if mental symptoms are constructs, i.e. their 'final' frame, form and content are derived from internal and external material, then is it correct to say that mental symptoms are only private affairs? The question we feel should rather be which element of the mental symptom is private and which external? Also, in what way does this affect the availability of the mental symptom to scientific scrutiny? The answer to the first question is not simple, for it is unlikely that mental symptoms have the same structure (for the question of symptom heterogeneity, see Marková and Berrios, 1995b). Thus, whereas in the case of 'hallucinations' it might be possible to say that there is a sizeable private component (namely the image) and that the formatting elements are not crucially important, in the case of 'formal thought disorder' or 'manipulation', meaning would seem to depend more upon the way in which it is constructed than upon the private or subjective contribution of the patient. There is no space here to develop this issue in any depth. Suffice it to say that current philosophy of mind is, in general, far more accepting of the fact that mental states exist (Rosenthal, 1991), that private access means self-intimation rather than infallibility, and that the epistemological validation of such states revolves around both internal and external elements (Burge, 1979; Fumerton, 1988; Alston, 1989).

The view that mental symptoms result from conceptual and linguistic sources qualifies the simplistic view that they are but morsels of information passed on from a source to a receiver, where the source is the psychopathological experience, and the receiver the cognitive system of the clinician. But it is also true that, at another level, mental symptoms contain information that has the power to increase or decrease the probability of a case falling into a given diagnostic category. One issue is, therefore, what aspects of mental symptoms can be modelled by neural networks? The first step when answering this question is to consider the factors that modulate the exchange of information between patient and clinician.

Multidimensional representation of symptoms

Current diagnostic systems tend to regard mental symptoms as dichotomous variables (that is, as either present or absent). The limitations of this approach have become obvious in relation to recent research (e.g. the neuroimaging of mental symptoms). It is thus increasingly recognized that multidimensional models are needed to capture more information about the symptoms, particularly because such dimensions may contain information that is biologically relevant. In this regard, it could be said that neural networks are inherently appropriate to model multidimensional information. The non-hierarchical representation of such dimensions should also facilitate the development of relatively neutral accounts, i.e. avoid assuming that certain features have supremacy over others.

Context dependence of pattern-recognition modules

In clinical situations, symptoms are never considered in isolation but as part of a presentation context. Given the same set of external data about a particular symptom, different conclusions may result, depending on preceding and/or ongoing contextual information. Thus, during a diagnostic run, clinical information tends to emerge sequentially, and hence the outcome of an earlier evaluation of symptoms (indeed, the order in which they are picked up) may become part of the context against which later symptom evaluations will take place (Berrios and Chen, 1993).

Modelling issues

Basic modelling of diagnosis

The use of neural network models redefines the diagnostic process as essentially a pattern-recognition task (Ripley, 1996), and fundamentally departs from the rigid algorithmic approach. What is really taken advantage of in this case is the neural network capacity for associative retrieval of a best-fit pattern. Because a diagnostic category, for example, is considered as a permutation of symptoms, different 'patterns' will be learned of combinations of symptoms encountered in real life. Information on symptom co-occurrence is then encoded as connection weights within the network. In this way, a number of different symptom patterns can be represented in the same set of units, and encoded in the same set of connections.

Figure 3.1 shows an example of an autoassociative network in which each processing unit is connected to all other units in the network through weighted connections. The matrix containing information on a combination of weights can thus be said to hold information about a co-occurrence pattern, i.e. on which set of units will be activated together. Weights are acquired during exposure to training patterns through learning algorithms such as the Hebb rule.

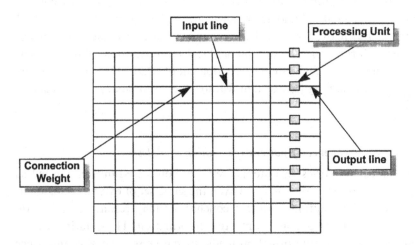

Fig. 3.1 Structure of an autoassociative network. Processing units receive input from junctions to their left. Their outputs are returned as input to other units through weighted connections in the next processing cycle. The connection weight between a unit and itself is set to zero.

$$W_{ij} = \frac{1}{N} \sum_{\mu=1}^{p} \sigma_i^\mu \sigma_j^\mu$$

where W_{ij} is the element in the weight matrix connecting unit i and unit j; N is the number of units in the network, μ refers to patterns to be stored in the network (numbered from 1 to p), and σ is the activity of the unit i and j in pattern μ (Amit, 1989a).

When the network encounters a new pattern, it takes on the activation values embedded in the pattern as its initial activation state. Units within the network then interact with one another in subsequent processing cycles. Figure 3.2 depicts a prototypical processing unit. Input to the unit is derived from the activation patterns in other units in the network at the end of the preceding processing cycle (upstream units). The activation of each unit is multiplied by the respective connection weight. The weighted activations are then summated by the current processing unit to yield an input that is instituted into an activation function in order to compute the current activation level of the processing unit. At the end of this processing cycle, the activation is communicated 'downstream' to the next cycle of processing (Fig. 3.3). Processing cycles are repeated until the state of the network becomes stable, i.e. further cycling results in the same pattern of activity. When this occurs the network is said to have settled into an attractor (Fig. 3.4). The final stable pattern reflects a best-fit solution between the presented pattern (external input) and the constraints written into the internal weights of the network. When this pattern corresponds to a previously specified pattern (presented during the learning stage), the network is considered to have mapped a current set of symptoms onto a known diagnostic category (Amit, 1989c).

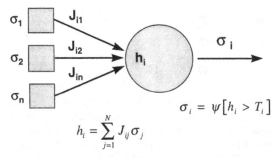

Fig. 3.2 A neurocomputation unit. J_{ij}, weight of connection between units i and j; h_i, input; Ψ, an activation function; T_i, threshold; σ, activation level (usually binary in Hopfield-type autoassociative networks).

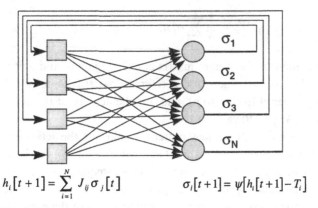

$$h_i\left[t+1\right] = \sum_{i=1}^{N} J_{ij}\sigma_j\left[t\right] \qquad \sigma_i\left[t+1\right] = \psi\left[h_i\left[t+1\right] - T_i\right]$$

Fig. 3.3 An autoassociative attractor network. $h_i[t+1]$, input at cycle $t+1$; $\sigma[t+1]$, output at cycle $t+1$; Ψ, an activation function; T_i, threshold; J_{ij}, weight of connection between units i and j; N, number of units.

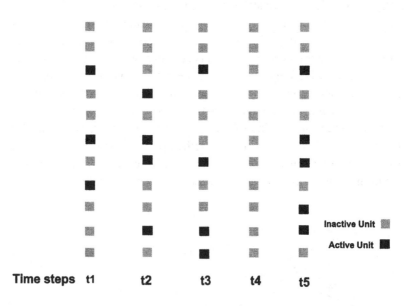

Fig. 3.4 Evolution of states of a network. Dynamic behaviour of a network could be visualized as in this example. A unit at any given time could be active or inactive. Which state it is in is determined by its activation level, computed as described earlier. This network has not yet settled into an attractor. (When this happens, there is no change in pattern of activation with further time-steps.)

The use in this manner of an autoassociative network corresponds to a 'prototype' view of diagnostic classification (Hampton, 1993). According to this view, individual instances of a diagnostic category (combinations of features) share a 'family resemblance'. (In the sense discussed by Wittgenstein (1958) that concept-words do not denote sharply circumscribed concepts, but are meant only to mark resemblance between the things labelled and the concept.) A newly encountered instance is then classified according to the extent to which it resembles pre-existing instances in that category. Individual features all contribute in a parallel fashion towards the recognition process, i.e. a large number of features are taken into consideration in every step. (It is not implied here that the features are weighted equally; indeed, it is permissible to set weights to zero.) Or to put it another way, no feature on its own is allowed exclusively to override the processing of other features, as would be the case when category membership is defined by the presence or absence of a small number of features. The latter corresponds to what has been known for a long time as the 'privileged features' method (see above) or as the 'defining features' type of classification (Howard, 1987). It goes without saying that this method is at the basis of the operationalized approaches to diagnosis.

The use of an autoassociative network to recognize diagnostic patterns is a straightforward application of neural networks. It is, however, dependent on the assumption that the arrays of clinical features are available as a ready set prior to the onset of processing. In other words, it is meant to depict a unidirectional, 'bottom-up' mapping from symptom to diagnosis. In view of what has been said above, it is clear that this idealization of the diagnostic process is incorrect. For one thing, it is not the case that in actual clinical practice issues pertaining to the diagnosis of the disease are withheld until all information pertaining to symptoms becomes available. Instead, diagnostic hypotheses constitute from the start the conceptual background against which symptom recognition takes place (Berrios and Chen, 1993). A more realistic model will have to take into account the effect of ongoing higher level processing (diagnostic hypothesis) as well as concurrent processing at a lower level (e.g. symptom processing) (Fig. 3.5).

Modelling issues pertaining to 'context effect'

The influence of top-down processing on the dynamics of a network's pattern recognition can be represented as information flowing from

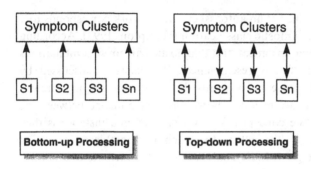

Fig. 3.5 Relationship between symptom and diagnosis processing. In bottom-up processing, symptom processing (S1 etc.) precedes symptom cluster (diagnosis) processing. In top-down processing, symptom cluster processing could affect symptom processing.

higher to lower level units. Through this flow, the ongoing pattern of activity in the higher level network (diagnosis) could be made to influence processing at a lower level, namely whether certain ambiguous features in the set are interpreted as meaning that a particular symptom is present or absent. For the sake of simplicity, this influence has been called 'priming' (Fig. 3.5). In actual computational terms, priming is implemented by the selective subthreshold activation of units corresponding to the primed pattern (Berrios and Chen, 1993).

To demonstrate the effect of such influence on the dynamics of the network, it is helpful to introduce the notion of 'energy landscape', which describes the stability of different possible activity patterns in a given network (Amit, 1989b). In a network of n units, any state of activity of the network can be expressed as a point in a n-dimensional state space. The change of activity pattern in the network over a period of time could be traced as a trajectory in the n-dimensional state space. Each point in the state space is associated with an index analogous to the notion of potential energy in physical systems. 'Energy' is a measure of how well internal and external constraints are satisfied in that particular pattern, given the set of connection weights, i.e. how well the co-occurrence patterns in the external input match the patterns stored in the network's memory. Points of high degrees of correspondence are assigned low energy levels, and vice versa. The dynamic behaviour of a network could be envisaged as a tendency to move from states of high energy (peaks) to states of lower energy (valleys) (Fig. 3.6).

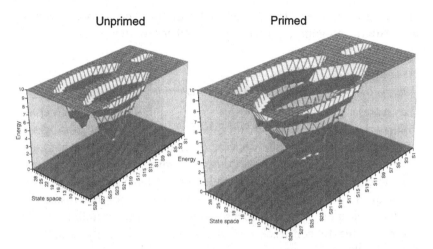

Fig. 3.6 Change in 'energy landscape' with priming. This schematic diagram illustrates the concept of energy landscape for a trained network. The vertical axis represents the energy function. The horizontal plane represents a projection of the state space onto the two-dimensional plane. In the unprimed state there are three attractors, two with larger basins of attraction, one with a smaller basin of attraction. When one of the attractors is primed, its basin of attraction increases. A set of points initially lying in between the two larger basins of attractions (therefore neutral) now falls within the basin of the primed attractor.

When a network is trained to recognize certain patterns, states of the network representing the target activity patterns develop into energy 'minima' (bottom of valleys in the energy landscape) so that patterns in the surrounding regions in the state space are likely to evolve according to a trajectory leading into the target pattern (leading to 'retrieval' of the pattern). The entire region in which any starting network state will converge to the same target pattern is called the 'basin of attraction' for the target pattern. In a given network, the energy landscape consists of a number of memory patterns and their basins of attraction. Together, they describe the path that the network behaviour is likely to follow given a particular initial state (which corresponds to an external input).

It can be demonstrated that priming systematically distorts the energy landscape of a network, effectively enlarging the basin of attraction of the primed pattern at the expense of other patterns. It is possible that given the same set of external features, outcome might depend on whether priming takes place (Fig. 3.6). In this sense, the context (priming from a higher level) interacts with the ongoing input to determine which

patterns are retrieved. This model highlights the dependence of lower
level pattern recognition on the state of higher level representations.

Construction of a multidimensional representation for symptoms

The representation of a symptom as a multidimensional structure
requires that additional information (about novel aspects of the symptom) be obtained from the patient. In clinical practice, the clinician
probes for only some salient aspects of the symptom. Often, this suffices,
and the clinician 'completes' – from his or her internal database – the
profile of the symptom. On other occasions, this may not be satisfactory
and the clinician will embark on a series of further probes until he or she
has been able to construct a final representation for the symptom.
Typically, this ascertainment procedure is sequential (Fig. 3.7).

In terms of the modelling strategy, the multidimensional structure that
represents a symptom is built up in stages. Successive quanta of information trigger revisions against a pre-existing representation that serves as the
background context. This process can be modelled by an attractor network
to which input information is presented in 'segmental codes', each covering
only a portion of the representation (Fig. 3.8). A segmental code,

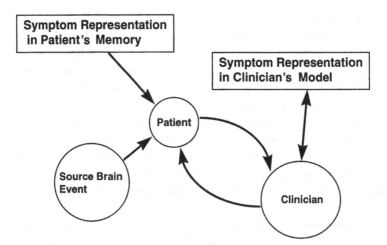

Fig. 3.7 The symptom construction process. When a symptom is experienced by
the patient, presumably as a result of a pathological brain signal, it is filed into the
patient's memory. The clinician strives to re-construct this experience by formulation in his or her own mind of a model of the symptom, and further elaborates
different dimensions of this model by repeated clarification with the patient.

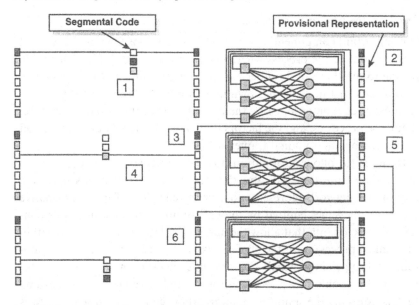

Fig. 3.8 Series processing of segmental codes. One segment of information addressing the first few units of the representation is transmitted from the source (patient report, left) to the receiver (clinician, right) (1). When the attractor network receives the information segment, it settles according to its internal dynamics into a 'provisional representation' (2). This provisional representation is then exposed to the arrival of the next segment of code (3, 4). The relative weight given to the provisional representation in relation to the incoming code is a measure of the extent of 'top-down' priming. After the arrival of the second code segment, the network is once again allowed to settle into a further provisional representation (5, 6). This cycle repeats itself until all the segmental codes have been presented.

therefore, specifies the pattern of activity for a subset of units in the network. At each processing stage, one segment is presented to the network. A segment corresponds clinically to a statement (or reply) made by the patient containing quanta of information on some aspect of the symptom. In the light of information presented as a segmental code, the network settles according to its own internal dynamics (guided by internal weights). The resulting network state is considered as a provisional representation of the symptom based on the information presented thus far. As the next segment of information arrives, the provisional representation becomes the starting point for further processing, following which the network is once again allowed to settle into a further provisional representation (now revised in the light of the new segment of information). This cycle repeats itself until all information segments have been presented.

Tracking the flow of information

One important component of symptom recognition is the monitoring and mapping out of the process whereby information is transferred from the patient to the clinician. In other words, an important aim for the clinician is to reconstruct in his or her own mind a representation of the pathological experience entertained by the patient. It is of the essence, therefore, that these processes, and the factors that affect them, are duly represented in the neurocomputational framework.

In order to follow information flow in the network, it is desirable to derive a measure that indicates the impact of code segments upon the provisional network representation, i.e. a reflection of how informative successive messages emitted by the patient are. Information in this context refers to quanta that allow the narrowing down of alternatives within the clinical process until the clinician is in the position to select a 'symptom prototype' into which the patient's description fits best. In this regard, Shannon's measure of entropy could be employed. According to this concept, the amount of information contained in a message is expressed as the amount of uncertainty in the system that is reduced upon the arrival of that message. Entropy can be measured in bits, one bit being the amount of information that corresponds to a binary decision. The entropy in a system (expressed as the number of bits) is therefore the average number of binary decisions required to reduce all uncertainty in the system. This quantity could be calculated as the negative sum of the product of the probability of each outcome times the logarithm of the probability to the base two:

$$H(A) = -\sum_{a \in A} p_a \log_2 p_a$$

where $H(A)$ is entropy of the system A; a represents possible states of system A; p_a is the probability of a occurring in A.

The amount of information associated with an event (such as the arrival of a verbal message) could thus be quantified in the system as the difference in entropy before and after the event. In the neural network model, the entropy in a given provisional representation could be measured by presenting the network with a large number of initial input vectors, covering randomly the entire state space. The frequency with which different prototypes are retrieved in response to such arrays of input probes is a measure of the probability associated with that prototype in the provisional representation. Accordingly, the entropy of the representation can be calculated. The difference in entropy in the representation before and after the event could thus be used to determine the informational impact of a particular event (such as the arrival of a code segment).

The effect of top-down influence

With the modelling method described, it is possible to explore the way in which the dynamics of a symptom recognition network interact with the amount of top-down priming (Fig. 3.9). In the extreme case of there not being any top-down influence, each code segment is processed entirely independently of previous codes, as if the network starts anew after each step. In this case, the information profile reflects the absolute amount of information in each code segment. On the other hand, with very high top-down weights, the system would settle very early on into a stable pattern.

Entropy

Retrieval

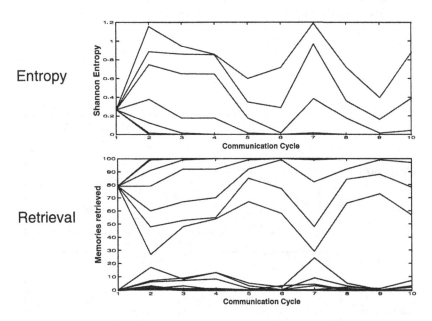

Fig. 3.9 Effect of top-down influence. The top figure depicts the changes in entropy in the system with time. In a network with a high degree of top-down priming, the entropy falls rapidly as the system quickly settles into a stable state. With decreasing levels of top-down priming, the entropy settles less readily. When there is no priming (top series), each code results in an entropy level independently of preceding codes. The bottom diagram shows the retrieval probability of the different learned patterns. A high level of priming ensures the early retrieval of a stable pattern.

The effect of the order of presentation

A further issue is whether it makes a difference to have highly informative segments presented earlier or later in the sequence. Simulation with this model has provided some initial ideas (Figs. 3.10 and 3.11). If highly informative codes are presented first, the network tends to settle earlier, even when top-down influence is relatively low. In contrast, if highly informative codes are presented late, the network tends to settle later, and top-down influence becomes important in determining the rate of settling. The higher the influence, the quicker the settling.

In situations in which there is high top-down influence, outcomes are not affected by the order of presentation, though decisions take longer to be arrived at if the highly informative codes are presented later. Interestingly, there is an intermediate range of top-down influence in which the outcome of processing crucially depends upon the order of presentation. In this situation, late arrival of high informational code segments would actually enable the network to escape from a previously held diagnostic hypothesis.

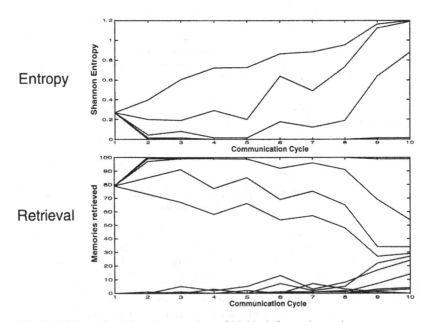

Fig. 3.10 Network with early reception of highly informative codes.

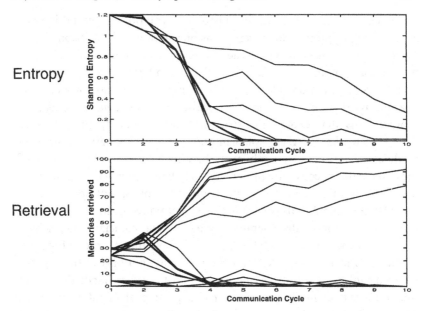

Fig. 3.11 Network with late reception of highly informative codes.

Summary

Neural networks are analogical representations of the way in which the human brain is assumed to approach cognitive tasks such as pattern recognition. This has led to the view that they are capable of multidimensional representation and parallel processing. It is also assumed that in real life clinicians tackle their diagnostic duties by making use of pattern recognition routines. It follows from this that neural networks might assist with clinical diagnoses. Moderate success in this enterprise has led others to model 'diagnostic reasoning' and, on occasions, to conceive of clinicians as 'embodied' neural networks. This chapter is about this modelling, its concepts, limitations, and the influence that it may have on the mapping and collecting of clinical information and even on the diagnostic constructs themselves. It also contends that pattern recognition of nosological (diagnostic) categories is crucially dependent upon the lower level processing of individual symptoms. Thus, the diagnostic process is conceptualized as a nest of hierarchical pattern-recognition processes involving symptom, syndrome and disease. Consideration of the rate and quality of information flow between these levels is important in understanding how, after all, the process of 'diagnosis' actually occurs in the mind of the clinician.

The chapter first discusses the historical evolution of the notions of disease and symptom, and current ideas on symptom construction. Then, ways are mentioned in which the problem of diagnosis and symptom recognition in psychiatry might be addressed in terms of neurocomputational models. At this early stage, these models were not proposed as quantitative descriptions of actual processes, but were considered as conceptual tools that exploit the structural and processing properties of neural networks for the implementation of basic pattern recognition modules. Using parallel modules as building blocks, realistic vistas of the diagnostic processes are presented, including context effects, information flow, and the recursive construction of symptom representation.

It also transpired that when studying symptom recognition, there is the need to focus upon the cognitive system of the clinicians themselves. Current reliance on structured interview and operational criteria for diagnostic assessment may have improved reliability, but only at the expense of losing information about symptoms. On the other hand, the use of multidimensional models requires that a great deal of information be collected; and this effort triggers into action the cognitive processes operating in the clinician's mind. Thus, unless these are properly mapped and modelled, there is the real danger that a rich vein of information and construction mechanisms is left unexplored. But what is worse is that we shall have no real method or knowledge to teach those who follow us, and each generation of psychiatrists will be condemned to the Sisyphean task of having to learn things all over again (i.e. they will have to format their own clinical experiences as best they can, without benefiting from the richness of the past). It is proposed in this chapter that neurocomputational models of symptom recognition and diagnostic processes might provide one of the frameworks (others will have to be sought in phenomenology, psychodynamic models, narrative theory, etc.) for the mapping of diagnostic skills, thereby rendering their teaching possible.

References

Aarsleff, H. (1982). *From Locke to Saussure. Essays on the Study of Language and Intellectual History*. London: Athlone Press.

Alston, W.P. (1989). *Epistemic Justification*. Ithaca: Cornell University Press.

Amit, D.J. (1989a). Symmetric neural networks at low memory loading. In *Modeling Brain Function: The World of Attractor Neural Networks*, pp. 155–213. Cambridge: Cambridge University Press.

Amit, D. (1989b). General ideas concerning dynamics. In *Modeling Brain Function: The World of Attractor Neural Networks*, pp. 97–154. Cambridge: Cambridge University Press.

Amit, D.J. (1989c). The basic attractor neural network. In *Modeling Brain Function: The World of Attractor Neural Networks*, pp. 58–96. Cambridge: Cambridge University Press.

APA (1980). *Diagnostic and Statistical Manual of Mental Disorders*, 3rd edn. Washington DC: American Psychiatric Association.

APA (1994). *Diagnostic and Statistical Manual of Mental Disorders*, 4th edn. Washington DC: American Psychiatric Association.

Baars, B.J. (1986). *The Cognitive Revolution in Psychology*. New York: Guilford Press.

Bailey, G.W.S. (1979). *Privacy and the Mental*. Amsterdam: Rodopi.

Berg, F (1956). Linné et Sauvages. *Lychnos*, **16**, 31–54.

Berrios, G.E. (1996). *The History of Mental Symptoms. Descriptive Psychopathology Since the 19th Century*. Cambridge: Cambridge University Press.

Berrios, G.E. & Chen, E.Y.H. (1993). Recognizing psychiatric symptoms: relevance to the diagnostic process. *British Journal of Psychiatry*, **163**, 308–14.

Bridgman, P.W. (1927). *The Logic of Modern Physics*. New York: MacMillan.

Burge, T. (1979). Individualism and the mental. *Midwest Studies in Philosophy*, **4**, 73–121.

Canguilhem, G. (1975). *Le Normal et le Pathologique*, 3rd edn. Paris: Presses Universitaires de France.

Cho, S. & Reggia, J.A. (1993). Multiple disorder diagnosis with adaptive competitive neural networks. *Artificial Intelligence in Medicine*, **5**, 469–87.

Davis, G.E., Lowell, W.E. & Davis, G.L. (1993). A neural network that predicts psychiatric length of stay. *Clinical Computing*, **10**, 87–92.

Faber, K. (1923). *Nosography in Modern Internal Medicine*. London: Milford.

Fumerton, R. (1988). The internalism/externalism controversy. *Philosophical Perspectives*, **2**, 442–59.

Gigerenzer, G., Swijtink, Z., Porter, T. et al. (1989). *The Empire of Chance*. Cambridge: Cambridge University Press.

Guimón, J., Mezzich, J.E. & Berrios, G.E. (eds.) (1988). *Diagnóstice en Psiquiatría*. Barcelona: Salvat.

Haigh, E. (1984). Xavier Bichat and the medical theory of the eighteenth century. *Medical History* (Suppl. 4), 1–138.

Hall, G.H. (1967). The clinical application of Bayes' theorema. *Lancet*, ii, 555–7.

Hampton, J. (1993). Prototype models of concept representation. In *Categories and Concepts: Theoretical Views and Inductive Data Analysis*, ed. I.V. Mechelen, J. Hampton, R.S. Michalski & P. Theuns, pp. 67–96. San Diego: Academic Press.

Howard, R.W. (1987). *Concepts and Schemata: an Introduction*. London: Cassell.

Jones, O.R. (ed.) (1971). *The Private Language Argument*, London: Macmillan.

Katz, M.M., Cole, J.O. & Barton, W.E. (eds.) (1965). *The Role and Methodology of Classification in Psychiatry and Psychopathology*. Washington DC: US Government Printing Office.

Kendell, R.E. (1975). *The Role of Diagnosis in Psychiatry*. Oxford: Blackwell.

Kendler, K.S. (1990). Towards a scientific psychiatric nosology. *Archives of General Psychiatry*, **47**, 969–73.

56   Eric Y.H. Chen and German E. Berrios

López-Piñero, J.M. (1983). *Historical Origins of the Concept of Neurosis*, translated by D. Berrios. Cambridge: Cambridge University Press.
Marková, I.S. & Berrios, G.E. (1995a). Insight in clinical psychiatry. A new model. *Journal of Nervous and Mental Disease*, **183**, 743–51.
Marková, I.S. & Berrios, G.E. (1995b). Mental symptoms: are they similar phenomena? The problem of symptom-heterogeneity. *Psychopathology*, **28**, 147–57.
Mezzich, J.E. & Solomon, H. (1980). *Taxonomy and Behavioural Science*. London: Academic Press.
Modai, I., Stoler, M., Inbar-Saban, N. & Saban, N. (1993). Clinical decisions for psychiatric inpatients and their evaluation by a trained neural network. *Methods of Information in Medicine*, **32**, 396–9.
Neale, M.C. & Cardon, L.R. (1992). *Methodology for Genetic Studies of Twins and Families*. Dordrecht: Kluwer Academic Publishers.
Newell, A. (1990). *Unified Theories of Cognition*. Cambridge, MA: Harvard University Press.
Plotinus (1996). *Ennead I*, translated by A.H. Amstrong. Cambridge, MA: Harvard University Press.
Ragin, C.C. & Becker, H.S. (1992). *What is a Case?* Cambridge: Cambridge University Press.
Riese, W. (1953). *The Conception of Disease*. New York: Philosophical Library.
Ripley, B.D. (1996). *Pattern Recognition and Neural Networks*. Cambridge: Cambridge University Press.
Rosenthal, D.M. (ed.) (1991). *The Nature of Mind*. New York: Oxford University Press.
Rumelhart, D.E. & McClelland, J.L. (1986). *Parallel Distributed Processing: Explorations in the Microstructure of Cognition*, Vols. 1 and 2. Cambridge, MA: MIT Press.
Sadler, J.Z., Wiggins, O.P. & Schwartz, M.A. (eds.) (1994). *Philosophical Perspectives on Psychiatric Diagnostic Classification*. Baltimore: Johns Hopkins University Press.
Saunders, J.T. & Henze, D.F. (1967). *The Private Language Problem*. New York: Random House.
Schwartz, M.A. & Wiggins, O.P. (1986). Logical empiricism and psychiatric classification. *Comprehensive Psychiatry*, **27**, 101–14.
Schwartz, M.A. & Wiggins, O.P. (1987). Diagnosis and ideal types: a contribution to psychiatric classification. *Comprehensive Psychiatry*, **28**, 277–91.
Stevens, P.F. (1984). Metaphors and typology in the development of botanical systematics, 1690–1960. *Taxon*, **33**, 169–211.
Vernon, K. (1988). The founding of numerical taxonomy. *British Journal for the History of Science*, **21**, 143–59.
Wittgenstein, L. (1958). *Philosophical Investigations*, 2nd edn, translated by G.E.M. Anscombe. Oxford: Blackwell.

4

Neural networks and psychopharmacology
S.B.G. PARK

Introduction

Psychopharmacological models have been developed from the two traditions now known as artificial neural networks and computational neuroscience. Artificial neural networks are based on primitive computing elements that are arranged to provide a brain-like architecture for information processing that contrasts with symbolic accounts of mental function. Computational neuroscience developed from mathematical models of phenomena at the level of the single neuron. Psychopharmacological models are on a spectrum between these two approaches, both of which have potential weaknesses. Artificial neural network models may include too many simplifying assumptions accurately to reflect pharmacological effects. Conversely, a model that incorporates too much cellular detail will be too complex to be useful in providing an explanation of network behaviour. This is reflected in the functions of these two types of model. Detailed models generally aim to replicate the causal mechanisms of a network and seek explanatory status through simplification. Artificial neural networks are used in a more limited fashion as hypothesis-generating tools. Available computing power leads to a trade-off between the size of a network and the amount of detail included. However, increasing power is leading to a convergence in the modelling process. The simplifications involved in model abstraction can be increasingly assessed against the behaviour of networks of much more detailed and biologically realistic neurons.

Psychopharmacology lacks a theoretical framework relating events at the level of the neuron to those at higher levels of central nervous system organization. Despite a wealth of detail on the cellular and behavioural effects of psychotropic drugs, the relation between the two remains obscure. Formulations of the role of different transmitter types frequently overlap (e.g. compare Spoont (1992) on serotonin (5-HT) and Callaway, Halliday and Naylor (1992) on acetylcholine) and the language used collapses across different levels of description. Thus, the effects of a neurotransmitter, for example, on signal to noise ratio are frequently not distinguished between cellular and attentional levels. Many current theories of monoamine action implicitly or explicitly assume a modular organization in function and describe a transmitter action in terms of a projection to a certain brain area. An example of the difficulties this leads to can be seen if Molliver's (1987) and Deakin's (Deakin and Graeff, 1991) theories of serotonergic function and mood are compared. In depression, the former theory argues for the importance of dorsal raphe projections to the frontal cortex, the latter for median raphe projections to the hippocampus. Neither hypothesis is able to discuss and contrast the function of the converse projections, i.e. dorsal raphe to the hippocampus and median raphe to frontal cortex. The immediate significance of neural network models is that they allow an explicit examination of neurotransmitter effects at both cellular and network levels within the same theoretical framework. In the case of serotonin, this allows an examination of the functional effect of the differential localization of the receptor types associated with these two projections within the same area of cortex.

Pharmacology in neural network models

Fast synaptic transmission

Fast synaptic transmission is modelled in biologically realistic simulations in terms of the specific receptor types. Thus, N-methyl-D-aspartate (NMDA), alpha-amino-3-hydroxy-5-methyl-4-isoxazole proprionic acid (AMPA), gamma-amino butyric acid receptor type A (GABA-A), and GABA-B receptors are regularly instantiated within such simulations as specific inputs to the postsynaptic cells with different time courses and amplitudes. These simulations typically allow an examination of the contribution of transmission through the different receptor types in the generation of different types of rhythmic network behaviour (e.g. Traven et al., 1993; Pinsky and Rinzel, 1994). The level of detail in these simulations can include models of the calcium-dependent link between presynaptic action potentials and transmitter release (Yamada and Zucker, 1992) and detailed kinetic schemes representing different conformational states and activities of the receptors (Standley et al., 1993; Destexhe et al.,

1994c). Interactions between transmitter types are modelled in terms of the contributions of different conductances to the firing behaviour of the target neuron (Kotter and Wickens, 1995).

Artificial neural networks distinguish between inhibitory and excitatory connections, though do not distinguish between inhibitory and excitatory cell types. This may be significantly unrealistic. Pyramidal cells within a layer of cortex are able to make specific excitatory contacts with other pyramidal cells, but only have inhibitory effects through interneurons that also receive input from many other pyramidal cells. Inhibitory effects are therefore much more diffuse. Inhibition within network models has a number of specific effects on network behaviour (Levene and Leven, 1991), as does its selective modulation as evidenced in the more biologically realistic models (Wilson and Bower, 1992; Liljenstrom and Hasselmo, 1993; 1995). Given that a number of neuromodulatory inputs have selective effects on inhibitory interneurons, this also requires models that aim to represent this to separate inhibitory and excitatory neuron types.

Activation (input–output) functions

The output of a neuron within neural network models ranges from a simple on–off switch to models in which the cells are able to generate complex spike trains. The activation function within an artificial neural network represents the mathematical translation of the inputs to a neuron into an output. Artificial neural networks typically use a sigmoid function. In addition to the properties of baseline and ceiling firing rates, their non-linear character adds to the computational power of neural networks. They are used to reflect an average firing rate of neurons. As part of the examination of neuromodulatory effects on the signal to noise ratio behaviour of networks of neurons, alteration of this input–output function has attracted particular interest. The part of the activation function that is altered is known as the gain; this determines the slope of the sigmoid at the inflection point and hence the differential response to inputs of varying strengths (Fig. 4.1). The baseline and ceiling rates remain the same, but in the presence of either inhibitory or excitatory stimulation with increased gain, the response of the unit is greater so that there is a decreased response to smaller inputs and an increased output to stronger stimulation. This approach is relatively recent (Servan-Schreiber, Printz and Cohen, 1990) but it has led to a number of simulations encompassing the changes in information processing in

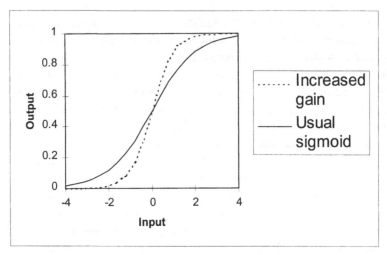

Fig. 4.1 Sigmoid input–output function and the effect of increased gain.

schizophrenia, and the response to various drug challenges in normal human volunteers. These simulations are examined in more detail later in the chapter.

An aspect of the input–output function which has been criticized as being absent from artificial network models is the adaptation and decrease in firing rate of a neuron that is observed in response to prolonged stimulation. This is relevant to the examination of the effects of neuromodulation given the large body of evidence that multiple neurotransmitters affect this property of neurons. Noradrenaline, dopamine, acetylcholine and 5-HT have all been shown to decrease adaptation. The difficulty in including this property within artificial neural networks is the static nature of the input–output function reflecting an average firing rate. The change in adaptation thus occurs within a time frame that is not included within these simulations, and hence a more detailed approach is required. Within biologically realistic simulations, this effect is readily represented (Barkai and Hasselmo, 1994). Among the effects of including this component are that learning rules that include a covariance component will show an increase in weight gain in connections with this change in cellular behaviour; indeed, changes in the rate of adaptation could by themselves be a limited component of the way in which memories are represented (Berner and Woody, 1991).

The time frame of simulations is also important in the generation of complex network phenomena. It has been argued that this complexity provides a further dimension to information processing in the brain that cannot be captured in simpler models (Globus, 1992). Models using simplified network components, with neuromodulation of these network dynamics through alterations in the gain parameter (Wu and Liljenstrom, 1994) and neuronal adaptation (Cartling, 1995), show a number of effects on the information-processing properties of the network. The biological significance of these effects is not clear, given the difficulties in characterizing these complex states.

Baseline firing rate

A further cellular effect of neurotransmitters is on the resting membrane potential. Within detailed simulations, the importance of this effect can be clearly seen in the models of Destexhe on the oscillatory properties of thalamic reticular neurons (Destexhe et al., 1994a) and networks of such neurons (Destexhe et al., 1994b), as discussed below.

Within artificial neural networks, general effects on the level of neuronal excitability are readily represented by altering the effect of a 'bias' unit or by more directly moving the unit input–output function sideways (Fig. 4.2). This provides the neuron units with an activity reflecting a longer time period and as such can be used to reflect both tonic neuromodulatory inputs and the level of activity of second messenger systems.

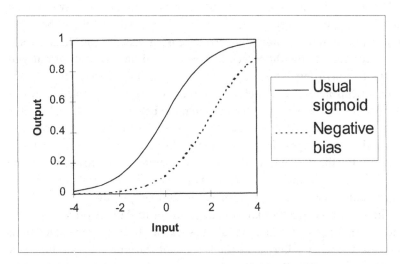

Fig. 4.2 The effect of decreasing the input from the bias unit on input–output function.

In addition, it can be used as a point of distinction between cell types in more detailed models (Berns and Sejnowski, 1996).

Learning

The discovery of the properties of the NMDA receptor provided an important impetus to neural network models in that it provided a basis for the most basic form of learning represented. Learning as represented by changes in synaptic strength reflecting long-term potentiation (LTP), with the extent of the changes being dependent on the product of pre-synaptic and postsynaptic activity, is known as Hebbian. Typically, such learning rules have an associated learning rate constant that can be modified to reflect neuromodulation. More detailed cell-level computational models of LTP induction (Holmes and Levy, 1990; Ambros Ingerson and Lynch, 1993) have yet to be reflected in abstract neural networks, which rarely distinguish the mechanisms of LTP from long-term depression (LTD). However, one aspect of the cellular basis of learning that has been examined at network level is the distinction between volume and wiring transmission (Agnati et al., 1995). This has been looked at in models of the role of nitric oxide in learning (Montague, Gally and Edelman, 1991). The computational consequences of volume learning rules have largely been explored in terms of cortical map formation and have not yet been applied to behaviour.

The most popular learning algorithm in artificial neural networks, the back-propagation of error, adds a non-physiological element in the explicit computation of an individual error term for each unit in the network. The error reflects the difference between actual and desired output and allows for environmental feedback in the learning process. The significance of this addition is unclear, as units in a network trained with this algorithm have responses that can match the behaviour of the cells in the biological networks they represent in a number of respects. One possibility is that error minimization occurs within cortical structures without the need for the computation of an explicit error term. However, despite this face validity, questions remain as to the impact of this non-physiological component on any pharmacological manipulations.

The most biologically plausible mechanism to date of providing feedback as an error signal to a neural network can be seen in the algorithms carrying out what is known as reinforcement learning. This learning rule is intended to reflect the combined effect of ascending noradrenergic and dopaminergic pathways and provides a general signal to the whole network or selected regions rather than specific signals to each unit. As a result, training in such networks can take significantly longer. This rule is discussed in more detail later in the chapter in terms of its relationship to what is known of dopaminergic function. Given that the time course of the therapeutic effect of both antidepressant and antipsychotic drugs is consistent with mechanisms involving learning, this is an area of psychopharmacological neural network modelling that will particularly benefit from more neurophysiological detail (Spitzer, 1995).

Network architecture

Important pharmacological differences occur at both cytoarchitectonic and modular levels. Artificial neural networks can readily accommodate modular distinctions in innervation (Callaway et al., 1994) by selectively changing aspects of identified groups of units representing different brain regions. However, this is not the case for cytoarchitectonic distinctions that are not represented in such models. In addition to the failure to distinguish excitatory and inhibitory cell types, often there is no representation of recurrent connections within a given layer. Given that the majority of the excitatory input to a layer comes from such intrinsic connections, this may be an important omission from more abstract models. Indeed, certain models posit functional effects that are dependent on this grain of detail (e.g. Hasselmo and Schnell, 1994; Niebur and Koch, 1994). Whereas it is argued that models at different levels of detail aim to describe different phenomena, this is not always the case, and hypotheses are at times in direct competition. Modular selectivity of neuromodulatory inputs is often a very relative phenomenon, whereas cytoarchitectonic distinctions can be much clearer. However, detailed knowledge of cytoarchitectonic pharmacology is limited and the development of these models requires further anatomical and neurophysiological characterization of the receptor distributions and effects.

Animal behavioural pharmacology

The importance of these studies arises from the fact that some of the invertebrate networks studied are the most completely characterized in terms of their neurophysiology and pharmacology. They can therefore be used to gain an understanding of those simplifications in neurophysiological detail that can be made that still leave a robust model of network behaviour. Additionally, they provide a number of examples of how network modelling and experimental studies have been combined to gain an understanding of the relationship between the network components and the resulting behaviour (Kepler, Marder and Abbot, 1990; Calabrese and de Schutter, 1992). A number of different pharmacological effects have been examined. They include the role of multiple receptors in the expression of neuromodulation by a single transmitter (Zhang and Harris Warwick, 1994), neuromodulation intrinsic to network function (Katz, Getting and Frost, 1994; Katz and Frost, 1996), and the effects of peptidergic and electrical neurotransmission (Kepler et al., 1990; Johnson, Peck and Harris Warrick 1993, 1994). In certain instances, they show that relatively detailed circuit models have difficulty in capturing major neuromodulator effects on rhythmic network behaviour (Rowat and Selverston, 1993). However detailed these models are, they too will make certain assumptions about network components for which there may be limited evidence, e.g. ion channel distribution within the neuron. Thus, increasing the level of detail in a model will not necessarily lead to a replication of the desired effect.

Some of the most detailed experimental and modelling work in vertebrates has been carried out on the neural basis of swimming movements in the lamprey. The relative contribution of NMDA and non-NMDA receptor-mediated excitatory transmission and the effect of serotonin (5-HT) on the frequency of the rhythmic burst pattern of the spinal network underlying locomotion have been studied, and the effects of experimental pharmacological manipulation on the behaviour have been replicated (Wallen et al., 1992; Traven et al., 1993). From a methodological perspective, a repeated statement is that the modelling was a necessary adjunct to the experimental work because of the complexity brought about by the number of elements in the networks. This statement remains true for artificial neural networks in that the non-linearity of the input–output functions of the multiple units renders them opaque to intuitive predictions as to their behaviour in response to manipulation.

Psychopharmacological simulations

Simulations of the generation of specific patterns of electrical activity in diverse brain areas include some of the highest level effects examined using biologically realistic neurons and neuromodulation. At the network level, it can be readily shown that the combination of short-range and long-range excitation with local inhibition leads to synchronized oscillations (Freeman, 1968; Wilson and Cowan, 1972; Wilson and Bower,

1991, 1992). Two groups of simulations that are of particular interest to psychopharmacology relate to the generation of hippocampal and thalamic rhythms in response to pharmacological challenge and their relationship to epilepsy, learning and sleep. The extension of this work to examine the neuropathology of Alzheimer's disease can be found in Chapter 12 of this book.

Hippocampal oscillations

A model of the hippocampal oscillations occurring in the disinhibited hippocampal slice has been developed by Traub and Miles (1992). In the slightly disinhibited slice long-duration after-hyperpolarization, slow GABA-B IPSPs and the recurrent pyramidal cell excitation were all critical in the generation of the population oscillation of 1–4 Hz. However, in extending the model to examine the mechanisms underlying synchronized multiple bursts, a phenomenon seen with the use of GABA-A blocker picrotoxin and that may reflect seizure activity, the authors generate the prediction that a dendritic calcium conductance was the critical component to the network behaviour. Two aspects of this simulation of a more general note are the use of the model to develop a hypothesis for subsequent experimental confirmation (see Traub and Wong, 1982; Miles and Wong, 1983) and the detail of simulation involved in this particular prediction.

Traub, Miles and Buzsaki (1992) have also presented a model of the rhythmic activity induced in the hippocampal slice by the muscarinic agonist carbachol as a method of examining the relationship between those rhythms and the hippocampal theta rhythm recorded in rodents in vivo. The effect of carbachol was simulated as a block in GABA-A-mediated and GABA-B-mediated inhibition, a block in NMDA postsynaptic activity, a reduction in the after-hyperpolarization conductance, and a tonic depolarization of the apical compartment of the pyramidal cell dendrites. The model produced oscillations at the observed frequencies of 5 Hz. A critical component in the generation of this effect was the recurrent excitatory connections between pyramidal cells. This was in contrast to their simulation of the theta rhythm in which the resonance of the CA3 network at the septal input frequency was not dependent on these connections. This model can be compared with that of Liljenstrom and Hasselmo (1993, 1995) of cholinergic modulation of the oscillatory activity of the structurally similar piriform cortex. Again, their model was able to replicate a number of experimental observations of the effects of cholinergic modulation on both the electroencephalogram (EEG) and evoked potentials. However, the inclusion in this model of data from their laboratory on the effect of acetylcholine to suppress intrinsic excitatory synaptic transmission led to a separate mechanism of rhythm production that was not dependent on intrinsic bursting activity in the pyramidal neurons as in the Traub model. The suppression of intrinsic connections was also proposed as the mechanism for the suppression of the faster gamma-type oscillations. These models show the interplay between experimental findings at the cellular level and the use of the models in understanding the interaction of the multiple components involved in the behaviour at the network level. The difference in mechanism proposed by the models attests to the fact that it is not just the amount of detail that determines the observed effects, but also which details.

A further important difference between the two models is that the later uses a much more abstract representation of the neural elements. In particular, the input–output function of the neurons used was an experimentally determined sigmoid in which a single parameter determined the threshold, slope and amplitude of the response to stimulation. The use of this abstraction that was developed in comparison with the performance of a more biologically realistic simulation of the oscillatory properties of piriform cortex (Wilson and Bower, 1992) can be viewed against the use of the sigmoid function as the input–output function of artificial neural networks.

Thalamic oscillations and sleep

The relay and reticular nuclei of the thalamus have an important role in generating some types of sleep oscillations. Realistic models of networks of thalamic reticular cells, interconnected with inhibitory synapses, show robust oscillations (Destexhe et al., 1994d, Golomb, Wang and Rinzel, 1994, 1996), reflecting their in-vivo behaviour. In vitro, however, such oscillations do not occur and it has been proposed that this is as the result of the absence of neuromodulatory inputs to the in-vitro preparation. This has been modelled in terms of the effect of noradrenergic and serotonergic inputs to depolarize thalamic cells by blocking a leak potassium current (Destexhe et al., 1994b). The change in resting membrane potential brought about by the neuromodulatory input was able to generate these two activity states of the thalamic reticular network. This is proposed as a means whereby the ascending neuromodulatory inputs from the brain stem control arousal.

This model included a representation of the transduction of the neuromodulator effects on the potassium current by G-proteins developed in earlier work (Destexhe et al., 1994a). The extent of pharmacological detail possible in these models is perhaps most clearly seen in a model that examines how the relationship between transmitter reuptake, synaptic concentration of transmitter and G-protein activation kinetics determines differences in inhibitory responses between the thalamus and hippocampus (Destexhe and Sejnowski, 1995). In addition to the equilibrium between active and desensitized GABA-B receptor states, the model includes multiple binding sites for the G-proteins on the potassium channel and a consideration of the effect of uptake blockade on synaptic currents. As yet, there are no equivalent network models of monoamine reuptake and receptor activation, but elements of such models are present in this work, with estimates for the parameters of the G-protein-mediated conductances for 5-HT1 (serotonergic), alpha-2 (noradrenergic) and D2 (dopaminergic) receptor subtypes (Destexhe et al., 1994a).

Models have also been developed examining the neuromodulatory control of the rhythmic behaviour of thalamocortical neurons. The status of the neuromodulatory inputs to these neurons in part determines the different firing patterns associated with EEG-synchronized sleep, and periods of arousal and cognition. One of the difficult problems posed for psychopharmacologists is how to disentangle multiple and apparently overlapping effects of the different transmitters. In the case of the thalamic relay neuron, three different ionic conductances are affected by a number of different neuromodulators, including acetylcholine, noradrenaline, serotonin and histamine. McCormick, Huguenard and Strawbridge (1992) have used simulations as a means of exploring the relative contribution of modulation of the three different conductances. As the authors point out, such an experiment would be difficult to perform either in vivo or in vitro. Through the modelling, they were able to clarify the relative effects of the conductances on neuronal activity and were able to replicate the marked effect of neuromodulation on firing mode. The models also suggested experimental tests of the effects of the neuromodulators on specific aspects of cell behaviour. This model can be compared with the higher level model of Lytton, Destexhe and Sejnowski (1996), which examined the behaviour of the cell in response to simulated repetitive cortical synaptic input and a more restricted representation of neuromodulation that suggested neither alone was sufficient to generate the range of oscillation frequencies seen in thalamocortical neurons.

As yet, there is no specific way of modelling the effect of 5-HT2 receptor blockade to increase slow wave sleep, though more general models of the respective influences of cholinergic and serotonergic inputs on slow wave sleep and REM sleep exist (Sutton, Mamelak and Hobson, 1992; Sutton and Hobson, 1993; Yamamoto et al., 1994). Sutton's model is based on a neocortical network with ascending aminergic and cholinergic inputs from the brain stem, thalamic inputs and intracortical excitation. The further abstraction within this model generates predictions that can be tested in human experiments. The model stores sequences of 'memories' that can be reliably reproduced by the network during the simulated wake state, but are output in a discontinuous and mixed fashion during simulated REM sleep as a reflection of dream bizarreness. In view of the limited information on cognitive processes during sleep, the predictions are made in terms of the respective effects of ponto-geniculooccipital burst cell activity in sleep and during waking on cortical activity assessed by combining functional magnetic resonance imaging (MRI) with EEG.

Dopamine and learning

The ascending diffuse inputs from the brain stem have been recognized for some time within the neural network literature as being of importance to learning (Hawkins and Kandel 1984; Gluck and Thompson, 1987). The aim of the earlier models was more to do with developing an understanding of learning than exploring the role of specific ascending inputs. However, as these models have developed, they are increasingly making explicit calls to the neuroscience literature as regards the behaviour of these inputs. Two recent examples (Montague and Sejnowski, 1994; Friston et al., 1994) support their simulations by reporting the match between their models and the electrophysiological data of Ljungberg, Apicella and Schultz (1992) on the firing behaviour of primate dopaminergic neurons during learning. The loss of the phasic response of the dopaminergic neurons once a behavioural response to a reward is acquired shows that the association between the reward and dopamine is not a simple linear relationship. The hypothesis suggested by these simulations is that the firing of the dopaminergic neurons reflects a prediction error (Quartz et al., 1992; Montague et al., 1993). This hypothesis about events at the level of the cell receives further face validity from simulations using the same type of learning algorithm showing the development and registration of activity-dependent neural maps in the superior colliculus (Pouget et al., 1993), and from the large body of work using a temporal difference learning algorithm to replicate many of the phenomena of associative learning (Klopf, 1988; Sutton and Barto, 1990; Donahoe, Burgos and Palmer, 1993). The selectionist framework of Friston et al. (1994), although it differs from the temporal difference learning algorithm in certain important respects, shares the use of the time derivative of the sensory signals. Despite the different theoretical derivation of the selectionist model, its convergence at this point adds important support to this explanation for the behaviour of dopaminergic neurons.

At an algorithmic level, one area that can be questioned as a reflection of dopaminergic function is the extent to which synaptic weights are differentially increased or decreased following the reinforcement signal. Evidence from both neocortex (Law Tho, Desce and Crepel, 1995) and striatum (Pennartz et al., 1993) suggests an effect of dopamine on LTD but not on LTP. However, reinforcement algorithms lead to both increases and decreases in weights, and in certain instances the effect of the reinforcement signal to increase weights is 10–100 times greater than the effect to decrease them. This may be reflected in the failure of some of the simulations of associative learning to replicate the effects of dopaminergic manipulation. The latent inhibition and Kamin blocking apparent in some of the models are not amenable to changes in the strength of the reinforcement signal in the same way as described for dopaminergic manipulation in the animal and human experiments (Joseph and Jones, 1991). Part of the difficulty may also arise from the fact that these phenomena are differentially dependent on a number of different brain structures (Gallo and Candido, 1995) not represented within the models. More anatomically detailed models have been developed (Gluck and Myers, 1992) that provide a more realistic representation of these interference effects, although as yet they have not been validated against such pharmacological manipulation.

The role of the basal ganglia in learning is examined in the significantly more detailed model of Berns and Sejnowski (1995, 1996). This model includes representations of the cortex, striatum (with separate matrix and striosomal neurons), internal and external segments of the globus pallidus, subthalamic nucleus and thalamus, with realistic connectivity and differences between the input–output functions of the different cell types. It incorporates the Montague–Dayan–Sejnowski model of dopamine and reinforcement learning (Montague et al., 1995) and additionally describes a mechanism whereby a prediction error is computed by the striosome to be sent to those units representing the dopamine neurons of the ventral tegmental area and substantia nigra. As a result, it provides one of the most biologically complete accounts of dopamine function yet developed that simulates a number of different behaviours. In addition to a consideration of the appearance of hemiballismus with lesions of the subthalamic nucleus, the model examines the performance on the Wisconsin Card Sorting Test and shows perseveration typical of Parkinson's disease when a dopaminergic deficit is simulated. This model is not specifically about dopamine, but rather aims to develop a model of the role of the basal ganglia in learning and selecting between sequences of actions. In part, it was motivated by the difficulty for more abstract connectionist models to learn sequential cognitive processes such as used in the Wisconsin Card Sorting Test (Parks et al., 1992). Thus, the effect of a pharmacological manipulation has been successfully used in the validation of this much more biologically constrained network.

Attention

An important series of models examining dopaminergic, noradrenergic and subsequently cholinergic effects on tasks involving the effects of neuromodulation on attention has been implemented by the addition of two features to artificial neural networks. The gain of the sigmoid input–output function of units within the network is altered to increase its sensitivity to the inputs, and only certain groups of units within the network are changed in this way to reflect a selective innervation of discrete brain areas by the neuromodulatory inputs.

The justification for the change in the shape of the sigmoid is based on the literature suggesting that the effect of dopamine and noradrenaline on neuronal firing is not to alter the baseline rate but rather to potentiate the responses to excitatory and inhibitory inputs. The seminal publications examined catecholamine effects through a comparison of their simulations with the effects of amphetamines in normal volunteers and the performance of patients with schizophrenia on a series of attentional tasks (Servan-Schreiber et al., 1990; Cohen and Servan-Schreiber, 1992). The use of this and more complicated single gain parameters in determining the shape of the neuronal input–output functions to represent neuromodulatory effects can be seen in subsequent publications from several different groups (Callaway et al., 1994; Sutton and Hobson, 1993; Jobe et al., 1994; Wu and Liljenstrom, 1994). The additional feature of the original simulations was to designate one group of units as representing the frontal cortex, and then to examine the effect of selectively modulating this group of units in order to reflect the relative dominance of the dopaminergic input to this area compared with other neocortical areas. The psychological component of the tasks was the working memory component that maintains representations of task-relevant information on line and that has been termed 'contextual' information.

The strength of these simulations is that despite their simplicity they are able to simulate many non-intuitive findings (e.g. Servan-Schreiber et al., 1994, Servan-Schreiber and Blackburn, 1995) from drug challenge studies affecting different neuromodulator systems. (Callaway et al. (1994) explore the differences between pimozide and clonidine on speed–accuracy curves in a signal detection task.) Also, by their explicit nature, they are able to generate falsifiable hypotheses. Difficulties arise, however, as a result of the degree of abstraction used in terms of both the representation of the psychological task and the neuromodulation. Typical criticisms would be the failure of the gain parameter to reflect the change in adaptation in neuronal firing that is a predominant effect of neuromodulators (e.g. Barkai and Hasselmo, 1994; Hasselmo, 1995), or that attention both involves multiple networks (Jackson, Marrocco and Posner, 1994) and is determined by phenomena at the level of the single cell (Niebur and Koch, 1994). Against this it is argued that at the level of description of the task performance, these models provide a coherent account, and modification is required when they do not match up to the observed effects at that level (Callaway et al., 1994). A more theoretical criticism reflects the falsifiability of the more general hypotheses derived from such models. When Cohen and Servan-Schreiber describe their models in terms of a predominant effect of dopamine on the 'internal representation of contextual information', it is not clear how one would specifically measure this type of context. However, this difficulty is not restricted to neural network models, as can be seen in comparison with, for example, the 'disconnection' hypothesis of median raphe function (Deakin and Graeff, 1991). Arguably, the more explicit nature of the network models increases their falsifiability in comparison.

Clinical psychopharmacology

General effects of neuromodulation on cortical behaviour

One of the earliest neural network models of psychopathology (Hoffman, 1987) examined possible neuromodulator effects in a model of flight of ideas and mania. In this model, parameters determining general network dynamics were altered and the behaviour of the network was then compared with clinical phenomena. One particular perturbation was to increase the general randomness of the neural responses to excitatory and inhibitory input. This led to a network that failed to stabilize and instead moved from one memory to the next in a manner suggestive of flight of ideas. In support for the model, evidence was cited of lithium effects to reduce randomness in neuronal firing patterns, and the effects of noradrenergic projections to alter randomness in terms of signal-to-noise effects, thus proposing mania as a hyponoradrenergic state. It is important to note that this was not a model designed to challenge the classical amine hypothesis of affective disorder, but rather an exploration of what network effects might be seen as a result of perturbations at the cell level that might reflect neurotransmitter actions. A similar perspective is useful in a more recent publication (Jobe et al., 1994) that looks at similar abstract neuromodulator effects, but in a more detailed cell model in which the primary effect is in terms of dendritic conductances, and relates this to a wide variety of psychiatric phenomena.

Dopamine and Parkinson's disease

A number of models exist that examine the dopaminergic deficit in Parkinson's disease (Borrett, Yeap and Kwan, 1993; Contrerasvidal and Stelmach, 1995; Contrerasvidal, Teulings and Stelmach, 1995; Berns and Sejnowksi, 1995, 1996). Points of comparison between the models include their relative detail, which aspect of the disturbance they are aiming to examine, and the type of predictions the models make. The most abstract model (Borrett et al., 1993) aims to find a simple explanation for certain aspects of the movement disorder using a four-layer recurrently connected artificial neural network to represent a cortical–basal ganglia–thalamic–cortical loop. The effect of dopamine depletion was modelled as a general reduction in activity of the layer representing the thalamus (equivalent to increased inhibition from the basal ganglia component of the network), thus taking a very functional approach to its representation. The network was able to reproduce prototypical activations in agonist and antagonist muscles that produce the displacement of a limb about a single joint, and the bradykinesia and inability to maintain repetitive movements seen in Parkinson's disease. The model thus supports the evidence from MPTP models of parkinsonism that the functional effect of the reduced dopamine is to increase the inhibitory input from the globus pallidus, and that this is sufficient to explain these aspects of the movement disorder. This simple abstract model thus provides a relatively simple explanation that is not obvious intuitively.

Dopamine and schizophrenia

Despite inconsistent evidence, the dopamine hypothesis of schizophrenia remains one of the most enduring in psychopharmacology. Similarly, there is an extensive literature on frontal deficits in schizophrenia. These two hypotheses have been linked in the growing body of evidence that frontal lobe function is impaired with deficits in dopaminergic transmission and that this is responsible for a number of the cognitive deficits seen in schizophrenia. Cohen and Servan-Schreiber (1992, 1993) have compared their simulations of decreased gain in 'context' units and found them to match the performance of schizophrenic patients in a number of psychological tasks – the Stroop Test, a continuous performance test, and a lexical disambiguation task. In each case, the simulation was able to capture the pattern of deficits seen in the clinical population, thus presenting a hypothesis with marked face validity and no small degree of construct validity. The authors acknowledge that disturbances other than a reduction in dopamine to the prefrontal cortex are involved in schizophrenia, and also provide a possible explanation for the apparently contradictory observation that thought disorder improves with neuroleptic medication. In an extended discussion, the model is contrasted with other neuropsychological models of schizophrenia and the deficits found in related disorders such as Parkinson's disease and specific frontal lobe lesions (Cohen and Servan-Schreiber, 1992).

A difficulty for the models is that a number of the components are still regarded as unproven hypotheses. Studies relating to and questioning some of the assumptions made, such as the distinction between specific and generalized psychological deficits in schizophrenia (Javitt et al., 1995), whether schizophrenia is associated with increased or decreased interference on the Stroop (Williams et al., 1996), and the role of mesocortical dopaminergic transmission in cognitive function (Roberts et al., 1994), continue to appear as active topics of research. However, the framework provided by the models allows testing against such new evidence by virtue of the explicit representation of the components. A separate issue is the status accorded to the hypothesis generated by this work. That it is at least similar to the status of hypotheses generated more directly from experimental observation can be seen in the diversity of experimental studies in which it is cited. These range from animal behavioural pharmacology (Brockel and Fowler, 1995) through genetic (Maier et al., 1994) and social studies (Penn et al., 1995) in schizophrenia.

The models so far described of the three major ascending dopaminergic inputs are to a large extent independent of each other. However, with the development of models of specific dopamine receptor types, the building blocks will be in place to examine questions such as why D2 blockade is relevant to the effects of abnormal frontal–temporal connectivity.

Serotonin and depression

The functions of serotonin on mood are often contrasted with those of dopamine, and a model is developed of this by Hestenes in Chapter 6 of this book. The hippocampus is an area of the brain with a limited dopaminergic innervation, but which has a pronounced input from serotonergic neurons. The most comprehensive theoretical account of the relationship between 5-HT neurotransmission and mood (Deakin and Graeff, 1991) has proposed that projections from the median raphe nucleus terminating on 5-HT1A receptors in the hippocampus mediate adaptive responses in the face of chronic aversive stimulation. Depression occurs when there is a failure of transmission in this pathway, which is rectified by treatment with antidepressants. The following model, whilst in general agreement with this hypothesis, aims to show the ways in which it can be developed further.

There is good evidence that the pathways of the two major serotonergic projections from the median and dorsal raphe nuclei are anatomically and functionally distinct. The thicker axons from the median raphe appear to be selectively associated with a subset of inhibitory interneurons subserving feedforward inhibition in predominantly dendritic fields (Hornung and Celio, 1992; Miettinen and Freund, 1992), with the finer projections from the dorsal raphe terminating on 5-HT2 receptors on a different set of interneurons located at a deeper cytoarchitectonic layer, which may modulate feedback inhibition. There is indirect evidence that the effects of median raphe transmission are inhibitory to their respective interneurons, in keeping with the anatomical association between the median raphe innervation and the 5-HT1A receptor. Conversely, the evidence supports a stimulatory role for the effects of dorsal raphe stimulation through 5-HT2 receptors. Architecturally, this is fairly straightforward (Fig. 4.3). At a coarser level of anatomical detail, there is an extensive overlap between the projections from the two serotonergic nuclei.

A number of questions can now be posed. What is the role of feedforward inhibition in depression? How do the functional effects of median raphe projections differ between frontal cortex and hippocampus? How do the functional effects of dorsal and median raphe projections differ in the hippocampus? These are not questions that can be currently answered, but with conventional accounts of serotonergic function it is also very difficult to generate hypotheses. As a result of the use of particular neurons as the target of an innervation within a given brain region, this is no longer the case for a neural net model. In order to implement representations of the two different serotonergic projections, the basic artificial neural network will not suffice. Inhibitory interneurons need to be distinguished from excitatory cells, along with different types of inhibitory interneuron. In addition, excitatory feedback and more excitatory units than inhibitory units are included in the network to

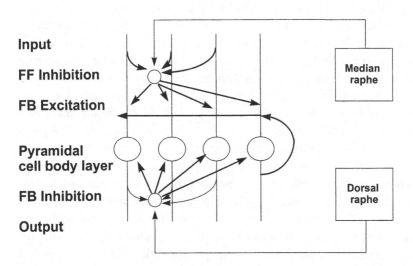

Fig. 4.3 Serotonergic innervation to a simplified archicortex as represented in simulation of antidepressant action. Inhibitory input to feed forward (FF) inhibitory interneuron from the median raphe nucleus; excitatory input from dorsal raphe nucleus to feedback (FB) inhibitory interneuron.

increase the extent to which it resembles archicortex. However, other than these architectural constraints, the neural network has the same components as an artificial neural network. Unlike dopamine, there is clearer evidence that changes in serotonergic transmission are associated with changes in the firing rate of the target neurons. Hence change in activity at the different 5-HT receptor subtypes is implemented as a change in the baseline firing rate of the respective interneurons through a change in the effect of the bias unit (see Fig. 4.2).

In order to simulate the depressed state, the network is first trained to discriminate two sets of inputs, one of which represents rewarding stimuli, the other punishing. The network is then trained on a set of patterns in which one of the previously rewarding inputs is paired with the punishment-type response. Previous punishment-type input–output pattern pairs continue to be presented, and reward-type pairs are excluded from the training set. This is intended to reproduce the effect of loss and a stressful environment. This leads to a generalization of punishment-type responding such that all reward-type inputs when now presented to the network are responded to as though they were punishing. In the final part of the simulation, the remaining reward-type input–output pattern pairs are returned to the training set. The extent to which the network continues to respond to reward-type inputs as punishing is taken as the measure of depression, and the time it takes the network to relearn the former reward responding is the measure of the time to 'recovery'.

Both tricyclic antidepressants and selective serotonin reuptake inhibitors are active at the terminals of both of the two serotonergic projections. They have similar effects to increase transmission at postsynaptic 5-HT1A receptors, but have opposite effects on dorsal raphe transmission, which can be seen clinically as part of their differing side-effect profiles. The effects of both types of antidepressant, placebo and a postsynaptic 5-HT1A antagonist were examined during the third phase of training the network. The results of the simulations can be seen in Figure 4.4. The simulated antidepressant treatment decreased the time the network took to return to the original non-depressed-type responding. This effect was not seen with the simulation of acute changes in serotonergic function however strongly implemented. The model supports Deakin's prediction that a postsynaptic 5-HT1A antagonist would delay the recovery compared with placebo (Deakin, Graeff and Guimaraes, 1993), and additional simulations showed a partial prophylactic antidepressant effect during the second stage of training.

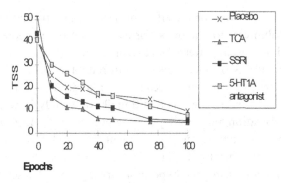

Fig. 4.4 Results of simulation of antidepressant activity. TSS (total sum of squares) reflects training error and level of 'depression' within the network; epochs are the number of presentations of the training set and reflect time. The TCA (tricyclic antidepressant) effect is implemented as decreased feedforward inhibition and decreased feedback inhibition; SSRI (selective serotonin reuptake inhibitor) decreased feedforward inhibition and increased feedback inhibition; 5-HT1A receptor antagonist increased feedforward inhibition. Results shown are the mean of ten simulations for each of the types of serotonergic manipulation.

The mechanism of antidepressant action within the simulation is through enhancing the learning at the connections between the input and middle layers. This is compatible with controlling a gating function by the feedforward inhibitory interneurons, as might be reflected in the predominant innervation of the dentate by the median raphe nucleus within the hippocampus, and the role of the dentate in the hippocampal–entorhinal circuitry (Jones, 1993). Further support for this aspect of the model can be seen in the effects of median raphe stimulation on LTP induction in the dentate (Klancnik and Phillips, 1991) and the 5-HT1A receptor specificity of the effect of 5-HT-releasing drugs to increase the sensitivity of the dentate gyrus to perforant path stimulation (Richter-Levin and Segal, 1990).

In terms of the behaviour of the network, the effect of the antidepressant is to reduce the interference resulting from the changed association of one of the input patterns. Effects such as generalization and interference are important properties of neural networks in the more general argument as regards the extent to which artificial neural networks can reflect brain functioning. Connectionist interference is not synonymous with that observed experimentally in interference learning paradigms; however, as the experimental form is thought to arise as a result of the hippocampally mediated context effects, the antidepressant effect may also be reflected in experimental interference effects. This then provides a potential explanation for the effect of decreasing serotonergic function in normal volunteers to impair performance on a paired associate learning task and not visual pattern short-term memory (Park et al., 1994; Fig. 4.5), and the effects of selective serotonin reuptake blockers to enhance recognition memory but not recall in an auditory list-learning task (Linnoila et al., 1993). There is additionally one study in which tryptophan administration improved performance on a list-learning task in depressed patients before an improvement in mood was noted (Henry, Weingartner and Murphy, 1973).

In more general terms, the hypothesis arising from this series of simulations is that the impaired serotonergic transmission in depressed patients prevents the unlearning of the depressed associations and hence leads to the persistence of the depressed state. This in a number of respects is not substantially different from Deakin's formulation (Deakin and Graeff, 1991) in terms of the disconnection hypothesis of median raphe function. However, the hypothesis generated by the model has a number of different implications. The mechanism of antidepressant action does not restrict serotonergic effects to stimuli of a particular emotional valence. This allows for modulatory effects of serotonergic transmission on both positively and negatively reinforced operant

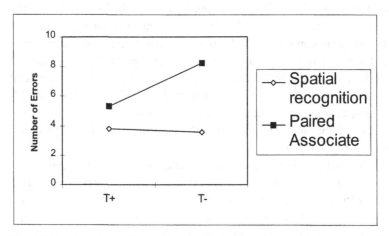

Fig. 4.5 Results of experimental manipulation of serotonergic function on learning in placebo-controlled, cross-over, within-subjects design in 12 healthy volunteers. T− condition, tryptophan (serotonin precursor) deficient amino acid mixture; T+, balanced amino acid drink control. Error rates for spatial recognition memory (F 0.17 d.f. 3,30, NS), paired associate learning (F 4.12 d.f 1,11, p = 0.07 with F 5.12, p < 0.05 for trials to criterion). (See Park et al. (1994) for further details.)

behaviour, as is observed experimentally (Wogar, Bradshaw and Szabadi, 1993). Neither is it restricted to effects at the hippocampus in that it can also operate in other areas with strong input from the median raphe nucleus, such as frontal cortex. As a neuromodulatory input that may enhance the learning of changed associations, this then provides a potential explanation for the input to the median raphe nucleus from the orbitofrontal cortex and the latter area's association with reversal learning. Perhaps the most significant difference between this model and other accounts of antidepressant action is the fact that the delay in treatment effect is related to the learning process and not to adaptive receptor changes, as is typically proposed. A further observation from this simulation is that an experience of reward from the environment is necessary for the antidepressant effect to occur. This may have as its clinical correlate the apparent resistance to treatment of patients who relapse whilst receiving treatment with antidepressants. It is in these differences that neural network models can be seen to deconstruct the psychological component of psychopharmacology. However, it is important to note that the model is not necessarily antecedent to any of these hypotheses or their falsifiability.

That this model is a tool rather than an explanation can be seen in a number of different ways. In common with other higher level models, elements missing as a result of the simplifications used may well be important. 5-HT1A receptors found outside of median raphe synapses on pyramidal neurons have not been included. The assumption that extrasynaptic 5-HT is not important in antidepressant effects is based on limited evidence. 5-HT–cholinergic interactions are well recognized in learning and at the level of cell function. There is some evidence that depression is a hypercholinergic state, and antidepressant responsiveness has been associated with presumably cholinergically mediated REM sleep suppression. This provides multiple possible confounds to the model. Such problems are potentially amenable to examination by more detailed models in which cholinergic and serotonergic effects are examined together. However, the effect of acetylcholine on learning has also been argued to occur through a reduction in interference (Hasselmo, 1993). This compounds the problem, in that the interference effects in the models of cholinergic function and this model are different in terms of network functions that do not map directly to psychological interference. This reflects the potential differences in information processing as carried out by the brain and the psychological means of description available.

Conclusion

Neural network models provide a method of directly integrating know-ledge of the cellular and receptor level effects of drugs and neurotrans-mitters into a model of higher mental function to examine psychopharmacological effects. Conversely, findings from experimental psychopharmacology provide an important source of data whereby neural network models can be tested for their robustness. The experience from the studies of the oscillatory properties of simple networks is that the functional significance of the cellular effects of pharmacological chal-lenge can only be understood when they are incorporated into network models. Models at this level can and have been directly assessed and validated against neurophysiological experiment and show predictive validity. Though the understanding of which simplifications in a network model maintain an accurate reflection of network dynamics is at an early stage, the amount of such information continues to accumulate and is increasingly being incorporated into more abstract simulations. Such abstract models share the property of being testable at different levels of organization, from the pattern of activity of identified cells to the behaviour of the network. As a tool for the clinical psychopharmacolo-gist, the techniques of neural network modelling remain in development. In addition to the delineation of a definitive cortical architecture, more experimental information is required concerning the effects of transmis-sion through different receptor types on cellular function. However, as a means of understanding the relationship between clinical observations and the effects of a transmitter on arrays of non-linear target neurons, neural network modelling shows the expected promise of a paradigm shift.

Summary

Neural network models can represent transmission through a number of different receptor types. This is achieved by implementing synaptic events and effects with differing time courses and specific anatomy within the network architecture. The effects on network behaviour as a whole are then examined. This provides a theoretical bridge between pharmacolo-gical effects observed at cellular and behavioural levels. At its simplest, a model can distinguish between the slow, diffuse neuromodulator effects that are directly modified by drugs such as neuroleptics and antidepres-sants, and the fast neurotransmission that occurs between the target neurons. At more detailed levels of simulation, individual receptor types with selective effects on ion channels and second messenger systems can be used. This chapter examines the different ways in which pharmacological detail has been included within neural network models, and describes the models that seek to explain the effects on observed behaviour.

References

Agnati, L.F., Zoli, M., Stromberg, I. & Fuxe, K. (1995). Intercellular communication in the brain – wiring versus volume transmission. *Neuroscience*, **69**, 711–26.

Ambros Ingerson, J. & Lynch, G. (1993). Channel gating kinetics and synaptic efficacy: A hypothesis for expression of long-term potentiation. *Proceedings of the National Academy of Sciences of the United States of America*, **90**, 7903–7.

Barkai, E. & Hasselmo, M.E. (1994). Modulation of the input/output function of rat piriform cortex pyramidal cells. *Journal of Neurophysiology*, **72**, 644–58.

Berner, J. & Woody, C.D. (1991). Local adaptation of 2 naturally-occurring neuronal conductances, GK + (A) and GK + (CA), allows for associative conditioning and contiguity judgments in artificial neural networks. *Biological Cybernetics*, **66**, 79–86.

Berns, G.S. & Sejnowski, T.J. (1995). A computational model of local memory in the primate pallidal–subthalamic circuit. *Society of Neuroscience Abstracts*, **21**, 678.

Berns, G.S. & Sejnowski, T.J. (1996). How the basal ganglia make decisions. In *The Neurobiology of Decision Making*, ed. A.R. Damasio, H. Damasio & Y. Christen, New York: Springer-Verlag.

Borrett, D.S., Yeap, T.H. & Kwan, H.C. (1993). Neural networks and Parkinson's disease. *Canadian Journal of Neurological Science*, **20**, 107–13.

Brockel, B.J. & Fowler, S.C. (1995). Effects of chronic haloperidol on reaction-time and errors in a sustained attention task – partial reversal by anticholinergics and by amphetamine. *Journal of Pharmacology and Experimental Therapeutics*, **275**, 1090–8.

Calabrese, R.L. & de Schutter, E. (1992). Motor-pattern-generating networks in invertebrates: modelling our way to understanding. *Trends in Neurosciences*, **15**, 439–44.

Callaway, E., Halliday, R. & Naylor, H. (1992). Cholinergic activity and constraints on information processing. *Biological Psychology*, **33**(1), 1–22.

Callaway, E., Halliday, R., Naylor, H., Yano, L. & Herzig, K. (1994). Drugs and human information-processing. *Neuropsychopharmacology*, **10**, 9–19.

Cartling, B. (1995). Autonomous neuromodulatory control of associative processes. *Network-Computation in Neural Systems*, **6**, 247–60.

Cohen, J.D. & Servan-Schreiber, D. (1992). Context, cortex and dopamine: a connectionist approach to behaviour and biology in schizophrenia. *Psychological Review*, **99**, 45–77.

Cohen, J.D. & Servan-Schreiber, D. (1993). A theory of dopamine function and its role in cognitive deficits in schizophrenia. *Schizophrenia Bulletin*, **19**, 85–104.

Contrerasvidal, J.L. & Stelmach, G.E. (1995). A neural model of basal ganglia–thalamocortical relations in normal and parkinsonian movement. *Biological Cybernetics*, **73**, 467–76.

Contrerasvidal, J.L., Teulings, H.L. & Stelmach, G.E. (1995). Micrographia in Parkinson's disease. *Neuroreport*, **6**, 2089–92.

Deakin, J.F.W. & Graeff, F.G. (1991). 5-HT and mechanisms of defence. *Journal of Psychopharmacology*, **5**, 305–16.

Deakin, J.F.W., Graeff, F.G. & Guimaraes, F.S. (1993). Altered 5-HT1A receptor mediated neurotransmission. Clincial implications of microdialysis findings. *Trends in Pharmacological Sciences*, **14**, 263.

Destexhe, A., Contreras, D., Sejnowski, T.J. & Steriade, M. (1994a). Modeling the control of reticular thalamic oscillations by neuromodulators. *Neuroreport*, **5**, 2217–20.

Destexhe, A., Contreras, D., Sejnowski, T.J. & Steriade, M. (1994b). A model of spindle rhythmicity in the isolated thalamic reticular nucleus. *Journal of Neurophysiology*, **72**, 803–18.

Destexhe, A., Mainen, Z.F. & Sejnowski, T.J. (1994c). An efficient method for computing synaptic conductances based on a kinetic-model of receptor-binding. *Neural Computation*, **6**, 14–18.

Destexhe, A., Mainen, Z.F. & Sejnowski, T.J. (1994d). Synthesis of models for excitable membranes, synaptic transmission and neuromodulation using a common kinetic formalism. *The Journal of Computational Neuroscience*, **1**, 195–231.

Dextexhe, A. & Sejnowski, T.J. (1995). G protein activation kinetics and spillover of gamma-aminobutyric acid may account for differences between inhibitory responses in the hippocampus and thalamus. *Proceedings of the National Academy of Sciences of the United States of America*, **92**, 9515–19.

Donahoe, J.W., Burgos, J.E. & Palmer, D.C. (1993). A selectionist approach to reinforcement. *Journal of the Experimental Analysis of Behavior*, **60**, 17–40.

Friston, K.J., Tononi, G., Reeke Jr, G.N., Sporns, O. & Edelman, G.M. (1994). Value-dependent selection in the brain: simulation in a synthetic neural model. *Neuroscience*, **59**, 229–43.

Freeman, W. J. (1968). Analog simulations of prepiriform cortex in the cat. *Mathematical Bioscience*, **2**, 181–90.

Gallo, M. & Candido, A. (1995). Dorsal hippocampal lesions impair blocking but not latent inhibition of taste aversion learning in rats. *Behavioral Neuroscience*, **109**, 413–25.

Globus, G.G. (1992). Toward a noncomputational cognitive neuroscience. *Journal of Cognitive Neuroscience*, **4**, 299–310.

Gluck, M.A. & Myers, C.E. (1992). Hippocampal function in representation and generalization: a computational theory. In *Proceedings of the 1992 Cognitive Science Society Conference*. Hillsdale, NJ: Erlbaum.

Gluck, M.A. & Thompson, R.F. (1987). Modelling the neural substrates of associative learning and memory: a computational approach. *Psychological Review*, **94**, 176–91.

Golomb, D., Wang, X.J. & Rinzel, J. (1994). Synchronization properties of spindle oscillations in a thalamic reticular nucleus model. *Journal of Neurophysiology*, **72**, 1109–26.

Golomb, D., Wang, X.J. & Rinzel, J. (1996). Propagation of spindle waves in a thalamic slice model. *Journal of Neurophysiology*, **75**, 750–69.

Hasselmo, M.E. (1993). Acetylcholine and learning in a cortical associative memory. *Neural Computation*, **5**, 32–44.

Hasselmo, M.E. (1995). Neuromodulation and cortical function – modeling the physiological basis of behavior. *Behavioural Brain Research*, **67**, 1–27.

Hasselmo, M.E. & Schnell, E. (1994). Laminar selectivity of the cholinergic suppression of synaptic transmission in rat hippocampal region ca1 – computational modeling and brain slice ₋hysiology. *Journal of Neuroscience*, **14**, 3898–914.

Hawkins, R.D. & Kandel, E.R. (1984). Is there a cell-biological alphabet for simple forms of learning? *Psychological Review*, **91**, 375–91.

Henry, G.M., Weingartner, H. & Murphy, D.L. (1973). Influence of affective states and psychoactive drugs on verbal learning and memory. *American Journal of Psychiatry*, **130**, 996–71.

Hoffman, R.E. (1987). Computer simulations of neural information processing and schizophrenia/mania dichotomy. *Archives of General Psychiatry*, **44**, 178–87.

Holmes, W.R. & Levy, W.B. (1990). Insights into associative long-term potentiation from computational models of NMDA receptor-mediated calcium influx and intracellular calcium changes. *Journal of Neurophysiology*, **63**, 1148–68.

Hornung, J.P. & Celio, M. (1992). The selective innervation by serotonergic axons of calbindin-containing interneurons in the neocortex and hippocampus of the marmoset. *The Journal of Comparative Neurology*, **320**, 457–67.

Jackson, S.R., Marrocco, R. & Posner, M.I. (1994). Networks of anatomical areas controlling visuospatial attention. *Neural Networks*, **7**, 925–44.

Javitt, D.C., Doneshka, P., Grochowski, S. & Ritter, W. (1995). Impaired mismatch negativity generation reflects widespread dysfunction of working memory in schizophrenia. *Archives of General Psychiatry*, **52**, 550–8.

Jobe, T., Vimal, R., Kovilparambil, A., Port, J. & Gaviria, M. (1994). A theory of cooperativity modulation in neural networks as an important parameter of CNS catecholamine function and induction of psychopathology. *Neurological Research*, **16**, 330–41.

Johnson, B.R., Peck, J.H. & Harris Warrick, R.M. (1993). Dopamine induces sign reversal at mixed chemical–electrical synapses. *Brain Research*, **625**, 159–64.

Johnson, B.R., Peck, J.H. & Harris Warrick, R.M. (1994). Differential modulation of chemical and electrical components of mixed synapses in the lobster stomatogastric ganglion. *Journal of Comparative Physiology A – Sensory Neural and Behavioral Physiology*, **175**, 233–49.

Jones, R.S.G. (1993). Entorhinal–hippocampal connections: a speculative view of their function. *Trends in Neurosciences*, **16**, 58–64.

Joseph, M.H. & Jones, S.H. (1991). Latent inhibition and blocking – further consideration of their construct-validity as animal-models of schizophrenia – commentary on animal-models with construct-validity for schizophrenia. *Behavioural Pharmacology*, **2**, 521–6.

Katz, P.S. & Frost, W.N. (1996). Intrinsic neuromodulation – altering neuronal circuits from within. *Trends in Neurosciences*, **19**, 54–61.

Katz, P.S., Getting, P.A. & Frost, W.N. (1994). Dynamic neuromodulation of synaptic strength intrinsic to a central pattern generator circuit. *Nature*, **367**, 729–31.

Kepler, T.B., Marder, E. & Abbott, L.F. (1990). The effect of electrical coupling on the frequency of model neuronal oscillators. *Science*, **248**, 83–5.

Klancnik, J.M. & Phillips, A.G. (1991). Modulation of synaptic plasticity in the dentate gyrus of the rat by electrical stimulation of the median raphe nucleus. *Brain Research*, **557**, 236–40.

Klopf, A.H. (1988). A neuronal model of classical conditioning. *Psychobiology*, **16**, 85–125.

Kotter, R. & Wickens, J. (1995). Interactions of glutamate and dopamine in a computational model of the striatum. *Journal of Computational Neuroscience*, **2**, 195–214.

Law Tho, D., Desce, J.M. & Crepel, F. (1995). Dopamine favours the emergence of long-term depression versus long-term potentiation in slices of rat prefrontal cortex. *Neuroscience Letters*, **188**, 125–8.

Levine, D.S. & Leven, S.J. (1991). Inhibition in the nervous system: Models of its roles in choice and context determination. *Neurochemical Research*, **16**, 381–95.

Liljenstrom, H. & Hasselmo, M.E. (1993). Acetyl choline and cortical oscillatory dynamics. In *Computation and Neural Systems*, ed. F.E. Eeckman & J.M. Bower, pp. 523–30. Boston: Kluwer Academic Publishers.

Liljenstrom, H. & Hasselmo, M.E. (1995). Cholinergic modulation of cortical oscillatory dynamics. *Journal of Neurophysiology*, **74**, 288–97.

Linnoila, M., Stapleton, J.M., George, D.T., Lane, E. & Eckardt, M.J. (1993). Effects of fluvoxamine, alone and in combination with ethanol on psychomotor and cognitive performance and on autonomic nervous system reactivity in healthy volunteers. *Journal of Clinical Psychopharmacology*, **13**, 175–80.

Ljungberg, T., Apicella, P. & Schultz, W. (1992). Responses of monkey dopamine neurones during learning of behavioural reactions. *Journal of Neurophysiology*, **67**, 145–63.

Lytton, W.W., Destexhe, A. & Sejnowski, T.J. (1996). Control of slow oscillations in the thalamocortical neuron: a computer model. *Neuroscience*, **70**, 673–84.

Maier, W., Franke, P., Kopp, B., Hardt, J., Hain, C. & Rist, F. (1994). Reaction-time paradigms in subjects at risk for schizophrenia. *Schizophrenia Research*, **13**, 35–43.

McCormick, D.A., Huguenard, J. & Strowbridge, B.W. (1992). Determination of state-dependent processing in thalamus by single neuron properties and neuromodulators. In *Single Neuron Computation*, ed. T. McKenna, J. Davis & S.F. Zornetzer, pp. 259–90. San Diego: Academic Press.

Miettinen, R. & Freund, T.F. (1992). Convergence and segregation of septal and median raphe inputs onto different subsets of hippocampal inhibitory interneurons. *Brain Research*, **594**, 263–72.

Miles, R. & Wong, R.K.S. (1983). Single neurons can initiate synchronized population discharge in the hippocampus. *Nature*, **306**, 371–3.

Molliver, M.E. (1987). Serotonergic neuronal systems: what their anatomic organization tells us about function. *Journal of Clinical Psychopharmacology*, **7**, 3S–23S.

Montague, P.R., Dayan, P., Nowlan, S.J., Pouget, A. & Sejnowski, T.J. (1993). Using a periodic reinforcement for directed self-organization. In *Advances in Neural and Information Processing Systems*, 5th edn, ed. C.L. Giles, S.J. Hanson & J.D. Cowan. San Mateo, CA: Morgan Kauffman.

Montague, P.R., Dayan, P., Person, C. & Sejnowski, T.J. (1995). Bee foraging in uncertain environments using predictive hebbian learning. *Nature*, 377, 725–8.

Montague, P.R., Gally, J.A. & Edelman, J.A. (1991). Spatial signalling in the development and function of neural connections. *Cerebral Cortex*, 1, 1–20.

Montague, P.R. & Sejnowski, T.J. (1994). The predictive brain: temporal coincidence and temporal order in synaptic learning mechanisms. *Learning and Memory*, 1, 1–33.

Niebur, E. & Koch, C. (1994). A model for the neuronal implementation of selective visual attention based on temporal correlation among neurons. *Journal of Computational Neuroscience*, 1, 141–58.

Park, S.B.G., Coull, J.T., McShane, R.H. et al. (1994). Tryptophan depletion in normal volunteers produces selective impairments in learning and memory. *Neuropharmacology*, 33, 575–88.

Parks, R.W., Levine, D.S., Long, D.L. et al. (1992). Parallel distributed processing and neuropsychology: A neural network model of Wisconsin card sorting and verbal fluency. *Neuropsychology Review*, 3, 213–33.

Penn, D.L., Mueser, K.T., Spalding, W., Hope, D.A. & Reed, D. (1995). Information-processing and social competence in chronic schizophrenia. *Schizophrenia Bulletin*, 21, 269–81.

Pennartz, C.M.A., Ameerun, R.F., Groenewegen, H.J. & Lopes da Silva, F.H. (1993). Synaptic plasticity in an in vitro slice preparation of the rat nucleus accumbens. *European Journal of Neuroscience*, 5, 107–17.

Pinsky, P.F. & Rinzel, J. (1994). Intrinsic and network rhythmogenesis in a reduced Traub model for CA3 neurons. *Journal of Computational Neuroscience*, 1, 39–60.

Pouget, A., Montague, P.R., Dayan, P. & Sejnowski, T.J. (1993). A developmental model of map registration in the superior colliculus using predictive Hebbian learning. *Society of Neuroscience Abstract*, 19, 858.

Quartz, S.P., Dayan, P.R., Montague, P.R. & Sejnowski, T.J. (1992). Expectation learning in the brain using diffuse ascending connections. *Society of Neuroscience Abstract*, 18, 1210.

Richter-Levin, G. & Segal M. (1990). Effects of serotonin releasers on dentate granule cell excitability in the rat. *Experimental Brain Research*, 82, 199–207.

Roberts, A.C., DeSalvia, M.A., Wilkinson, L.S. et al. (1994). 6-hydroxydopamine lesions of the prefrontal cortex in monkeys enhance performance on an analog of the Wisconsin Card Sort Test – Interactions with subcortical dopamine. *Journal of Neuroscience*, 14, 2531–44.

Rowat, P.F. & Selverston, A.I. (1993). Modeling the gastric mill central pattern generator of the lobster with a relaxation-oscillator network. *Journal of Neurophysiology*, 70, 1030–53.

Servan-Schreiber, D. & Blackburn, J.R. (1995). Neuroleptic effects on acquisition and performance learned behaviors: A reinterpretation. *Life Sciences*, 56, 2239–45.

Servan-Schreiber, D., Callaway, E., Halliday, R. et al. (1994). Amphetamine can slow reaction-times, *Biological Psychiatry*, 35, 665–6.

Servan-Schreiber, D., Printz, H. & Cohen, J.D. (1990). A network model of catecholamine effects: gain, signal-to-noise ratio, and behaviour. *Science*, **249**, 892–5.

Spitzer, M. (1995). Neural networks and the psychopathology of delusions – the importance of neuroplasticity and neuromodulation. *Neurology, Psychiatry and Brain Research*, **3**, 47–58.

Spoont, M.R. (1992). Modulatory role of serotonin in neural information processing: implications for human psychopathology. *Psychological Bulletin*, **112**, 330–50.

Standley, C., Norris, T.M., Ramsey, R.L. & Usherwood, P.R. (1993). Gating kinetics of the quisqualate sensitive glutamate receptor of locust muscle studied using agonist concentration and computer simulations. *Biophysics Journal*, **65**, 1379–86.

Sutton, J.P. & Hobson, J.A. (1993). State dependent sequencing and learning. In *Computation in Neurons and Neural Systems*, ed. F.H. Eeckman, pp. 275–80. Boston: Kluwer Academic Press.

Sutton, J.P., Mamelak, A.N. & Hobson, J.A. (1992). Modelling states of waking and sleeping. *Psychiatric Annals*, **3**, 137–43.

Sutton, R.S. & Barto, A.G. (1990). Time-derivative models of Pavlovian reinforcement. In *Learning and Computational Neuroscience: Foundations of Adaptive Networks*, ed. M. Gabriel & J. Moore, pp. 497–537. Cambridge, MA: MIT Press.

Traub, R.D. & Miles, R. (1992). Synchronized multiple bursts in the hippocampus: a neuronal population oscillation uninterpretable without accurate cellular membrane kinetics. In *Single Neuron Computation*, ed. T. McKenna, J. Davis & S.F. Zornetzer, pp. 463–75. San Diego: Academic Press.

Traub, R.D., Miles, R. & Buzsaki, G. (1992). Computer simulations of carbachol-driven rhythmic population oscillations in the CA3 region of the in vitro rat hippocampus. *Journal of Physiology*, **451**, 653–72.

Traub, R.D & Wong, R.K.S. (1982). Cellular mechanism of neuronal synchronization in epilepsy. *Science*, **216**, 745–7.

Traven, H.G.C., Brodin, L., Lansner, A. et al. (1993). Computer simulations of NMDA and non-NMDA receptor-mediated synaptic drive: sensory and supraspinal modulation of neurons and small networks. *Journal of Neurophysiology*, **70**, 695–709.

Wallen, P., Ekeberg, O., Lansner, A. et al. (1992). A computer based model for realistic simulations of neural networks. II. The segmental network generating locomotor rhythmicity in the lamprey. *Journal of Neurophysiology*, **68**, 1939–50.

Williams, J.H., Wellman, N.A., Geaney, D.P. et al. (1996). Schizophrenics show reduced Stroop interference if long-latency responses are excluded. *Schizophrenia Research*, **18**, 230.

Wilson, H.R. & Cowan, J.D. (1972). Excitatory and inhibitory interactions in localized populations of model neurons. *Biophysics Journal*, **12**, 1–24.

Wilson, M.A. & Bower, J.M. (1991). A computer simulation of oscillatory behaviour in primary visual cerebral cortex. *Neural Computation*, **3**, 498–509.

Wilson, M. & Bower, J.M. (1992). Cortical oscillations and temporal interactions in a computer simulation of piriform cortex. *Journal of Neurophysiology*, **4**, 981–95.

Wogar, M.A., Bradshaw, C.M. & Szabadi, E. (1993). Effect of lesions of the ascending 5-hydroxytryptaminergic pathways on choice between delayed reinforcers. *Psychopharmacology*, 111, 239–43.

Wu, X.B. & Liljenstrom, H. (1994). Regulating the nonlinear dynamics of olfactory cortex. *Network-Comuptation in Neural Systems*, 5, 47–60.

Yamada, W.M. & Zucker, R.S. (1992). Time course of transmitter release calculated from simulations of a calcium diffusion model. *Biophysics Journal*, 61, 671–82.

Yamamoto, M., Nakao, M., Mizutani, Y. et al. (1994). Pharmacological and model-based interpretation of neuronal dynamics transitions during sleep–waking cycle. *Methods of Information in Medicine*, 33, 125–8.

Zhang, B. & Harris Warrick, R.M. (1994). Multiple receptors mediate the modulatory effects of serotonergic neurons in a small neural-network. *Journal of Experimental Biology*, 190, 55–77.

5

A connectionist view of psychotherapy[1]

FRANZ CASPAR

The state of the art in psychotherapy

Psychotherapy is the discipline of treating psychological (including soma-
toform) disorders with psychological means in a planned, professional
way. Psychotherapy has made considerable progress since the days of
unsystematic, although sometimes very effective, stimulation of psychological change by gifted and charismatic individuals. The elaboration of
unconscious mechanisms by Freud, the formulation of learning mechanisms by the behaviourists, and the plea for the power of human relationship by Rogers, are just a few of the many steps in this development. A
better understanding of the mechanisms underlying the development and
maintenance of disorders, as well as the principles of change, has been
achieved. More is known both about the effects of psychotherapeutic
procedures and about the factors that are significant in the process of
psychotherapy. Under the scrutiny of empirical data, some approaches,
such as (cognitive) behaviour therapy, have experienced considerable
change. Today, depending on the type of disorder, psychotherapy offers
success rates of 70–85 per cent.

Studies of cost-effectiveness show that high-quality psychotherapy is
such an excellent investment that the question is not whether society can
afford psychotherapeutic services, but whether society can afford to
renounce psychotherapy if the limited costs of psychotherapy are compared with the almost unlimited costs of untreated psychological problems (Grawe, Donati and Bernauer, 1998). Books such as the
Handbook of Psychotherapy and Behavior Change (Bergin and Garfield,
1994) give testimony to the progress we have made and the position we
have reached. Such books contain a wealth of knowledge, too extensive
to be stored and handled by any one individual. We have reason to be
proud of what we have achieved so far.

Despite the undoubted success of psychotherapy in many areas, there are still many types of disorder (and individuals whose problems do not fit into any simple category of disorder) for which psychotherapy has not been so successful. Success rates of 45 per cent for state of the art treatment for eating disorders still leave a majority who are not helped to a satisfactory degree. Even high success rates of around 70 per cent for psychotherapy in general (Grawe et al., 1998) means that almost a third of clients are investing time and money into therapy without a satisfactory outcome. Undoubtedly, there is still a need to improve psychotherapy, and one way to do this is to look for deficits in the existing basic concepts and try to overcome them.

The development of an integrative movement is certainly an important factor in improving psychotherapy, but it is very unlikely that simply combining existing concepts will eventually lead to the development of new, sufficiently powerful concepts (Norcross and Wogan, 1983). There are several specific frontiers where we need to make progress beyond integrating the most valuable elements developed by representatives of the current approaches.

One such frontier is the development and use of models for understanding the mechanisms underlying disorders, change, and the functioning of psychotherapists. Such an understanding is needed for practice: it would be of purely academic interest if psychotherapy was considered to be a mere cookbook application of techniques. However, if psychotherapy is more realistically considered to be a highly individualized process in which therapists may use standard procedures and techniques – as described in manuals – as *prototypes*, but generally develop a new, optimized procedure for every individual patient, a deeper understanding of patients is needed to guide the process of constructing the therapeutic procedure (Caspar, 1995). Similarly, a deeper understanding of therapists is needed as a basis for reflecting and improving their action.

The view taken here is that: (1) an individualized model of each patient and an individualized procedure are needed, and (2) although in some instances traditional models of cognitive–emotional functioning are very practical, they are not a suitable basis for understanding a number of other important aspects of psychopathology, of change, and of psychotherapists' functioning.

The main focus of this chapter is on connectionist concepts and their potential to serve as a basis for understanding and planning individual change. The potential of these concepts to guide research related to aspects that are difficult to deal with using traditional models is also discussed. Because of space constraints, it was necessary to decide whether to discuss few aspects in depth or to give an overview of numerous issues for which connectionist concepts may be relevant. The decision was for the latter, since the main goal of this chapter is not only to stimulate further interest in reading (e.g. Caspar, Rothenfluh and Segal, 1992; Stinson and Palmer, 1991) but also to stimulate the reader's own ideas related to a variety of phenomena. Possibilities of psychotherapy with patients with impaired neural systems cannot be addressed here, even though, from a connectionist point of view, this would be a particularly interesting issue. It is assumed that readers already have some familiarity with connectionism (see, for example, Stinson and Palmer, 1991; Caspar et al., 1992).

Limits of traditional concepts in founding an understanding and planning of psychotherapy

Therapists impose limits on their own thinking, on the one hand due to a one-sided adherence to specific therapeutic orientations, and on the other hand due to more fundamental limitations residing in the basic concepts used by several orientations. Such restrictions and deficiencies are discussed in more detail in Caspar et al. (1992). The question here is whether connectionism could provide concepts suitable for overcoming the limitations which characterize most psychotherapy approaches. The importance of some disadvantages of traditional models to psychotherapy may be small *in general*, but higher in specific cases (e.g. difficulties in thinking about the relation between 'software' and 'hardware' in a dynamic way for schizophrenia, or brain lesions).

One important function of adequate theoretical concepts is that they make sense of clinical observations. Traditional concepts are unable to help with many phenomena observed in therapy. In therapy practice, the aspects neglected by traditional models can therefore be taken into account only incompletely and unsystematically. Although the patient's self-organizational forces often bring about change *in spite* of our insufficient understanding, it is obvious that not only would most professionally minded therapists feel more comfortable if they understood their patients and the process of therapy better, but also they would work more efficiently.

The difficulty symbolic cognitive models have in dealing with some obviously important aspects of human functioning has had another effect: it has contributed to the enduring appeal of psychoanalysis.

Although psychoanalysis is not well founded in contemporary empirical psychology and has may problems in explaining postulated mechanisms *in detail*, it does at least address phenomena such as ambiguity, ambivalence, simultaneous conscious and unconscious processing, multiplicities of selves, latent contents, etc. (Stinson and Palmer, 1991).[2] It is desirable to develop concepts that at the same time address these and other clinically relevant issues *and* are based on modern scientific psychology and other important fields.

The appeal of connectionist models

It would be foolish to pretend that only a connectionist approach could deal with all the phenomena addressed below, but in many cases a connectionist approach does so in a more natural or flexible way. The relevance of connectionist points of view for psychotherapy is not always made explicit if it can be assumed that it is obvious.

Distributed representation, interconnectedness, and the distinction of aspects of human functioning

In the most typical connectionist models, it is assumed that information is represented in a distributed (as opposed to localist) manner. In addition, different domains of a person's functioning (work, family, leisure, etc.), as well as different aspects (cognition, emotion, etc.) are heavily interconnected. There is, however, variation in the density of connectedness, and the system may even be built up in a way that could be described as modular (e.g. Bechtel, 1993). As a matter of fact, complete connectedness only works as long as networks remain relatively small.

There are several consequences of distributedness and interconnectedness. Although the aim of this section is to introduce the basic concepts and not the clinical consequences, some macrolevel clinical analogies are used for reasons of illustration.[3]

1. A limited impact from outside tends only to reach a part of the elements responsible for adaptive or maladaptive patterns of behaviour and experience directly. For example, criticism of a person's defensiveness usually triggers arousal and stimulates greater defensiveness, but has no direct impact upon the reasons for the defensiveness.

2. Interconnectedness guarantees that parts that are not reached directly can be reached by their connections to other elements. They are then not changed under the direct influence of an input from the environment, but because other, connected elements inside the system have changed. For example, it may not be possible to change a person's wish to kill himself or herself directly, but it may be possible to establish a cognitive dissonance by stating that killing oneself would mean doing a favour to the person one most hates.

As long as connected elements are in the old state, they work against change in a part of the structure that is under the direct influence of therapy. For example, a person may learn to say 'no', but may feel bad for some time because of the old belief that other people would reject such a person.

3. Because interconnectedness is limited in larger systems, among other things by modularity, in the sense of different components performing different tasks, the spreading out of activation is to some extent channelled (see discussion below). For example, a new attitude related to work may not easily generalize to private relationships.

4. Interconnectedness prevents behaviour and experience from simply obeying the will of a person (in an everyday language sense). Although will (e.g. the will to change) is one important factor, there are other factors preventing will from having perfect control. Furthermore, a person's will is itself influenced by many factors. From a connectionist point of view, much of the debate on determinism is obsolete. Temporary states, as analysed in free association, are also determined by a multiplicity of factors: 'The neural net theory could have been invented to explain free association' (Olds 1994, p. 598): Thoughts generally function according to free association, but freedom is normally restricted by perceptions from the external world as well as internal attention processes. In particular, states such as moods and associations can be channelled in certain directions beyond an individual's will, which is very relevant for mood disorders (e.g. Teasdale and Barnard, 1993).

According to a connectionist view, different elements of human functioning such as cognitions, behaviour and emotions, should not be seen as entities actually existing in a patient. They are rather constructions by the observer that serve to describe emergent properties of a system's functioning. People behave and feel 'as if' they had particular cognitions, emotions etc., but as these are patterns produced by innumerable densely connected, small, meaningless units, there is no need to distinguish between these elements as if they existed in reality. The idea that one can trace schemata in a patient's mind in a real sense has to be abandoned (Henningsen, 1996): connectionist models are inherently constructivist.

Connectionist models cannot only deal more easily than traditional models with the relation between 'psychological' aspects such as behaviour, cognitions and emotions, but also with the relationship between the biological and psychological aspects. For example, the effects of changes related to neurotransmitters can easily be understood as setting learning parameters to different values. Needless to say, the newer insights related to the temporary impact of psychological factors on neurotransmitters and their more enduring impact on the brain can be understood with no additional assumptions.

Much of the old discussion of what comes first, cognition or emotion, of whether or not there are basic emotions (Ortony, Clore and Collins, 1988), of whether one should concentrate on emotions, cognitions or behaviour in psychotherapy, etc., seems overly simplistic if one assumes that these elements exist primarily in the observer's mind, and that they are all heavily interconnected. Based on the latter assumption, one could argue both ways: because a change on one level, e.g. the behavioural, would unavoidably introduce changes on the other levels, e.g. the cognitive and emotional levels, it is sufficient to concentrate on one level in the therapeutic procedure and just be aware of the other levels. The other argument would be: we should use all levels and channels in a systematically planned strategy, because if we have direct access to only one level, the other levels will work against change, and true change should, after all, involve all levels (Stiles et al., 1990). Probably both arguments are true to some extent, but we have not even begun to study the issue beyond the single case in a differentiated way, as would be suggested by connectionist models.

Even in the absence of any precise knowledge of how different parts of an individual's functioning influence each other, a much broader range of 'side' effects needs to be considered when thinking about therapeutic procedures. For example, behavioural interventions and practice may not primarily or exclusively work on the behavioural level, but rather by causing repeated contact with the environment: they lead to new cognitive and emotional experiences, which can then be integrated into the whole system. Behaviour may, in addition, cause changes in the environment. Of these effects on the environment, it is not only the immediate 'objective' advantages that count (such as a rise in salary after an assertive dialogue with the boss), but also the fact that a changed environment provides changed input to a system,[4] with the possibilities of reinforcing or inhibiting healthy as well as dysfunctional trends within it. This dynamic interplay is certainly used by good therapists but, as yet, we possess by far too little systematic knowledge about it. A connectionist view makes the deficit obvious, and could serve as a basis for investigating the phenomenon in the future.

One general observation can be made regarding psychotherapy research findings: namely, that therapies are more successful if previously existing strengths and preferences of a particular patient are taken into account and used (Grawe et al., 1998). The widespread idea that in therapy one should mainly identify deficits and work on them is in line with a mechanistic approach. In contrast, a dynamic approach such as connectionism would suggest that desirable, adaptive patterns can be achieved in many ways and by a variety of different patterns – even systems that from a narrow normative point of view have severe deficits – as long as one takes advantage of the existing strengths.

Understanding parallel processing: a variety of factors in a process of multiple constraint satisfaction

People function in a holistic way. According to connectionist models, no central steering unit is necessary to account for this. Connectionist models are 'more democratic' than traditional models, as Olds (1994) stresses. This is guaranteed by a process of parallel satisfaction of multiple constraints. These constraints can be 'soft', i.e. they need not be defined and assessed in a precise fashion. They can be very different in character (e.g. a temporary mood *vs* a lasting ethical value *vs* a particular aspect of a situation), and they can have different weights, which in addition can vary over time and situations. A consequence is that people do not need to decide between distinct alternatives if they are to act in an optimal way. Psychological problems, if seen as 'solutions', may be unreasonable from a rational point of view, but when the internal and external situations of a client are considered more comprehensively, their development may make considerable sense. For example, painful obsessive–compulsive thoughts may distract from threatening insights.

Parallel multiple constraint satisfaction is a principle by which a system settles in a state of minimal tension. Rogers' (1951) tendency to grow can be seen as a tendency towards the integration of new experiences and the internal development towards increasingly better functioning (Greenberg, Rice and Elliott, 1993), which is perfectly in line with connectionism. Another way of thinking of minimizing tension is that a system tends to increase coherence of its elements. Coherence is indeed a principle found to be an essential basis for 'good solutions' throughout many domains, such as theory building, law, etc. (Thagard, 1989). It can be thought of and simulated in a very convincing way using connectionist models (see below).

In a process of parallel constraint satisfaction, many of the outputs and properties of a system that meet the eye of an observer must be seen as emerging from the whole functioning, rather than as tangible parts of it. As an illustrative analogy, the property of being humid cannot be located in a single O or H atom, nor in an H_2O molecule. Humidity, which is a very obvious property of water, emerges as a property of a large accumulation of H_2O molecules. As a clinical parallel, Ramzy and Shevrin (1976, p. 15) write in relation to psychoanalytic theorizing: 'there may be many conscious and unconscious communications involved in the formation of a symptom but the symptom itself need not be a communication. . . it is a trace left behind by these processes.' To view such phenomena as emergent is very much in the mind of connectionism. It would help to overcome simplistic views if therapists would think in such a way more often. Consciousness, just as other aspects of a system's functioning, is a feature dependent on many factors, none of which determines in isolation whether something is conscious or unconscious.

Perception, expectations and the impact of the past on present functioning

The ability to use patterns formed under the influence of earlier input when processing present input is crucial for survival. This assumption is shared by traditional (e.g. schema) and connectionist approaches. Connectionist models have the advantage that the process can take place without a supervising unit ('homunculus'). The old patterns do their job 'by themselves', and are themselves incrementally changed by incoming information. Deficient input is completed and expectations are formed because patterns have a built-in tendency to complete themselves. A small piece of information (e.g. aspects of a current situation) corresponding to an old pattern is sufficient to activate the whole pattern, including associated emotions and action tendencies. The stronger the old pattern as an attractor, the less the new, activating information needs to fit, in terms of similarity and completeness.

Although the traditional concept of 'default values' in traditional frame concepts working with 'slots' and 'fillers' (Minsky, 1975) was useful, connectionist models are more convincing in their effortless way of filling 'holes' and completing themselves, and in their ability to do this with soft, fuzzy information. Constructions with a heavy use of analogies occur all the time. Transference of old to new situations is a natural phenomenon, and not something particular to therapies. It is obvious that perception in this sense, filling in missing information, be it adaptive or maladaptive, and other aspects of information processing play a crucial role in patients' as well as psychotherapists' functioning. For this reason, realistic models of how these processes work are of great interest. Connectionism could be a basis for considering under which conditions analogies and other forms of pattern completion are used, and under which conditions they are or are not useful. An example of immediate clinical relevance is a connectionist model that is able to replace missing parts of stories (Golden and Rumelhart, 1993). This corresponds closely to what patient and therapist do when reconstructing the past.

Connectionist models make clear that an interactionistic view is needed: traditionally, psychoanalysis emphasized the old 'programs' within a person (Olds, 1994), and behaviourism emphasized the current stimulus situation. It is obvious that a system's (re)actions can only be understood if the interaction of person and situation is the focus of attention.

The role of the past is to provide remembered contents as well as learned structures (which are not separate in connectionist models) assisting the current performance of a system, including the processing of new inputs. Remembered content as well as existing structures are relatively stable, but are also changed by new input. Looking more closely, we can never have the same memories twice, because memories are always produced anew, although they may look identical on the surface. Only to the extent that the relevant parts of the producing system remain identical can memories be identical. As there is always some change, all states and outputs of a system continuously change to some extent. This is utilized in therapy to bring patients gradually into more favourable states, which often includes altering memories. Permanent change may be problematic though, for example when in sexual abuse cases it is pivotal to remember accurately what a person has actually done. It is obvious that the input by a therapist working on a patient's sexual abuse experiences over some time speeds up changes within abuse memories for better or worse.

Seemingly in contrast to such continuous change of memories, experiences that are related to strong, in particular traumatic, experiences tend to be stabilized against change. Conscious counterparts would be a conscious decision 'never to trust men', 'always to hide one's feelings, whatever happens', etc. We would thus need a model accounting not only for change but also for the maintenance of old patterns, even if in a weakened fashion, over long periods. Even if old patterns seem to have disappeared or lost their impact, the activation of other parts, or the setting of parameters, may lead to their activation, e.g. flashbacks in post-traumatic stress disorder.

Adaptive as they are, at first sight connectionist models seem less suitable to model such stability than traditional models. In connectionist models there are, however, mechanisms serving the resistance against change.

Change, the ability of systems to compensate irritating input and resistance to psychotherapy

A system may be ready for change, that is, in a state in which very little input can have a strong immediate effect, or incoming information may be embedded in such a way that it has a steady impact over a long period of time. An example of the latter is a manager of a well-known, malign sect who once came to see me. For a long time he identified totally with the sect and served it in many ways. When he witnessed how they treated members who had clearly psychologically decompensated, this impression did not have an immediate visible impact on him, but it haunted him, and gradually it eroded his formerly stable positive attitude towards the group, until he finally left and helped to fight the sect.

Although connectionist models have many built-in mechanisms making them flexible and prone to change (which is an obvious advantage in comparison to traditional models), it would be wrong to focus onesidedly on the adaptability of connectionist systems. They also have a remarkable self-protective ability of compensating disturbances and disagreeable input. This makes them tolerant to faulty and noisy input, and thus reliable. However, very often it also makes systems resistant to therapeutic input that is not compatible with the existing system.

The extent to which a system is resistant to change depends on the state of a particular system, such as the strength of the relevant attractors, and the setting of learning parameters. The clinical observation that a therapeutic input needs to be strong enough not to be neutralized can easily be simulated in connectionist models. The same is true of the observation that too strong and threatening an impact can lead to rigidity, caused by less favourable setting of learning parameters. These phenomena are general, built-in properties of connectionist systems, which are also in line with general concepts of change. In particular, Piaget (1954) assumes that in assimilation, individuals try to process incoming information in such a way that change to the existing structures is not necessary. This can include distortions of the input to resist change. Only if assimilation fails, accommodative processes lead to a change in the existing structures to re-establish congruence between individual and environment. Several clinical authors (among others Schneider, 1989; Stiles et al., 1990; Grawe, 1992) have referred to Piaget.

Beyond general conservative tendencies, the particular persistence of some patterns, which is well known and acknowledged by many clinical approaches,[5] needs specific explanation. Yates and Nashby (1993) postulate that attempts to access dissociated material activate inhibitory mechanisms. Other approaches assume special mechanisms that isolate some learning experiences from the new input (Grossberg, 1986, 1987; Brousse and Smolensky, 1989; Caspar et al., 1992).

Several approaches, rather than focusing all power on the elements to be changed, concentrate on creating favourable conditions in order to improve learning conditions in general, and to improve access to especially stable parts of an individual's functioning (Rogers, 1951; Erickson, 1968; Stiles et al., 1990; Mahoney, 1991; Caspar, 1995; Hayes, 1996; Grawe et al., 1998). The goal is to enable a system to become more flexible and allocate resources to adaptive change processes. Considerable thought has been given to the question of how a therapist can create favourable conditions for accommodation, in particular by providing a safe, assimilative basis within the therapeutic relationship (see below). Approaches to influence inhibitory mechanisms directly, such as hypnosis, are interesting but need to be studied more comprehensively to be understood properly.

It should also be noted that much stability is caused not so much by *compensating* existing input, but rather by avoiding it completely. This is the case with phobic patients. Connectionist models learn avoidance behaviour as easily as organisms learning in the sense of behaviouristic learning rules do. In addition, instead of having to wait for accidentally occurring avoidance to be reinforced, connectionist models can be active 'inventors' of 'creative' avoidance strategies, just as we observe with real patients. For example, based on behavioural learning principles, it would be hard to imagine how a sociophobic student could devise a strategy of speaking first in a seminar in order to prevent his or her tension from building up.

Emotions

Emotions have already been mentioned as being heavily interconnected to cognitions and other elements of human functioning. It is plausible that there is an old emotional system with at least partly innate reactions, and there is a more differentiated, modern emotional regulation with even more connections to cognitions etc. (Greenberg and Safran, 1987; Greenberg et al., 1993). In addition to links within the individual, emotional regulation is closely intertwined with the environment. Although emotions can be defined as a particular kind of schema or node (e.g. Bower, 1981; Grawe, 1992), it is difficult to understand the dynamic interplay of emotions with other elements from a schema point of view (Teasdale and Barnard, 1993).

Greenberg et al. (1993, p. 5) state that 'emotion schemes are internal synthesizing structures that preconsciously process a variety of cognitive, affective, and sensory sources of information to provide our sense of personal meaning. This will help us to present a view of people as wholistic, organismic beings in whom affect, cognition, motivation, and action are continually integrated in everything they do'. It can be assumed that Greenberg et al.'s referral to a scheme model is justified by the fact that such a model is better known to readers, whereas it would be difficult to show how a schema model can actually function in the way described by the authors on a microlevel. The example of depression shows how models that make intuitive sense on a macrolevel need to be revised when their functioning is traced empirically, as done by Teasdale and Barnard (1993). Although Teasdale and Barnard do not decide clearly for a connectionist approach, their model is a big step in this direction.

The fact that it is possible to distinguish between different systems (cognitive *vs* emotional, old *vs* new, etc.) is compatible with the connectionist view that elements such as cognitions, emotions, etc. can be used as constructs by the observer, but this does not mean they are real entities. They are emergent products of dynamic systems, in which neither cognitions nor emotions exist as real entities. This view makes it much

easier to account for the fact that in psychotherapy we often have to deal
with cognitive emotions (e.g. surprise), physical emotions (e.g. nervous-
ness), emotionally loaded action tendencies, etc. The boundaries are not
at all clear in clinical reality but, fortunately, from a connectionist point
of view, this does not pose a problem.

Implicit, unconscious aspects

From a connectionist standpoint, the fact that much of human functioning remains unconscious requires no explanation. This is related to the
subsymbolic nature of connectionist models, their ability to process
implicit information, and their ability to function without a central steering unit. Parts of the whole functioning become conscious only when
special activities of a system bring about such consciousness, and this
happens mostly with stable, persisting states (Stinson and Palmer, 1991).
The fact that as a common feature of many psychological problems,
patients tend to focus their attention on their own state (Ingram, 1990)
contributes to making some aspects of the problem conscious.[6] The fact
that spontaneous consciousness is limited to parts of the whole functioning contributes to patients' inability to change the situation.

There is no clear distinction between conscious and unconscious, and
between knowing and not knowing something, but rather a continuum:
'The process is completely gradual and there is no special point at which
we would say the network now knows, and before this, it did not know.'
(McClelland, 1994, p. 63). This corresponds closely to observations in
clinical practice.

Whereas conscious processing – which is in the foreground in traditional cognitive approaches but can also be simulated by connectionist
models – has advantages for some tasks, there are clearly other tasks
which, apart from greater speed of processing without conscious control,
can be done more easily by unconscious, subsymbolic processes. An example is pattern recognition, which typically involves parallel processing of
soft constraints, e.g. when processing non-verbal information. Another
related example is the framing of non-symbolic raw information to make
it accessible to conscious processing. Intuitive processing is a third issue
that connectionist models handle more easily. Obviously, all this is highly
relevant for the understanding of patients' as well as therapists' functioning. The list could be continued, with the functioning of dreams as
attempts by the system to spread activation with the aim of arriving at
a better state through processes of integration (Olds, 1994), etc.

One consequence of the dominance of the unconscious and implicit is that it would – as clinical practice shows – be naive to assume that human functioning can be controlled in a straightforward way by conscious, semantic thinking. At present, focusing attention is one of the most important principles in therapy (Greenberg et al., 1993). From a connectionist point of view, however, this is only one possible approach to changing people. In future practice, explicit cognitive learning will probably become less important in psychotherapy, and implicit forms of learning more important. The increased clinical interest in unconscious processing (Meichenbaum and Gilmore, 1984; Mahoney, 1991; Dowd and Courchaine, 1992), together with a wish to ground an approach on modern models of cognitive–emotional regulation, will most probably contribute to the appeal of connectionism in the future.

The environment and situations

Schema theories (e.g. Piaget, 1954; Neisser, 1976; Gallagher and Reid, 1981; Grawe, 1992) emphasize that the relationship between schemata and the environment is interactional, but only a few authors draw consequences from the notion that learning does not take place in isolated brains (Norman, 1986). The actual interface between individual and environment, incremental change, and other aspects that seem important for an adequate conceptualization of system–environment interaction have always been a problem for traditional approaches. Traditional models typically assume that the learning parts of a system need some kind of external control. In connectionist models, the person–environment interaction is crucial from the outset, and it happens in a continuous, smooth and autonomous manner. One important aspect of person–environment interaction is that goals, beliefs etc. are not fixed, but their activation and impact vary over time, largely under the influence of a changing environment (Ingram and Hollon, 1986; Ingram and Kendall, 1987).

It would be unfair to blame the neglect of the environment only on traditional models. There seems to be a built-in human mechanism to attribute psychological phenomena mainly to the individual (Caspar, 1995). Even when clinical approaches, such as systemic family therapy, pay more attention to the interpersonal environment, they usually concentrate on enduring and predictable aspects. A connectionist foundation of dealing with the environment could support a more dynamic approach in which a continuous interaction with the environment is presupposed and utilized, and in which stable parts are the exception rather than the rule. This would lead to a greater concentration on the less predictable parts, and on the on-line monitoring of the interaction (Pfeifer and Verschure, 1992). The consequences for specific psychotherapies are obvious: much more effort would be invested in the monitoring of ongoing processes by patients and therapists. When talking about a person, one would not focus on stable properties but on fluctuations, and how they can be monitored and used.

One aspect of a connectionist view is that, just like in Prigogine's (1977) dissipative structures, change to a higher order is stimulated by exchange with the environment. Learning is based on discrepancies between the expected and the observed: 'adjust each connection weight in the network in proportion to the extent that its adjustment will reduce the difference between the output of the network and the actual next event' (McClelland, 1994, p. 62). The question is, then, how the environment needs to be shaped, and how the individual needs to be exposed to the environment to maximize its stimulative impact. Clinically, one would put much more emphasis on between-session effects than many approaches do currently (Hayes, 1996). Repeated confrontation with the environment is needed to reach a stable new state, and 'noisy' input, which plays a specially important role in acquiring stable, reliable new patterns, can best be provided by a natural environment. For example, it is easy to provide exciting group experiences in a workshop 'on the island'; but in connectionist models, just as clinical experience suggests, fast change is not stable if it is not integrated by repeated experience, preferably in a patient's regular environment.

One justified criticism of psychotherapies and outcome research is their concentration on short-term outcomes. The more one is interested in the development of an individual in the long run, the less one can afford to concentrate on a brief phase with a strong impact from one source, such as therapy. In the long run, more factors, and especially factors in the environment, become relevant and need to be considered.

Specific and non-specific factors

From a connectionist point of view it would be unreasonable to distinguish between specific and non-specific factors of psychotherapy, as is done explicitly or implicitly in much of the literature. As a consequence, the question of what contributes more to change – favourable learning conditions brought about by 'unspecific' factors (e.g. a property of the therapist, or even the weather at a particularly important moment), or specific input by specific factors (e.g. exposure to a phobic situations) – is obsolete.

When analysing the impact of 'unspecific' factors, such as the therapeutic relationship, a connectionist view suggests that the dynamic character of a system should be taken into account to a greater extent. For example, some needs of a patient in the therapeutic relationship may be typical, i.e. relatively stable, corresponding to relatively stable attractors, but on closer investigation there may be a fluctuation in the moment-to-moment activation of needs. A concentration on fluctuations will help a therapist to increase the frequency of favourable states and to utilize them in the therapeutic procedure by timing interventions appropriately.

One of the most developed clinical approaches to tuning the system into a state favourable to change has been used by Erickson (1968). It was characteristic for him to use non-threatening entries to the system. Some therapists seem to be very gifted with such strategies, but research is needed to find out whether impressive intuitive strategies only work for a selection of patients, and whether and how the strategies can be made explicit and learned by therapists. Generally, a recommendation may be to base an individual therapeutic offer, composed of 'unspecific' and 'specific' parts, on more explicit approaches of individual case conceptualizations (Caspar, 1995). A generally useful rule is to support a patient in all important goals, and to create or maintain tension only in a restricted area in which one wants to work at a given moment (see below).

Understanding disorders in a dynamic way

The understanding of an individual patient's psychopathology is an important basis for every psychotherapy. In spite of this, a connectionist view of diverse disorders is addressed only very briefly here, as it is the topic of other contributions to this volume. A number of considerations have already been presented that, in sum, suggest a dynamic view of psychological disorders.

An earlier paper (Caspar et al., 1992) addressed in greater detail repetition compulsion as a common phenomenon underlying many psychological problems, and which exists independently of the concepts and terminology used to describe it. In brief, phenomena related to repetition compulsion are listed as described in the psychoanalytic literature (p. 730):

Repetition compulsion actions are accompanied by suffering, yet a person experiences a nearly inescapable compulsion to execute them. The actions themselves and the forces controlling them are usually not in direct awareness. A person experiences the suffering as destiny and often, their contribution to the situation is not or not accurately acknowledged. If a person has an explanation, it is usually limited to factors in the present. Mostly, however, a person is merely confused by the divergence between conscious awareness and what seems to actually determine the behavior.

Not only behaviours, but also cognitions (e.g. the view of oneself and other individuals) and emotions are part of such patterns, or, in other words, determined by as well as determining repetition compulsions.

Often, therapists are able to see parallels between patterns in the past and in the present, without being able to explain these patterns by positive goals, and often (but with the significant exception of personality disorders), the patterns are experienced as ego-dystonic by the patient. Nevertheless, the patient seems to invest great amounts of energy, in spite of the pain related to it, to re-establish problematic experiences and situations similar to the past situation in which the pattern had been learned. To speak of repetition compulsion, the situation in the present must be similar enough to the situation in the past to trigger the repetition, yet dissimilar enough to speak not simply of an 'appropriate use of knowledge acquired in the past'. A broad range of patterns can be viewed as repetition compulsions, from very concrete repetitive actions (e.g. compulsive cleaning) to patterns lasting over a long time (e.g. marrying a spouse similar to one's father or mother, and becoming gradually unhappy over the years), including the therapeutic relationship (e.g. pressuring the therapist into patterns familiar from people in the patient's earlier life). Strong emotions – experienced or avoided – are an obligatory part of repetition compulsions, going from strong negative feelings to sulky satisfaction when one finds out that one's view of the world has once again turned out to be right. Repetition compulsions are not characteristic of one particular disorder (e.g. obsessive–compulsive disorder), but are the basis of many psychological problems, also experienced by individuals without clinically significant disorders.

Explanations of repetition compulsion include discharge of affects, relaxation of tensions, mastering traumata, integrating traumatic experiences, undoing traumatic experiences, vicarious mastery by the therapist, distraction, and need for security guaranteed by the familiarity of patterns. These explanations are elaborated in greater detail in Caspar et al. (1992).

Most therapists would agree that whatever name is given to the phenomenon, repetition compulsions need to be dealt with because they can be seen as underlying clinical problems and/or as posing difficulties to the therapeutic relationship. Therefore, a connectionist therapist would need to find an explanation as a basis for developing therapeutic strategies. The ideal would be to explain repetition compulsion parsimoniously, to explain the involved mechanisms at the same time as precisely as possible, and to explain the pathological phenomenon with the same models used to explain adaptive functioning. If, as other approaches cannot, a connectionist view cannot provide all the answers, it should at least help in formulating the remaining questions in such a way that fruitful research is stimulated. To what extent do connectionist models live up to these demands?

Some properties of connectionist systems clearly have a direct correspondence to repetition compulsion phenomena.

Systematic patterns of behaviour and experience can be produced without awareness. As emphasized by psychoanalysis, hidden elements can have a strong impact without being visible on the surface.

Control cannot easily be established, for instance by replacing old, maladaptive, unconscious parts by adaptive, conscious parts of a structure.

New elements, such as insights, need to be well integrated if they are to determine behaviour and experience. This does not mean that a single piece of new information cannot have a strong impact, but a system needs to be prepared to react strongly upon it.

New information is interpreted in terms of the existing structure. There is no clear boundary between adaptive and maladaptive processes.

If the existing attractors are strong, the input can be distorted to an astounding degree, and the reactions of a system become strongly predictable. At best, there are several typical perceptive and behavioural patterns (local minima) but no comprehensive, balanced reactions. For example, a man can only be seen as either a rapist or as a 'regular guy', but nothing in between.

Variation in the reaction to similar input can be caused by variation of the states in which the system can be. An obvious example is the different behaviours of an alcoholic in a sober *vs* drunk state, but different states can also be induced in a merely psychological way (e.g. 'states of mind' concept by Horowitz, 1979).

Input has a stronger impact if the existing structures are 'ready' for it, typically when attractors determining the interpretation are already activated.

Long-lasting but not very strong stressors as well as brief, traumatic
experiences are able to build up strong, lasting attractors.

Patterns stabilize particularly well if they are interlocked with the environment in such a way that there is a mutual reinforcement.

The idea of mastering traumata by integrating them into the existing
structure is a very natural one from a connectionist point of view.
The observation that integration of an individual in a social network
has a protective effect and that talking through the experiences with
friends and relatives helps enormously with mastering traumata is very
much in line with what one would expect from a connectionist point of
view. Of course, it is not the integration on a macrolevel per se that
helps, but the ongoing integration of new and old experiences due to
permanent activation and exchange in the human interaction.

Problem solving can be an unconscious moving around in a space of
possible solutions until the one with a minimum of tension is found,
which may be only a local as opposed to a global minimum. The
possibility of getting stuck in a state that is far from an optimal state
('global minimum') is built in.

An important question is, of course: why do repetition compulsions
persist? First of all, many persist just long enough to be diagnosed, but
not over a very long period of time. Some may persist because they are
very isolated and have only few connections to the rest of the system,
therefore the impact of new experiences is minimal. Furthermore, from a
longitudinal perspective, it may make sense to assume sensible and less
sensible phases in which learning parameters are set differently. From a
cross-sectional perspective, the same may apply to different domains of
life. In addition, input seemingly suited to change repetition compulsions
may be disempowered already at the surface of the system by powerful
attractors that transform the original challenging information into
neutral or confirmatory information.

Figure 5.1 illustrates some aspects of a connectionist view of the functioning of repetition compulsions in terms of an energy landscape.
Although it is possible to model such a landscape strictly based on mathematical formulae (e.g. Rumelhart et al., 1986), at this point readers are
invited to look at it in an intuitive manner.

The question is what kind of impact therapeutic interventions can have
in such a system. It makes immediate sense that a variety of psychotherapeutic interventions 'heat up' the system, either in general or in some
parts. Therapeutic interventions can help – randomly or more targetedly

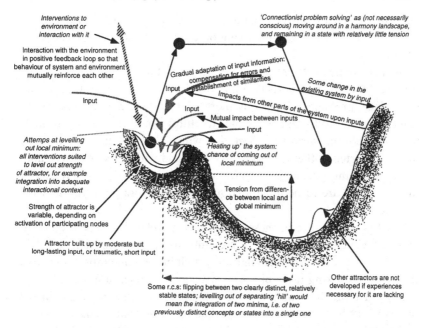

Interventions to environment or interaction with it

Interaction with the environment in positive feedback loop so that behaviour of system and environment mutually reinforce each other

Input

Attemps at levelling out local minimum: all interventions suited to level out strength of attractor, for example integration into adequate interactional context

Strength of attractor is variable, depending on activation of participating nodes

Attractor built up by moderate but long-lasting input, or traumatic, short input

'Connectionist problem solving' as (not necessarily conscious) moving around in a harmony landscape, and remaining in a state with relatively little tension

Gradual adaptation of input information: compensation for errors and establishment of similarities

Input

Some change in the existing system by input

Impacts from other parts of the system upon inputs

Input

Mutual impact between inputs

Input

'Heating up' the system: chance of coming out of local minimum

Tension from difference between local and global minimum

Some r.c.s: flipping between two clearly distinct, relatively stable states; *levelling out of separating 'hill' would mean the integration of two minima, i.e. of two previously distinct concepts or states into a single one*

Other attractors are not developed if experiences necessary for it are lacking

Fig. 5.1 Aspects of repetition compulsion (r.c.) and possible treatments, represented as an energy landscape. Roman text: state of maximal r.c.; *italic text*: *interventions, change.* (From Caspar et al., 1992.) For further explanation, see text.

– to bring systems into different states, in the sense of 'connectionist problem solving' as described above, to find more favourable states representing solutions. A wonderful example is Kelly's (1955) fixed role therapy in which different roles are tried out by patients.

Therapy can concentrate on building up additional connections, be it on a more conscious level as in cognitive therapy, or on a less conscious level by interventions, e.g. to integrate traumatic experiences by repeated contact with previously avoided situations. Corrective experiences, in particular, can contribute to changes in the connections traumatic experiences, as well as dysfunctional strategies, have to other elements. Two points are important from a connectionist point of view. First, old patterns hardly ever disappear completely. However, by strengthening new, competitive connections, and by weakening old ones, the probability is lowered that old patterns maintain a strong impact on behaviour and experience. Second, changes in connection strengths represent in themselves solutions, even if there is no explicit solution in the sense of traditional problem solving. Therapy should not be seen as replacing a distinct old state by a distinct new one, but rather as a gradual attempt to change the probabilities of a system moving on to different types of states as the situations change.

Because many parts are unconscious, it is not an easy task to establish better control. Even if parts become conscious, or if it is possible actually to 'replace' problematic parts by more adaptive alternatives, one would still expect that well-established old structures would resist integration of these new alternatives. An expectation would thus be that patients need to be supported in therapy over some time and with some intensity, and, most important, in concrete applications of the new patterns in reality, if the new parts are to be integrated and become more powerful than the old parts.

What is the balance of these considerations related to repetition compulsion? Connectionist models are able to account for all clinically important aspects; several are naturally built in. Few assumptions beyond the general working principles of connectionist models are needed.

Beyond repetition compulsion the list of similarities between clinical observations and connectionist concepts could be continued.

Comorbidity is an issue of high relevance in current discussions on psychopathology. Although enormous effort has always been put into placing different disorders in distinct categories, there is the observation that disorders co-occur, overlap, and develop into each other (Ingram and Kendall, 1987; Clarkin and Kendall, 1992; Caspar and Grawe, 1996). For example, the experience of anxious arousal in a particular situation, to which a caffeine overdose may have contributed, leads to avoidance (normally with an absence of high levels of actual anxiety). After some time, the avoidance leads to a loss of social contacts and other reinforcement, which is the beginning of a depression. Alternatively, the loss of energy and abilities caused by severe depression leads to anxiety about socially demanding situations, if they cannot be avoided.

Although for some purposes it may make sense to stress the distinction between anxiety and depression, for other purposes it may be better to acknowledge that they share many elements (negative affectivity, among others; Watson and Clark, 1984), and concentrate on a description of the aspects that actually differ, such as the type of physiological hyperarousal (Clark and Watson, 1991), without conceptualizing them as really separate phenomena. From a connectionist view, it is easy to imagine how a maladaptive development begins with a small 'hole' in the energy landscape (accidental anxious arousal) that gradually becomes larger and deeper (by avoidance) so that an individual gets into the hole from a greater variety of states, and gets out less easily. Then the loss of positive experience erodes a valley towards a 'depression hole' which, after some time, becomes deeper than the original anxiety hole. This increases the relative chance of an individual getting into and remaining in this depressive local minimum for longer periods of time, although the local minimum of anxiety has not disappeared yet. The interplay of multiple soft constraints, including the interaction with the environment, plays a greater role in this development than any single causal factor.

Such a view also reminds us of the fact that anxiety and depression are actually not homogeneous states: the individual goes through a series of states, including 'normal' ones, which can be distinguished, although they may share some properties causing one to summarize them as 'anxiety' or 'depression'. The aim of this way of thinking about disorders is not to invent yet another psychopathological model, but to ground a heuristic view of therapeutic procedure on it, as outlined below.

Understanding therapies in a dynamic way

A connectionist view of psychotherapy has a number of consequences. First of all, if psychological problems are viewed as described above, therapy must be conceptualized as introducing input into a system to change the landscape in such a way that desired states become more probable and undesired states become less probable. We would need to accept that no direct impact is possible but that we can only try to stimulate a system to self-organize itself in a more favourable direction. One could also say that we can provide only soft constraints that, in the right combination and in the right moment, can have a strong, but never a direct, impact. We would have to accept and utilize all properties of a dynamic system as described above. This shifts much of the therapist's attention away from applying a previously developed plan to monitoring the patient's present state, and to using the continually changing state of a patient (and the patient–therapist relationship) in a flexible way. The induction of good learning states – setting learning parameters appropriately for the whole system or particular domains – will become more important. The idea is not so new; Grawe (Grawe et al., 1998), among others, has given considerable thought to the question of how a therapist can create favourable conditions for accommodation, in particular by providing a safe, assimilative basis within the therapeutic relationship. Even earlier in modern psychotherapy, Rogers was an advocate of this approach, and now we have models to work it out in a much more detailed, individualized fashion. We should not shy away from (critically!) studying experts, such as sect leaders, successful salespeople, and politicians. Some of them are better practitioners of connectionist principles than the average psychotherapist!

Emphasizing learning conditions means that therapy should not be seen as an application of techniques. The situations with which patients are brought into contact (for example, in behavioural exposure) together with the therapist are a complex and changing input pattern. If therapists want to optimize this input pattern to maximize effectiveness and efficiency, they need to construct their action anew in every situation to take into account all lasting and temporary factors. Such factors are aetiological knowledge about a disorder, knowledge about prototypical procedures for a particular disorder (as described in treatment manuals), but also hypotheses about the patient's structure, including, but also going beyond, a particular problem (e.g. referring to individual resources). In addition, a connectionist view gives a special weight to constraints related to the particular situation, which is also dynamically related to the therapist's interventions (e.g. the therapeutic relationship), and the environment. Such a construction process is, of course, based on explicit or implicit predictions of effects the interventions will have. It is, however, obvious that at best, a *direction* of development can be anticipated, *not a precise state*. This does not mean that in the majority of cases we have to expect a development analogous to the fascinating observation that in chaotic systems the movement of a butterfly's wing can trigger a hurricane. In psychotherapy it is more common that realistically possible developments are limited and, although there are small surprises in every therapy, surprises on a larger scale are much less frequent.

There are a number of consequences related to such a view of therapy, which can only briefly be mentioned here.

Therapists should not strive for 'perfect' performance according to static rules, because a precise effect cannot be predicted, but rather *monitor* their action as well as patients' reactions, and permanently *adapt and correct* the procedure (Norman, 1986; Foppa, 1990) without overreacting (Vogel, 1994).

Because the therapist has important, but limited, possibilities of *directly* providing new input to the patient, an important task is to *mediate* input from a broader environment (Guidano and Liotti, 1983; Hayes, 1996).

Therapists should be ready to deal with both stability and sudden change, and try to understand and utilize them on an individual basis.

When thinking about effective principles, one should pay attention to aspects of *self-organization* and *timing*, and generally see therapy more as a 'sequential flow' (Orlinsky, Grawe and Parks, 1994). There are many references to dynamic models in the rather traditional psychotherapy literature, such as Piaget's assimilation/accommodation model (Gallagher and Reid, 1981), Waddingtons 'epigenetic landscape' (Waddington, 1974), and Prigogine's dissipative structures (Prigogine, 1977). In addition to rather metaphoric references to such dynamic models, we should try to use them more systematically, including precise modelling and simulating (Hayes, 1996; Schiepek et al., 1997; Tschacher, Scheier and Grawe, in press).

States with *disorganization* and increased variance should be expected, as several traditional concepts have suggested already. It seems that some therapies go through a phase of stagnation or even deterioration before deeper change takes place (Grawe, 1992; Newman and Martinovich 1996; Hayes, 1996). However, although overall temporary destabilization seems to be correlated with positive outcome (Hayes, 1996), it would be a relapse into causal-linear thinking to assume that change is related to destabilization in all cases, or 'the more destabilization the better'. Destabilization can also lead to deterioration. Connectionist modelling has the potential of helping to trace in detail developments observed with specific patients.

Strong attempts at changing a system often activate strong resistance. The secret of good therapy, if there is any, is to find a balance between too much and too little strength and persistence of input, or, in Piagetian terms, to compose an offer with a balance of parts that can be assimilated (to keep a patient open and flexible) and parts requiring accommodation (not to leave him or her in the maladaptive old state).

An assimilation of problematic experiences in such a way that they no longer have a maladaptive impact must *involve all levels* (cognitive, emotional, behavioural; Stiles et al., 1990). In the future, it may be possible to fine-tune therapeutic action based on even better elaborated dynamic models.

Input between therapy sessions can have a strong impact on the system, and easily outweigh the input by a therapist in one session a week. This may be a reason for some therapists to see their patients more frequently, or to do in-patient therapy. If we pay more attention to using a patient's natural environment systematically, as behaviour therapists and systemic therapists tend to do, we may be able to save time and money, and in addition minimize the patient's dependence on a therapist.

A connectionist perspective suggests a *neutral, functional view* of what different traditional approaches of psychotherapy can contribute. If we take – for reasons of space limitations as well as lack of empirical foundation for a more subtle view – *stereotypes* of different approaches as points of departure, one could speculate that, among others:

Psychoanalysis helps to develop insight and to inhibit old patterns consciously by such insights. It also helps to 'decentre', which, from a Piagetian point of view, supports change, and motivates the development of new patterns (for more information, see Turkle, 1988; Olds, 1994).

Cognitive therapy has a relatively direct impact on some cognitive premises of problematic behaviour and experiences. Not accidentally, however, cognitive therapists generally put a heavy emphasis on integration by paying due attention to emotions and behaviours.

Behaviour therapy provides new experiences by which new links are established and the weights of old structures become relatively less important (see Tryon, 1993).

Gestalt therapy or *experiential therapy* activates emotions: new experiences are provided so that the patient can survive strong emotions; an integration of more peripheral cognitive and behavioural learning experiences is furthered.

Rogerian therapy primarily creates favourable learning conditions by an accepting, warm relationship; insight and integration are furthered by deepening experiencing.

Focusing (Gendlin, 1978) uses non-symbolic access to implicit knowledge, etc.

A common element of different therapies, although with great differences in weight, is their encouragement and direct provision of new experiences, or help in getting into contact with new experiences. Thus, new input is introduced that has the potential of incrementally changing the existing landscape. Therapies providing strong, in general emotionally laden, experiences can be considered as 'heating up the system'. It is striking to what extent a quote by the cognitive scientist D. Norman (1986, p. 538) sounds psychotherapeutic: 'You have to shake up the system, heat up the temperature. Don't let it freeze into position. New interpretations suddenly arise, with no necessary conscious experience of how they came about; a moment of nothing and then clarity, as the system heats up, bounces out of one stable configuration and falls into a new configuration'.

Although clear main effects can be highlighted, the fact that therapy course and outcome are also, if not mainly, determined by the 'unspecific' effects of any intervention also needs to be highlighted. A more systematic consideration of side-effects can be postulated on the basis of traditional models as well (Caspar, 1995), but connectionism provides a more compelling general basis for thinking about the issue of main *vs* side-effects. A view of therapy resulting from a combination of little factors rather than one main factor corresponds much more to the view most patients as well as therapists have. If patients can single out one or two factors that they think are responsible for the change they have experienced, this often has more the character of a *construction* serving to organize their experience, than corresponding to the *experience itself*. Therapists often seem to think they did something wrong if therapy success just emerges from a variety of factors and only in some cases seems related to main factors – such as a particular technique – in a straightforward way. Side-effects should receive more attention, and they should be used more systematically.

The functioning and development of therapists

The question of how therapists function, and how this functioning is developed, is in itself interesting. It becomes all the more interesting if the perspective of applying a technique correctly is replaced by a perspective of developing an individualized therapeutic procedure that satisfies multiple constraints in parallel, and is continuously adapted based on the reaction of the system (patient). The question becomes even more exciting if we see therapists as managers of highly complicated dynamic processes, in which – to make things even more complicated – they also are involved as people. Traditional models deal well with a limited set of clear rules; connectionist systems with a multiplicity of soft rules.

Therapists' functioning has already been referred to above, and many of the principles addressed apply not only to patients but also to therapists. Issues of particular relevance are intuition, framing and handling of soft information, implicit knowledge, the ability to recognize non-obvious patterns, empathy, 'clinical wisdom', noise and fault tolerance, the ability to use defaults, automatization, the ability to process great amounts of information, graceful deterioration of performance ('graceful degradation') when working under bad conditions, automatic error compensation, the fact that processes running in parallel already have an impact on the whole before they are completed (Cohen, Dunbar and McClelland, 1990), and the need for a constructivist view.

The fact that traditional models have difficulties in accounting for intuition, whereas practitioners know how important intuition is, may be the most important single factor for the regrettable reluctance of practitioners to maintain contact with academic psychology, or whatever other scientific background they have. Three models seem particularly relevant in this context: the model describing frequency and adequacy of intuitive processing as depending on familiarity and difficulty of tasks and subtasks (Hammond, 1988; Hamm, 1988); the model of intuitive processing as depending on expertise (Dreyfus and Dreyfus, 1986); and the model of rapid switching back and forth between rational–analytic and intuitive processing, to use the respective advantages and compensate disadvantages in relation to varying subtasks (Pascual-Leone, 1990). The last-mentioned model is supported by research showing that therapists are able to be intuitive in the sense of holistic processing, and at the same time rational–analytic in the sense of conscious, reflected processing (Itten, 1994; Caspar, 1997). These approaches, among others, support the position that it is not acceptable to treat intuition as a non-scientific phenomenon. To the extent that traditional models have difficulties dealing with intuition, the need for models by which the phenomenon is treated as a regular form of processing grows. A related issue is the enormous capacity for processing large amounts of information very fast, for which connectionist models can also account (Shaastri and Ajjanagadde, 1993).

Traditional models are a good basis for teaching contents (diagnostic categories, techniques, etc.), but not sufficient for training internal processes (hypothesis generation, flexible use of knowledge, multiple constraint satisfaction) in a satisfactory way. An example of issues that need reflection, and for which a connectionist basis could be useful, is the development of automatization. Automatization is desirable because automatized processing is less vulnerable to capacity limitations (Shiffrin and Schneider, 1977; Cohen et al., 1990). However, it not only has advantages but disadvantages, as the automatized 'reflex' is not always the best reaction, and 'wisdom' includes the ability to resist automatization to some extent (Hanna and Ottens, 1995). Another example is the observation that patients fitting neatly into familiar concepts, with expert models performing therapy in an ideal way, are not ideal to learn from. Trainees also need 'noisy' input, that is, 'strange' patients, models that are not performing ideally, etc. But what are the right combination and timing?

As far as the therapist *as a person* is concerned, we need to think much more about conditions under which therapists can learn and perform well. For example, the concept of negative affectivity (Watson and Clark, 1984) should be considered from a connectionist perspective. It describes a type of person who is very introspective, self-reflexive, ready to discuss with others, dreaming and daydreaming more than others, and tending to focus on the negative side of others. Is this typical for therapists? If it is, how can we tune the systems (therapists) into more favourable states to use the positive and minimize the negative parts (negativity, lack of optimism)?

As far as diagnostic processes are concerned, we could, as Berrios and Chen (1993) do, view them in terms of energy landscapes, in which the therapist as a person is intertwined with the diagnostic system and with information from an individual patient. Different styles of relating symptoms to diseases could be identified and, if suboptimal, changed on the basis of a connectionist model.

The control of attention is another very important issue neglected by traditional approaches. Although elaborate connectionist models of attention are also lacking, it is relatively easy to imagine how a partly conscious, partly unconscious *competition* of different contents and processes *for attention*, as well as the *impact attention has on these processes*, could be modelled in a spreading activation model.

It is not arbitrary whether or not we have realistic models of therapists' performance and learning; we need them not only for research, each therapist should have them available, because otherwise they cannot systematically choose those conditions that favour optimal learning and performance. For example, the gain of expertise by experience strongly depends on the availability of feedback, which is not automatically provided by daily practice. Trainers, in particular, should base their practice on appropriate models: although supervision already now appears as a 'slow process of multiple corrections and rewards, similar to the "training" in a connectionist system' (Olds, 1994, p. 608), there is certainly much we can optimize based on explicit, dynamic learning models. As far as efficiency of training is concerned, we are still far from an optimal offer (Caspar, 1997).

Communication with the patient and with colleagues

Communication *with a patient* should reflect the assumptions that:

whatever is said reaches the patient only indirectly because it is interpreted by him or her at the periphery.
the patient has only limited introspective abilities.
what and, especially, the way we communicate have an impact on the
patient's ability to learn.

Many patients would prefer models that simplify a complex reality.
For example, they prefer to believe that their therapist 'knows' what is
wrong with them (instead of a constructivist view), that they 'have an
anxiety' (as a clearly distinguishable disorder, instead of thinking of
something always floating, which may be difficult to separate from
other disorder categories), that their therapist can change them or solve
their problems (instead of just providing some input to the system that
may or may not help the system to change itself).

Other patients, however – and we believe this group would be even
larger if we used existing possibilities of explaining models better –
develop justified resistance against simplistic, monocausal interpretations. They prefer a model in which a therapist would show awareness
that his or her hypotheses are of constructivist nature, that many factors
in therapy are in interaction and should be used, although nothing can be
predicted precisely, that the patient's functioning is something very complicated and that categories like 'anxiety', 'repression', 'reinforcement',
'threatening experience', etc. are only crude and imperfect descriptions of
what is actually going on, that change is normally incremental, that
conflicts and the tendency of a system to fight back against disturbances
caused by the therapist are something very natural. Needless to say, the
way such ideas are conveyed needs to be adapted to the intellectual
abilities of the patient (a resource often underutilized in therapy due to
the misconception that an intellectual approach is incompatible with the
often desired strengthening of emotions, and intuition). All, or most, of
the elements addressed above are not unique to connectionist thinking,
but a connectionist view implies them in a stringent, comprehensive way.

Many elements of a connectionist approach can be conveyed in a very
simple, concrete manner. An example would be to draw a picture similar
to that in Figure 5.2. As the therapist talks, he or she would point frequently to the drawing (pointing can be indicated here with numbers in
the figure only in a very imperfect way). The therapist could say:

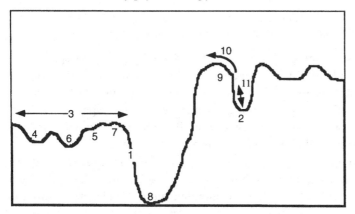

Fig. 5.2 Illustration of a patient's situation as a simplified version of Fig. 5.1. The numbers indicate where in the graph the therapist points when giving his or her comments. For further explanation, see text.

Let's for a moment see your problem in terms of a landscape. Of course, that's not how it really works, but it may help to think about a certain aspect. See this curve (1); it stands for the different states you can be in. For example, this hole (2) on a high overall level represents your anxiety. These (3) would be more pleasant states, during work; this (4) is, for instance, your excitement about the success you recently had with that sale. This part (5) stands for anxiety-free states when you are in your family; here (6) you are excited about what your son Ricky said yesterday to you. Here (7) you are a little upset, as was the case on Saturday, when you did not win the lottery. The line represents something like negative tension; the closer the line comes to the ground, the better off you are. Here (8) would be complete, desire-free happiness, if that's ideal at all. Got it?

Later on, one could continue:

The way I have drawn it here you see a crucial difference between the negative state due to the lottery and an anxiety state. The anxiety state is relatively lower, that is, more positive *compared to the immediate environment*. To come out of this state you would need to climb over (10) the hill. The hill (9) represents, for example, going out to places you are avoiding now, or confronting yourself in your mind with traumatic situations in the past. The situation we have now is that, following my suggestions, you always climb a little bit, and then, as tension increases, fall back into old patterns (11). You are disappointed, you develop doubts about therapy, etc. As we know, you are not always in anxiety states, but you have little control over whether you get into a panic or not. As long as this 'anxiety hole' exists, it works like a trap when you wander between different states over time. What I want to illustrate is, in order to move permanently into a new, really better state, you need to develop ways to overcome this hill, and that's painful. I wish I could spare you from that, but there is no way. So what do you think we can do, instead of getting desperate half way up and falling back, to be strong enough and eventually master the hill, steep and high as it may be?

Of course, what we have concentrated on here, due to space constraints, should ideally be developed in a dialogue with somewhat shorter therapist statements (although, if presented in a suitable way, many patients prefer to listen and get some conceptual input more than many therapists seem to believe). Also, if intellectual capability is low, the ideas conveyed may need to be even more simple.

In the communication with *colleagues*, a connectionist background can contribute to the awareness that it is never possible to make a colleague 'copy' one's view 100 per cent. Communication provides input patterns that are processed by the colleague's system, with many factors participating (including a hungry stomach, rivalry, personal biographic memories stimulated by a patient, sexual attraction to the colleague or the patient, the role played in an institution, to mention only a few). It is sometimes frustrating how limited our ability is directly to reach a colleague in a congress paper, an article, or even in a very close communication in daily work. To maximize our impact we should be aware, in particular, that:

how well we reach him or her depends on our ability to establish favourable learning conditions (current setting of parameters), and

whatever input we produce, its processing depends on existing knowledge (more enduring structures). When trying to address a colleague's knowledge base, we should be aware that most knowledge is not represented in readily available, explicit form, but is rather fuzzy, implicit and dynamic.

The development of new heuristic rules of therapy

A connectionist view of how theoretical concepts can be used by a practitioner suggests that a model like the connectionist model should be stored in several ways in a therapist's memory. It should be stored in a complex way to serve as background for thinking in depth about clinical observations and problems, and there should be some 'primitives' (Hofer, 1993; Caspar, 1995) closer to the surface and readily accessible, in the form of heuristic rules. In the above considerations, several statements had the character of such heuristic rules already. It may be useful, however, to collect and complete the list here. Again, to invent these rules, a connectionist background is not needed, but it makes them especially plausible.

Plan your interventions on several levels simultaneously (cognitive, affective, behavioural, somatic; Hayes, 1996).

Before starting an intervention, consider if the patient is in a favourable learning state.

Bring the system (the patient's as well as your own) into a favourable learning state.

Heat up the system to make it flexible.

Do not heat up the system too much in order to avoid decompensation and resistance.

Keep a balance between strong enough impact (not to be neutralized by the system) and not too strong impact (not to stimulate strong resistance).

Expose the patient repeatedly to natural input.

Further the integration of input to prevent it from getting stuck at the periphery.

Never intervene in a mechanistic way and always take the self-organizing abilities of the patient into account.

Keep in mind that, whatever you think about your patient, it is a construction.

Find coherent new solutions ('good gestalt'), in which different domains (e.g. private, work), goals (e.g. autonomy, closeness) and levels (cognitive, emotional, behavioural) are in a balance, or at least consider whether a patient has the possibility of developing coherence after the therapy.

If a relevant phenomenon does not make sense from the perspectives considered so far, keep looking for additional bio-psycho-social determinants. Maybe the phenomenon emerges from a variety of forces of which none alone would be strong enough.

Construct your procedure as parallel multiple constraint satisfaction (Caspar, 1995).

Pay attention to side-effects: therapy process as well as overall outcome are usually largely determined by a multiplicity of soft side-effects.

Rather than trying to be perfect in your therapeutic procedure, concentrate on learning from feedback and correcting your errors (Norman, 1986; Foppa, 1990).

To develop such a list further, many open questions need to be studied. For example, under what conditions is it better to concentrate on one problem or one aspect of a problem for a period of time? When is it better to work on its surroundings simultaneously?

Simulating the effects of planned intervention

Traditional models have their strength in capturing structure in a simple way, connectionist models in modelling change. The dynamics of change are considered less intensely than would be ideal in therapy planning, and this is largely due to our inability to model them (a) more precisely, and (b) in a sufficiently simple way to be utilized in practice, or at least in training. There are ideas in the literature of how connectionist simulations could be used to model phenomena relevant for psychotherapy. Park and Young (1994) refer to connectionist simulations of different psychodynamic defences in the recall of traumatic memories by altering the arousal state of the network during learning.

As part of an ongoing project on the training of inner processes in therapists (Caspar, 1997), a program by Mross and Roberts (1992) to simulate the construction–integration model by Kintsch (1988) is used. The program simulates connectionist spreading of activation, although the nodes are localist (symbolic). This way, not all advantages of the most typical distributed connectionist models are used. The advantage of such a hybrid model is that the networks are much easier to feed and it is much easier to trace what happens in them. Here, we give a simplified example of how a therapist's view of a case is represented (Fig. 5.3a), and how then the impact of an intervention can be simulated. The program does not actually simulate a real therapy course, but the impact an intervention should have, according to the view previously declared to the computer by the therapist. Space limitations do not allow all details to be explained here, but it is hoped that this gives at least an impression of what could be done on a larger scale.

The goal is to reduce social anxiety (as expressed by its activation value in the list) by using an intervention sending input to elements related to anxiety. Figure 5.3b illustrates how cognitive–behavioural interventions (needless to say they are simplified here), used to attack some underlying beliefs (as expressed by negative, dotted links), have hardly any effect: they are neutralized by the system – after 11 iterations their activation value is at zero, without noticeable traces in the remaining system. What impact would it have to bring the system into a more favourable state by appealing to the resources (positive aspects) of the patient's functioning? Several additional elements and links represent this approach (Fig. 5.3c). As the activation values show, most elements of this approach are also neutralized, but they leave traces: there is some reduction of the 'social anxiety's' activation. The simulation gives a flavour of how difficult it is,

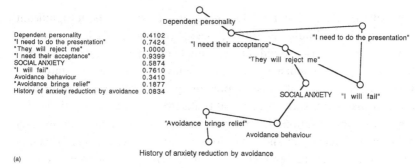

Dependent personality	0.4102
"I need to do the presentation"	0.7424
"They will reject me"	1.0000
"I need their acceptance"	0.9399
SOCIAL ANXIETY	0.5874
"I will fail"	0.7610
Avoidance behaviour	0.3410
"Avoidance brings relief"	0.1877
History of anxiety reduction by avoidance	0.0834

(a)

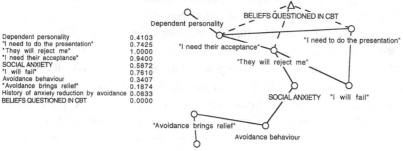

Dependent personality	0.4103
"I need to do the presentation"	0.7425
"They will reject me"	1.0000
"I need their acceptance"	0.9400
SOCIAL ANXIETY	0.5872
"I will fail"	0.7610
Avoidance behaviour	0.3407
"Avoidance brings relief"	0.1874
History of anxiety reduction by avoidance	0.0833
BELIEFS QUESTIONED IN CBT	0.0000

(b)

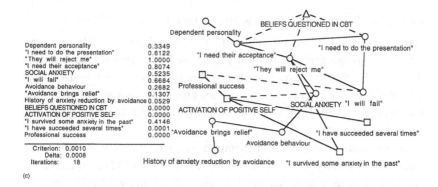

Dependent personality	0.3349
"I need to do the presentation"	0.6122
"They will reject me"	1.0000
"I need their acceptance"	0.8074
SOCIAL ANXIETY	0.5235
"I will fail"	0.6684
Avoidance behaviour	0.2682
"Avoidance brings relief"	0.1307
History of anxiety reduction by avoidance	0.0529
BELIEFS QUESTIONED IN CBT	0.0000
ACTIVATION OF POSITIVE SELF	0.0000
"I survived some anxiety in the past"	0.4146
"I have succeeded several times"	0.0001
Professional success	0.0000

Criterion:	0.0010
Delta:	0.0008
Iterations:	18

(c)

Fig. 5.3 Simplified networks representing a therapist's view of a patient's problem and two types of intervention. The solid lines represent a positive, the broken lines a negative (inhibitory) link. CBT: cognitive–behaviour therapy. For further explanation, see text.

not only in simulation but also in reality, to bring about significant change. When simulating difficult cases (e.g. a borderline case) we have, however, also found the phenomenon that a system may flip from a state with much parasuicidal behaviour to a stable state with very low activation of nodes representing such behaviour. Even with difficult disorders, such as personality disorders, such observations correspond to observations in reality, and connectionist simulations may help us to understand the conditions under which such change takes place. In the author's research group, important parts of an entire therapy with a bulimic patient have been successfully simulated and it was possible to simulate the flipping between bulimic and non-bulimic states by merely varying the degree of self-esteem dependent on the quality of interpersonal relationships, just as had been observed in reality.

Needless to say, such modelling does not contain any truth, and many technical as well as psychological aspects would need discussion. However, it can already be used in simple forms to guide reflection and, it is to be hoped, better planning by therapists. A pilot study shows that therapists' acceptance and interest are very high (Caspar and Torhorst, 1996), and connectionist modelling is used in current psychotherapy training (Caspar, 1997).

Problems of connectionist models and possible solutions

As Norman (1986, p. 546) states about connectionist models: 'A large number of issues are now naturally addressed that were difficult to deal with before. In turn, a large number of things that were easy to do before are now difficult'. However, just as not all advantages of connectionist models are relevant for a use in the domain of psychotherapy, this is also true of disadvantages.

A first point is that, with distributed representations, it is difficult to trace what actually happens in connectionist models. There is increased research that may help remove the 'black box' image of connectionist processing. Nevertheless, at the moment the limited transparency is indeed a great disadvantage. Several reactions are possible.

A recommendation to use traditional models (e.g. Plan Analysis; Caspar, 1995) is justified if they allow a good enough approximation to 'reality' for the purpose for which they are used.

For many reflections about the functioning of people and psychotherapy,
we do not need to trace developments in concrete detail, but can utilize
models in a more abstract way.

Some problems can be treated with hybrid models, as illustrated in the
last section.

An important step to make connectionist models more surveyable is the
more recent approach of building them in a modular way (Cohen et al.,
1990).

A second point is that connectionist models have many degrees of
freedom (which is a criticism levelled against information-processing
models in general; Cohen and Servan-Schreiber, 1992). This insight
should prevent us from trying to prove anything based on such models,
but we can still use them as a heuristic tool to give us new ideas about
psychotherapy and ultimately to *contribute* to true explanations. In addition, we should rather strive for simplicity than for too complex models.
However, if we want to simplify in a rational way, we need background
models that are sufficiently complex to imagine the effects a simplification
in one or another aspect may have (Elliott and Anderson, 1994).

As Miller, Galanter and Pribram (1960, p. 182) write: 'a good scientist
can draw an elephant with three parameters, and with four he can tie a
knot in its tail', but 'no benign and parsimonious deity has issued us an
insurance policy against complexity'. When looked at in detail, things are
often complex, but in order to take advantage of a model, not all details
need to be understood. As Olds (1994) argues, psychoanalysts were also
able to utilize a steam-engine model without understanding steam engines
in detail. To be useful practically, models need to be simple enough to be
used by practitioners without daily dependency on technical experts, even
if these are needed to question and improve models from time to time.

We should also be aware that, due to the number of degrees of freedom
in reality, in the field of psychotherapy generally a posteriori constructions of 'how something could happen' are more typical than true explanatory models. If connectionist models are too complex to be judged for
their quality as explanatory models, at least they allow a precise modelling and a tracing of the impact of variations in the structure and parameter setting.

A third point is the stability–plasticity dilemma, as addressed above.
Although there are some relatively simple mechanisms suited to explain
the persistence of some patterns in a dynamic system, the problem is not a
trivial one and should be kept in mind. Again, this difficulty exists not

only for connectionist models. McClelland (1994) points out that the graduality with which individuals learn, according to Piaget, is a need from a connectionist point of view. A system needs confrontation with a sufficient sample of an environment to develop well-integrated changes, which, of course, is a clinically relevant point. How is it possible that such an incremental system can also produce fast qualitative learning steps?

In part, the apparent problem may be a product of difficulties in tracing a system's development in sufficient detail (McClelland, 1994). It could be that the system does not really change so suddenly, but that there are all kinds of subtle, incremental changes in parts of the system that are less accessible to the therapist's observation and the patient's introspection, but significant for a later change on a larger scale. The change in a single, more accessible variable may then appear as a sudden shift, whereas, if seen relative to all other changes that have already taken place, or follow, it is a relatively small change. For example, a significant 'sudden' insight may have been preceded by several changes on the emotional level, which paved the way to the insight. In addition, to persist and gain clinically relevant influence on the whole system, the insight may need to be followed by changes in behaviour and in the environment. Important and sudden as it may be, if seen as a part of the whole, the insight is only part of a series of incremental changes. Possible conceptual solutions to the stability–plasticity dilemma have been mentioned above.

A temporary solution, at least to some of the problems stated above, is the use of hybrid models (Kintsch, 1988; Anderson, 1990; Ueberla and Jagota, 1993; Horgan and Tienson, 1994). If one uses them, it is important to maintain relevant properties of connectionist models, such as the dynamic functioning and the ability to deal with multiple soft constraints. From an economic point of view, hybrid models have advantages (Gutknecht, 1993), as pure models explaining the same range of phenomena tend to be much more complicated. In addition, it seems possible to use different models simultaneously. Physicists, for example, seem to be able to think of light as being a *stream of particles* and a *wave* at the same time, although, logically, these views contradict each other. The use of hybrid models is also a good way of mastering the difficult shift from thinking traditionally to thinking in a connectionist way in several steps.

Conclusions

Do we need connectionist models? Tietel (1991) presents the interesting argument that, in the view of some psychoanalysts, psychoanalysis has

rather the role of criticizing developments in society, including compu-
terization. This would be a role *above* models such as connectionism, and
indeed, if the role of approach A is to judge approach B, it should not let
itself be infiltrated by approach B. Other authors argue that connectionism may not go far enough in that it remains within the boundaries of
rationalism (Pfeifer and Verschure, 1992). Further, there are many examples of models that are in line with relevant aspects addressed in this
chapter without being connectionist. An example is Stiles et al. (1990),
using Piagetian schemata as a base. Another example would be M.
Horowitz's (1979) 'states of mind' concept. It seems, however, that
often authors open up to connectionist models when they keep looking
at their phenomena in detail (Caspar et al., 1992), or they leave open the
question of which basic models are more advantageous (e.g. Greenberg,
Rice and Elliott, 1993).

Obviously, the interest in and acceptance of new approaches depend to
a large degree on their ability to account for phenomena that were hard
to account for by existing approaches. This is, however, not an all-or-
nothing issue, and it would be naive to believe that connectionism should
simply replace other approaches ('scientific reductionism'; Smolensky,
1988).

From the perspective of connectionist approaches, each (or most) of
the existing approaches to psychotherapy is able to contribute unique
aspects to understanding and stimulating change. None is, on its own,
comprehensive enough to provide a flexible, individualized approach
using all the opportunities to give every patient an optimal and efficient
psychotherapy – or to state clearly and reliably that psychotherapy is not
the means to help a patient in a particular situation. A connectionist
perspective can contribute to an unbiased evaluation and utilization of
the respective advantages and at the same time make clear where an
integration of the existing (as opposed to developing new) concepts is
not sufficient, as discussed throughout this chapter. In addition, connectionism can contribute to developing a common language (Tryon, 1993).

The utilization of connectionism in psychotherapy should be furthered
by case studies similar to those by Stiles et al. (1991) for the assimilation
model, and by comparing real therapies with simulations. Already, connectionism can be used as 'a framework in which to develop models or
theories' (Bechtel, 1993, p. 149). Traditional models favour thinking in
terms of a limited number of main factors, working in isolation or
together in a simple way. Such a view prevents us from looking into
the dynamic interaction of many soft factors, each of minor importance,

which, however, seem to be responsible for a great deal of outcome variance. The general development is away from seeing all that remains unexplained by a limited number of simple factors as 'error variance' (Mahoney, 1991).

One last argument in favour of connectionism is that it has gained ground in cognitive science, and psychotherapy needs to maintain contact with basic science: 'One reason that psychoanalysis lost some of its scientific respectability in recent decades is that it lost touch with the rest of science' (Olds, 1994, p. 605). This should not happen to psychotherapy in general.

If this chapter has not been successful in convincing the reader to believe in the advantages of a connectionist approach to psychotherapy, it is to be hoped that it has had at least one effect: that schemata should no longer be seen as static entities, but as active, dynamic processes.

Summary

The field of psychotherapy has clearly made progress over the past decades. Nevertheless, some patients have not been helped as much as would be desirable, and some phenomena are still hard to conceptualize based on traditional models. The potential of connectionist models to contribute to further development is discussed and exemplified. Their potential lies mainly in the dynamic process of satisfying a multiplicity of soft constraints in parallel, which is typical in clinical practice. The role of past experiences, resistance to change, the interplay of cognition, emotion, behaviour, and environment, the functioning of psychotherapists, and a constructivist position are also addressed from a connectionist perspective. Finally, inherent problems of a connectionist approach to psychotherapy and possible solutions are discussed.

Endnotes

1 Just as in Caspar, Rothenfluh and Segal (1992), the term 'connectionist' is preferred over 'neural networks' because the still much discussed issue of whether these models actually correspond more to the biological basis is of minor importance for the points made in this chapter. Additional arguments in favour of the term 'connectionism' are used by Henningsen (1996). Rather than reproduce the points made in an earlier, more comprehensive paper on 'the appeal of connectionism for clinical psychology' in general (Caspar et al., 1992), this chapter focuses on psychotherapy, and tries to add some new aspects.

2 See Stinson and Palmer (1991) and Caspar et al. (1992) for a more complete list of deficiencies of traditional approaches.

3 The use of a different level for reasons of illustrations does not imply that the author believes in simple continuity between levels.

4 Unless specified otherwise, the term 'system' is used for the functioning of an individual patient, not a multiperson system.

5 Grawe (1992): 'sore spots'; Stiles et al. (1990, p. 412), refer to Gendlin (1978): felt referent; Rice (1983): problematic reaction point; Horowitz et al. (1975): warded off content and conflictual ideas, object-relational notions of experiences that are split off from awareness to maintain a sense of self-coherence and connection with an idealized internal object; interpersonal notions of 'not-me' experiences that are selectively inattended to in an attempt to avoid anxiety; Kelly (1955): anxiety when events occur that fall beyond the range of convenience of the individual's construct system, etc.

6 Connectionist concepts may also be a good basis for thinking about the interesting contradiction that, on the one hand, increased self-attention is a vehicle of several approaches to therapy (e.g. psychoanalysis, schema theory; see Grawe, 1992), and, on the other hand, there are indicators that 'effective change mechanisms of therapy are those methods that induce a decrease in self-focused attention' (Ingram, 1990, p. 165).

References

Anderson, J.A. (1990). Hybrid computation in cognitive science: neural networks and symbols. *Applied Cognitive Psychology*, **4**, 337–47.

Bechtel, W. (1993). Currents in connectionism. *Minds and Machines*, **3**, 125–53.

Bergin, A.E. & Garfield, S.L. (eds.) (1994). *Handbook of Psychotherapy and Behavior Change*. New York: Wiley.

Berrios, G.E. & Chen, E.Y.H. (1993). Recognising psychiatric symptoms: relevance to the diagnostic process. *British Journal of Psychiatry*, **163**, 308–14.

Bower, G.H. (1981). Mood and memory. *American Psychologist*, **36**, 129–48.

Brousse, O. & Smolensky, P. (1989). Virtual memories and massive generalization in connectionist combinatorial learning. In *Proceedings of the 11th Annual Conference of the Cognitive Science Society*, pp. S380–7. Hillsdale, NJ: Erlbaum.

Caspar, F. (1995). *Plan Analysis, Towards Optimizing Psychotherapy*. Seattle: Hogrefe.

Caspar, F. (1997). What goes on in a psychotherapist's mind? *Psychotherapy Research*, **7**, 105–25.

Caspar, F. & Grawe, K. (1996). Was spricht für, was gegen individuelle Falkonzeptionen. In *Psychotherapeutische Problemanalyse*, ed. F. Caspar, pp. 650–86. Tübingen: DGVT.

Caspar, F., Rothenfluh, Th. & Segal, Z.V. (1992). The appeal of connectionism for clinical psychology. *Clinical Psychology Review*, **12**, 719–62.

Caspar, F. & Torhorst, F. (1996). How to think about your patient? Computer Assisted Training of Coherence. Paper presented at the Conference of the Society for Psychotherapy Research. Amelia Island, Florida.

Clark, L.A. & Watson, D. (1991). Tripartite model of anxiety and depression: psychometric evidence and taxonomic implications. *Journal of Abnormal Psychology*, **100**, 316–36.

Clarkin, J.F. & Kendall, P.C. (1992) Comorbidity and treatment planning. *Journal of Consulting and Clinical Psychology*, **60**, 904–8.

Cohen, J.D., Dunbar, K. & McClelland, J.L. (1990). On the control of automatic processes: A parallel distributed processing model of the Stroop effect. *Psychological Review*, **97**, 332–61.

Cohen, J.D. & Servan-Schreiber, D. (1992). Context, cortex, and dopamine: a connectionist approach to behavior and biology in schizophrenia. *Psychological Review*, **99**, 45–77.

Dowd, E.T. & Courchaine, K. (1992). Implicit learning, tacit knowledge, and implications for stasis and change in cognitive psychotherapy. Paper presented at the World Congress on Cognitive Therapy, Toronto, Canada.

Dreyfus, H.L. & Dreyfus, S.E. (1986). *Mind Over Machine: The Power of Human Intuition and Expertise in the Era of the Computer*. New York: Free Press.

Elliott, R. & Anderson, C. (1994). Simplicity and complexity in psychotherapy research. In *Reassessing Psychotherapy Research*, ed. R.L. Russell, pp. 65–113. New York: Guilford Press.

Erickson, M.H. (1968). *Advanced Techniques of Hypnosis and Therapy*. New York: Grune.

Foppa, K. (1990). Topical progression and integration. In *The Dynamics of Dialogue*, ed. E. Markova & K. Foppa, pp. 176–200. New York: Harvester Wheatsheaf.

Gallagher, J.M. & Reid, D.K. (1981). *The Learning Theory of Piaget and Inhelder*. Monterey, CA: Brooks/Cole.

Gendlin, E.T. (1978). *Focusing*. New York: Everest House.

Golden, R.M. & Rumelhart, D.E. (1993). A parallel distributed processing model of story comprehension and recall. *Discourse Processes*, **16**, 203–37.

Grawe, K. (1992). *Schema Theory and Heuristic Psychotherapy*, Report No. 1–1992. Bern: Psychologisches Institut der Universität Bern.

Grawe, K., Donati, R. & Bernauer, F. (1998). *Psychotherapy in Transition*. Seattle: Hogrefe.

Greenberg, L. & Safran, J. (1987). *Facilitating Emotional Change: The Moment-by-Moment Process*. New York: Guilford Press.

Greenberg, L.S., Rice, L.N. & Elliott, R. (1993). *Emotion in Psychotherapy. Affect, Cognition, and the Process of Change*. New York: Guilford Press.

Grossberg, S. (1986). Adaptive pattern classification and universal recording: I. Parallel development and coding of neural feature detectors. *Biological Cybernetics*, **23**, 121–34.

Grossberg, S. (1987). Competitive learning: From interactive activation to adaptive resonance. *Cognitive Science*, **11**, 122–63.

Guidano, V.F. & Liotti, G. (1983). *Cognitive Processes and Emotional Disorders*. New York: Guilford Press.

Gutknecht, M. (1993). Adaptive hybrid artifacts: three perspectives on designing artificial systems. Dissertation, Zürich.

Hamm, R.M. (1988). Clinical intuition and clinical analysis: expertise and the cognitive continuum. In *Professional Judgment*, ed. J. Dowie & A. Elstein, pp. 78–108. Cambridge: Cambridge University Press.

Hammond, K.R. (1988). *Information Models for Intuitive and Analytical Cognition*. Report 281. University of Colorado, Center for Research on Judgment and Policy.

Hanna, F.J. & Ottens, A.J. (1995). The role of wisdom in psychotherapy. *Journal of Psychotherapy Integration*, **5**, 195–219.

Hayes, A.M. (1996). Dynamic systems theory as a paradigm for studying the process of change in psychotherapy for depression. *Constructive Change*, **1**, 9–12.

Henningsen, P. (1996). Mental states in a connectionist world. The conceptual impact of cognitive neuroscience on psychiatry. Unpublished manuscript. Department of Psychosomatic Medicine, Heidelberg.

Hofer, H. (1993). Die Rolle von Theorien im Klinischen Erstinterview. Unpublished thesis, Bern.

Horgan, T. & Tienson, J. (1994). Representations don't need rules. *Mind and Language*, **9**, 38–55.

Horowitz, L.M., Sampson, H., Siegelman, E.Y., Wolfson, A. & Weiss, J. (1975). On the identification of warded-off mental contents. *Journal of Abnormal and Social Psychology*, **84**, 545–58.

Horowitz, M.J. (1979). *States of Mind: Analysis of Change in Psychotherapy*. New York, London: Plenum Press.

Ingram, R.E. (1990). Self-focused attention in clinical disorders: review and a conceptual model. *Psychological Bulletin*, **107**, 156–76.

Ingram, R.E. & Hollon, S.D. (1986). Cognitive therapy of depression from an information processing perspective. In *Information Processing Approaches and Clinical Psychology*, ed. R.E. Ingram, pp. 259–81. Orlando: Academic Press.

Ingram, R.E. & Kendall, P.C. (1987). The cognitive side of anxiety. *Cognitive Therapy and Research*, **11**, 523–36.

Itten, S. (1994). Intuitives Informationsverarbeiten in klinischen Erstgesprächen. Unpublished thesis, Universität Bern.

Kelly, G.A. (1955). *The Psychology of Personal Constructs*. New York: Norton.

Kintsch, W. (1988). The role of knowledge in discourse comprehension: A construction–integration model. *Psychological Review*, **95**, 163–82.

Mahoney, M. (1991). *Human Change Processes*. New York: Basic Books.

McClelland, J.L. (1994). The interaction of nature and nurture in development: a parallel distributed processing perspective. In *Current Advances in Psychological Science: Ongoing Research*, ed. P. Bertelson, P. Eelen & G. D'Ydewalle, pp. 57–88. Hillsdale, NJ: Erlbaum.

Meichenbaum, D. & Gilmore, J.B. (1984). The nature of unconscious process: a cognitive–behavioral perspective. In *The Unconscious Reconsidered*, ed. K. Bowers & D. Meichenbaum, pp. 273–98. New York: Wiley.

Miller, G.A., Galanter, E. & Pribram, K.H. (1960). *Plans and the Structure of Behavior*. New York: Holt.

Minsky, M. (1975). A framework for representing knowledge. In *The Psychology of Computer Vision*, ed. P.H. Winston, pp. 211–77. New York: McGraw-Hill.

Mross, E. & Roberts, J. (1992). *The Construction–Integration Model: A Program and Manual*. Technical Report 92–14. Boulder: Institute of Cognitive Science, University of Colorado.

Neisser, U. (1976). *Cognition and Reality*. San Francisco: Freeman.

Newman, F.L. & Martinovich, Z. (1996). Interpreting results: alternatives and supplements to traditional hypothesis testing. Paper presented at the

Congress of the Society for Psychotherapy Research, Amelia Island, Florida.

Norcross, J.C. & Wogan, M. (1983). American psychotherapists of diverse persuasions: characteristics, theories, practices, and clients. *Professional Psychology: Research and Practice*, **14**, 529–39.

Norman, D. (1986). Reflections on cognition and parallel distributed processing. In *Parallel Distributed Processing. Explorations in the Microstructure of Cognition*, ed. J.L. McClelland, D.E. Rumelhart & P.R. Group, pp. 531–46. Cambridge, MA: MIT Press.

Olds, D.D. (1994). Connectionism and psychoanalysis. *Journal of the American Psychoanalytic Association*, **42**, 581–611.

Orlinsky, D.E., Grawe, K. & Parks, B.K. (1994). Process and outcome in psychotherapy-Nocheinmal. In *Handbook of Psychotherapy and Behavior Change*, ed. A.E. Bergin & S.L. Garfield, pp. 270–376. New York: Wiley.

Ortony, A., Clore, G.L. & Collins, A. (1988). *The Cognitive Structure of Emotions*. Cambridge: Cambridge University Press.

Park, S.B.G. & Young, A.H. (1994). Connectionism and psychiatry: a brief review. *Philosophy, Psychiatry & Psychology*, **1**, 51–8.

Pascual-Leone, J. (1990). An essay on wisdom: toward organismic processes that make it possible. In *Wisdom: Its Nature, Origins, and Development*, ed. R. Sternberg, pp. 244–78. New York: Cambridge University Press.

Pfeifer, R. & Verschure, P. (1992). Beyond rationalism: symbols, patterns and behavior. *Connection Science*, **4**, 313–25.

Piaget, J. (1954). *The Construction of Reality in the Child*. New York: Basic Books.

Prigogine, I. (1977). *Self Organization in Nonequilibrium Systems: from Dissipative Structures to Order through Fluctuations*. New York: Wiley.

Ramzy, I. & Shevrin, H. (1976). The nature of the inference process in psychoanalytic interpretation: A critical review of the literature. *International Journal of Psychoanalysis*, **57**, 151–9.

Rice, L.N. (1983). The relationship in client-centered therapy. In *Psychotherapy and Patient Therapist Relationships*, ed. M.J. Lambert. Homewood, IL: Dow Jones-Irwin.

Rogers, C.R. (1951). *Client-Centered Psychotherapy*. Boston: Houghton Mifflin.

Rumelhart, D.E., Smolensky, P., McClelland, J.L. & Hinton, G.E. (1986). Schemata and sequential thought processes in PDP models. In *Parallel Distributed Processing. Explorations in the Microstructure of Cognition*, ed. J.L. McClelland & D.E. Rumelhart, pp. 7–57. Cambridge, MA: MIT Press.

Schiepek, G., Kowalik, Z.J., Schütz, A. et al. (1997). Psychotherapy as a chaotic process I. Coding the client–therapist interaction by means of sequential Plan Analysis and the search for chaos: A stationary approach. *Psychotherapy Research*, **7**, 173–94.

Schneider, H. (1989). Toward a more detailed understanding of selforganizing processes in psychotherapy. In *Selforganization in Psychotherapy*, ed. A.L. Goudsmith, pp. 72–99. Berlin: Springer-Verlag.

Shaastri, L. & Ajjanagadde, V. (1993). From simple associations to systematic reasoning: A connectionist representation of rules, variables and dynamic bindings using temporal synchrony. *Behavioral and Brain Sciences*, **16**, 417–94.

Shiffrin, R.M. & Schneider, W. (1977). Controlled and automatic human information processing: II. Perceptual learning, automatic attending, and a general theory. *Psychological Review*, **84**, 127–90.
Smolensky, P. (1988). On the proper treatment of connectionism. *Behavioral and Brain Sciences*, **11**, 1–74.
Stiles, W.B., Elliott, R., Llewelyn, S.P. et al. (1990). Assimilation of problematic experiences by clients in psychotherapy. *Psychotherapy*, **27**, 411–20.
Stiles, W.B., Morrison, L.A., Haw, S.K., Harper, H., Shapiro, D. & Firth-Cozens, J.A. (1991). Longitudinal study of assimilation in exploratory psychotherapy. *Psychotherapy*, **28**, 195–206.
Stinson, C.H. & Palmer, S.E. (1991). Parallel distributed processing models of person schemas and psychopathologies. In *Person Schemas and Maladaptive Interpersonal Patterns*, ed. M.J. Horowitz, pp. 334–78. Chicago: University of Chicago Press.
Teasdale, J. & Barnard, P.J. (1993). *Affect, Cognition, and Change: Re-modelling Depressive Thought*. Hillsdale, NJ: Lawrence Erlbaum.
Thagard, P. (1989). Explanatory coherence. *Behavioral and Brain Sciences*, **12**, 435–502.
Tietel, E. (1991). Künstliche Intelligenz und Psychoanalyse: Eine Mesalliance? *Psychologie und Gesellschaftskritik*, **15**, 41–54.
Tryon, W.W. (1993). Neural networks: I. Theoretical unification through connectionism. *Clinical Psychology Review*, **13**, 341–71.
Tschacher, W., Scheier, C. & Grawe, K. (in press). Order and pattern formation in psychotherapy. *Nonlinear Dynamics, Psychology, and Life Sciences*.
Turkle, S. (1988). Artificial intelligence and psychoanalysis: a new alliance. *Daedalus*, **117**, 241–68.
Ueberla, J.P. & Jagota, A. (1993). Integrating neural and symbolic approaches: a symbolic learning scheme for a connectionist associative memory. *Connection Science*, **5**, 377–93.
Vogel, G. (1994). *Planung und Improvisation im therapeutischen Prozess*. Münster: Waxmann.
Waddington, C.H. (1974). A catastrophe theory of evolution. *Annals of the New York Academy of Sciences*, **231**, 32–42.
Watson, D. & Clark, L.A. (1984). Negative affectivity: the disposition to experience aversive emotional states. *Psychological Bulletin*, **96**, 465–90.
Yates, J.L. & Nashby, W. (1993). Dissociation, affect, and network models of memory: an integrative proposal. *Journal of Traumatic Stress*, **6**, 305–26.

6

Modulatory mechanisms in mental disorders
DAVID HESTENES

This chapter proposes a theoretical framework for biological psychiatry founded on the following general principles derived from neural network theory and empirical neuroscience.

1. *Cardinal principles of neuropsychology*:
   (a) the brain has a modular structure,
   (b) information is represented by neural activity patterns in each module,
   (c) all psychological functions, including perception, cognition, learning, memory and motor control, are modes of neural activity pattern processing.
2. *Central brain state control*:
   Pattern processing in the various brain modules is coordinated by a central control system. Control variables include the monoamines (dopamine, noradrenalin and serotonin), acetylcholine and possibly others. These variables modulate pattern formation, stabilization, biasing, mixing, matching and switching in the modules.
3. *Mental disorders from control malfunctions*:
   Manic–depressive illness and related mental disorders are malfunctions of the modulatory mechanisms for pattern processing. The particular symptoms of a disorder depend on the kind of malfunction and the specific module(s) in which it occurs.

The proposed cardinal principles are probably acceptable to most neuroscientists today, so it is unnecessary to justify them here. Indeed, they are so widely accepted that they are often taken for granted. However, the need for an explicit formulation of the cardinal principles is evident when one realizes that they have surprisingly rich implications that emerge when one tries to design brain architectures to implement them.

132

One of the premier theoretical neuropsychologists, Stephen Grossberg, has provided an analysis of these implications leading to a host of design principles for specific mechanisms and architectures. This chapter reviews a number of his results, with particular relevance to psychiatry.

Following Grossberg, the cardinal principles are elaborated into elementary network designs for the most basic pattern-processing capabilities: reliable pattern registration and short-term memory, competitive selection, long-term associative memory and recall, recognition and classification. Then gain control variables necessary to control pattern processing are classified. Later, these variables are identified with neuromodulators known to play a primary role in mental disorders, and an explanation is given of how symptoms of these disorders can be attributed to gain control malfunctions. This provides us with a theoretical framework for understanding the roles of neuromodulators within a central system for integrating and controlling whole brain function.

The clinical implications of this framework are extensive. First, it is a theoretical framework for psychiatric diagnosis – for analyzing psychiatric symptoms and their genesis in specific gain control malfunctions, and for identifying the loci of these malfunctions in brain modules or control centers for targeted treatment. Second, the framework can serve as a guide for research into neurobiological mechanisms in mental illness. The clinical utility of the framework is limited by uncertainties about neural correlates of the theoretical constructs. This uncertainty can only be reduced by basic research, but research is most productive when it is targeted toward crucial theoretical issues.

As the main concern of this chapter is to outline a theoretical framework, it cannot do justice to empirical issues. Hestenes (1992) reviews the enormous literature on monoamine neurotransmitters for evidence supporting identification of their roles as gain control variables. That article can therefore be regarded as an empirical partner of this chapter. The final section of the chapter reviews and updates some of the clinical evidence and implications.

Pattern-processing principles and mechanisms

The main objective of neuropsychology is to explain psychological functioning in terms of brain structure and activity. This calls for a definitive answer to the fundamental question: 'How is information represented and processed in the brain?'

According to our cardinal principles, the brain is a pattern-processing machine. This is to say that information is represented by spatially distributed patterns, and it is processed by dynamic mechanisms governing pattern formation. This should be contrasted with the alternative view that the brain is a symbol-processing machine, that is, information is represented by symbols and processed algorithmically – a view that still has a wide following within the disciplines of artifical intelligence, cognitive psychology, and psychiatry.

The brain certainly does process symbols, as they are essential elements of language. However, the question is whether symbols are basic elements of cognition or whether they emerge from more basic pattern-processing activity (Smolensky, 1989). Whereas the propositional structure of natural language has often been construed as evidence for the symbol-processing view, accumulated evidence from linguistics and neuroscience portrays language as a window to more fundamental mental processes (Pinker, 1994).

The pattern-processing view has been given its most definitive formulation by Stephen Grossberg (1982) in studies extending over several decades. He has elevated the subject to the status of a genuine scientific theory, with a rich network of robust general principles incorporated in mathematical models with testable empirical consequences. A qualitative formulation of Grossberg's ideas will suffice for the purposes of this chapter. However, it should be understood that these ideas are interrelated by (often sophisticated) mathematical arguments that lose much of their logical force when described qualitatively.

Some of Grossberg's insights have been arrived at independently by others and are fairly commonplace in neuroscience and connectionist theories of information processing. Connectionist theories are often said to be 'neurally inspired' because processing is distributed over networks analogous to real neural networks, and they employ a Hebbian learning law that may describe essential features of synaptic processes believed to be the mechanisms for long-term memory in real brains. The term 'connectionist' is often used as a disclaimer of any responsibility to model real neural networks accurately. Grossberg never makes this blanket disclaimer when he tries to model real brain function. However, like any good theoretician, he is careful to delineate the limitations and problematic features of his models.

Neuroscience has supplied mounting evidence in support of the pattern-processing principles and mechanisms described below. It should be understood, however, that these ideas were not extracted from empirical knowledge about real neural networks and so do not find their primary justification there. Instead, Grossberg derived them from a deep study of behavioral psychology (Grossberg, 1982). This is why they are so robust, which is to say that they have not been invalidated by the accumulating data of neuroscience, and they supply a secure framework for more detailed models to account for new data.

Our task now is to elaborate the cardinal principles, flesh them out with empirical results from neuroscience, and examine their implications. To bring the most important ideas to the fore, many details and subtleties of neural modeling will be ignored, but they can be incorporated by consulting the references.

Each module of the brain is, like a retina, a layered structure that can be modeled as a two-dimensional slab of identical computational units called nodes. Each node represents a neuronal population supporting a single output neuron. For example, the nodes of a cortical module may represent cortical minicolumns attached to a single pyramid cell. The internal state of a node is described by a single variable called its activity, which can be interpreted as the electrical generating potential of the output neuron. The activity has a limited dynamic range set by the minimum potential of the output neuron and the maximum potential at the firing threshold when the neuron discharges.

As depicted in Figure 6.1, the internal state of a module with n nodes is an *activity pattern* $x = \{x_1, x_2, \ldots x_n\}$, where x_i is the activity of the ith node. Two different levels of pattern activation can be distinguished. First, there is a subliminal pattern, for which the activation of each node is below its firing threshold; psychologically, this can be interpreted as a preparatory set or priming in both sensory and motor modules. Second, there is an output pattern, when the nodes are activated above firing threshold; the information in such a pattern is transmitted to other modules.

Nodes are connected by axons interacting with other nodes through synaptic connections which, according to biological evidence, can be

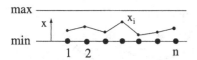

Fig. 6.1 Activity pattern in a module. For simplicity, the nodes are depicted as a string instead of a two-dimensional array, and their minimum/maximum activities are assumed to be identical.

either excitatory or inhibitory. The signal transmitted along an axon reflects the internal state of the generating node and, accordingly, has a numerical value (representing the firing frequency of the output neuron).

The pattern-processing capabilities of a module are determined by the structure of its nodal interactions. The following is a review of the structures necessary for some of the most important processing capabilities.

Pattern registration and storage

Since a neuron has a limited dynamic range, its sensitivity is limited by noise at low activity and saturation at high activity. How then can neurons maintain the sensitivity to wide variations in input intensities necessary for accurate pattern registration? Grossberg calls this the noise-saturation dilemma and has noted that it is a universal problem that must be solved by every biological system. He has proved under very general assumptions that for accurate pattern registration a module must be a cooperative–competitive network of particular type.

Interactions among nodes in the same module are called lateral interactions. Nodes linked by excitatory interactions are said to be cooperative because the interactions mutually enhance the activities of the nodes. Similarly, nodes linked by inhibitory interactions are said to be competitive. As illustrated in Figure 6.2, for stable pattern registration the excitatory interactions must be short range (on-center) while the inhibitory interactions are long range (off-surround). That explains why the on-centre/off-surround network structure is so common in real biological modules from the retina to cortex.

Cooperative–competitive networks have some remarkable information-processing capabilities. It is well known, from both empirical and theoretical studies, that they can enhance contrasts in input patterns. They also provide a means of implementing a competitive selection principle which works as follows. Simultaneous inputs from different sources

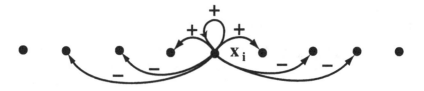

Fig. 6.2 Lateral interactions for one node in an on-center/off-surround network with short-term memory.

compete through lateral interactions to determine the activity pattern on a module; the resulting pattern eliminates any ambiguities or inconsistencies among the inputs. When 'sharply tuned,' the competition is so strong that only a few nodes can survive as winners. As described later, this is a fundamental mechanism for neural code compression.

To maintain activity patterns for periods of the order of seconds in biological systems, the structure of a module must be recurrent, i.e. the nodes must have excitatory self-interaction (feedback), as indicated in Figure 6.2. This type of pattern storage is called short-term memory (STM) by Grossberg, though it is not precisely equivalent to the usual definition of STM in cognitive psychology.

Associative learning recall

The most plausible biological mechanism for long-term memory (LTM) storage in the brain is alteration of transmissibility at modifiable synapses which *gate* signals from one neuron to another. In the simplest model of this mechanism, the transmissibility is represented by a numerical factor, called the synaptic weight, which alters the presynaptic signal multiplicatively to produce the postsynaptic input. Modification of the synaptic weight is governed by *Hebb's law*, which asserts that it increases when the two interacting neurons fire simultaneously. In psychological terms, this means the association strength between activities of the two neurons is increased. Variants of Hebb's law allow the synaptic weights to decrease as well.

Since the information to be stored in LTM is represented in activity patterns distributed across many nodes in a module, it cannot be stored in a single synapse. Another mechanism is required and, as depicted in Figure 6.3, that is supplied by the treelike structure of the output axon from a node. An essential property of this structure is that the *same* signal is transmitted simultaneously along all branches of the tree. This makes it possible, under appropriate conditions, to store (learn) an activity pattern in modifiable synapses of the tree. This minimal network for associative learning of a spatial pattern is called an outstar by Grossberg.

An outstar works like this: suppose that, as depicted in Figure 6.3, an input pattern $(I_1, I_2, \ldots I_n)$ is registered as an activity pattern in the module M_1. At the same time a signal I_0 activates a node in module M_2 which broadcasts a 'sampling signal' S_i to the nodes in M_1. This drives a change in the synaptic weights w_{ij} until they are proportional to the I_j. As only relative values of the variables have information content, this constitutes

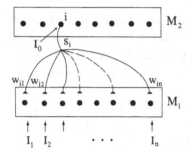

Fig. 6.3 Outstar connectivity enables a node in one module (M_2) to store and replay an activity pattern in another module (M_1). Every node in M_2 has outstar connectivity with M_1, but only one is shown. Each node in M_2 is therefore able to learn a different pattern on M_1. Only the simplest model is considered, in which a single node is activated to learn each pattern.

storage of the input pattern in the pattern of weights. The stored pattern can be regarded as a template or prototype of what the outstar has 'learned from experience.'

The outstar has truly learned the activity pattern on M_1 in the sense that it can *recall* it exactly, as follows. Suppose that, at some time after learning, the initial input to M_1 has vanished but the input I_0 reappears to activate a signal S_i from the outstar to read out, across the nodes of M_1, a subliminal pattern proportional to the synaptic weights. When the signal is strong enough to drive the nodes of M_1 above threshold, it is called a performance signal.

The outstar is a universal learning device for every kind of learning in the brain. Kinds of learning are distinguished by the different interpretations given to modules in which the outstar appears and how the modules fit into the central nervous system (CNS) as a whole. The following are three important examples.

1. *Top-down expectancy learning.* Suppose that nodes of module M_1 in Figure 6.3 represent sensory feature detectors in cerebral cortex. A visual (or auditory) event is encoded as an activity pattern across the module, with the activity x_i of the ith node representing the relative importance of the ith feature. The outstar node in M_2 can learn this pattern, and when the LTM pattern is played back on M_1, it represents a prior expectancy of a sensory event.

2. *Motor learning and control.* Suppose that the nodes of module M_1 in Figure 6.3 represent motor control cells, so that each node excites a particular muscle group and its activity determines the rate of con-

traction. Then the outstar command node can learn to control the synchronous performance of a particular motion with rate modulated by the strength of the performance signal.

3. *Temporal order encoded as spatial order.* If the nodes of module M_1 in Figure 6.3 represent items on a list (such as a phone number) and their activities represent the temporal order of the items, then the outstar can learn the temporal order.

Pattern recognition, classification, and code protection

Although the outstar can learn to recall a given pattern, it cannot recognize the pattern. Pattern recognition requires a different network configuration, called the instar by Grossberg. As illustrated in Figure 6.4, the instar consists of axonal projections from 'feature nodes' in M_1 with 'synaptic gates' at a single 'category node' in M_2. According to Hebb's law, when the category node is active the instar synaptic weights from active feature nodes increase in proportion to the node activities. In this way the node is sensitized to the features in the pattern.

To recognize a pattern is to distinguish it from alternatives. When a pattern appears on M_1 initially, it activates many nodes on M_2 through instar connections. Now suppose that M_2 is a competitive–cooperative network so sharply tuned that only the most strongly activated node survives the competition (winner-take-all). The winning node then becomes more strongly associated with the pattern. All patterns that select the same node by this competetive mechanism form a category –

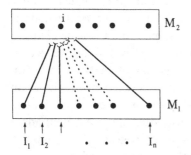

Fig. 6.4 Instar connectivity enables a node in M_2 to recognize a pattern in M_1. Every node in M_2 has instar connectivity with M_1, but only one is shown. Each node is able to recognize a different class of patterns on M_1, namely, those patterns that activate it more strongly than other nodes. The node responding to a given pattern is selected by competition through lateral interactions in M_2.

justifying the term 'category node.' The category could represent an object characterized by a set of its features.

Each node in M_2 can be sensitized to a different category of patterns. hence the two-module network in Figure 6.4 serves as a pattern classifier. It is, in fact, an adaptive pattern classifier because each category is defined by the instar synaptic weights that are tuned to the patterns it has 'experienced' (say, through sensory inputs to M_1).

The adaptive classifier is a general purpose device. It can be 'trained' to classify an arbitrary set of patterns by repeatedly activating samples of those patterns on M_1. In other words, it can learn to 'classify patterns presented by experience.' However, the number of patterns it can 'distinguish' is limited by the number of category nodes in M_2, and when this limit is approached the system begins massive recoding, which destroys categories it has already learned. This raises a profound issue of neural network design that Grossberg calls the stability–plasticity dilemma: how can a pattern classifier be plastic enough to learn from experience but stable enough to retain what it has learned?

Grossberg (1982) has shown that the stability–plasticity dilemma can be solved for an 'instar classifier' (See Fig. 6.4) by introducing 'outstar feedback' (see Fig. 6.3) from every category node. To grasp the crux of his solution, suppose that the nodes of M_1 are visual feature detectors. After filtering through the visual system, external sensory input from the retina is registered in M_1 as a 'bottom-up' input pattern. At the same time, a node in M_2 may be activated internally to read out its outstar template into M_1. This template can be interpreted as a 'top-down' expectation – the pattern that the module M_2 'expects to see.' This expectation is superimposed on the sensory input pattern in M_1. If the match between them is sufficiently close, then the instar signal to the active node is amplified and fed back by the outstar to amplify the template. Thus, a feedback loop of sustained resonant activity is set up, and it drives recoding of both instar and outstar in the direction of the input pattern. Grossberg calls this state of resonant activity between two modules an adaptive resonance. Of course, the visual system involves more than two modules, so an act of visual recognition would involve a coherent adaptive resonance among all modules of the system. Even so, the two-module system exhibits the essential features of the resonance mechanism.

Adaptive resonance holds great promise as a key to understanding the mind as a function of the brain. Grossberg himself suggests that it is 'the functional unit of perception and cognition,' and 'only the resonant state enters consciousness.' Sure enough, even the simplified model of the resonant process described above does much more than recognition. In accord with the deepest insight of Gestalt psychology, the resonant state has the hallmark of a percept: it is a *fusion* of 'bottom-up' sensory input with a 'top-down' expectation. More than that, it is a fusion of recognition and recall that adaptively recodes the template during every perceptual act. Since the sensory input is never quite the same for different 'sightings' of the same object or object category, the template will learn an average of the sensory patterns from different sightings. Moreover, features that are most frequently present on different sightings will be most strongly represented in the synaptic weights of the template, so the template tends to become a kind of cartoon emphasizing the most prominent features. It is not too far-fetched to suggest that this mechanism underlies the extraordinary human ability to identify people from simple cartoons.

In this mathematical formulation, the adaptive resonance idea is so rich in variations and implications that it has become a subject in its own right, which Grossberg calls Adaptive Resonance Theory (ART). The theory will continue to develop by incorporating empirical results from neuroscience into increasingly realistic models. Unfortunately, there seems to be no experimental means for verifying the existence of adaptive resonances in vivo at the present time. However, there are many possibilities for indirect tests of the theory. For example, ART provides the most coherent theoretical framework available for explaining empirical data on event-related potentials, and research in this direction has made significant progress (Banquet, Smith and Guenther, 1992). This greatly enriches the possibilities for using evoked potentials in psychiatric research and evaluation. In the absence of definitive empirical tests, the strongest evidence for ART is the theoretical coherence it gives to brain science. There seems to be no alternative to ART with such potential for explaining the mechanisms underlying perception and cognition.

ART has equal potential for explaining disorders of perception and cognition. Before considering this in the next section, the theory needs to be elaborated more fully. Adaptive resonances process only expected events. An unexpected event is characterized by a mismatch between template and external input. In that case, the node of the mismatched template must be shut off immediately to avoid inappropriate coding (code protection). Then the other nodes can compete to determine the one whose instar activation most strongly matches its outstar template (competitive search). To accomplish this, several new network mechanisms are needed. First, there must be a means for comparing 'top-down' and 'bottom-up' inputs at M_1. This can be achieved by introducing extra processing layers or interneurons in M_1. Second, there must be a rapid on–off switch at each node. This can be achieved neurally by opponent processing, which may explain why opponent cells are so common in the brain. Finally, there must be a special type of signal to shut off *all* the active nodes in the 'category module' M_2 when a mismatch has been detected in M_1. This is one of several mechanisms needed to control activity in a module, to which we now turn.

Gain control functions and malfunctions

Psychotic symptoms, such as hallucinations and delusions, appear in the conscious processes of perception and cognition. The association of these processes with mechanisms of adaptive resonance suggests that we look there for an explanation of psychotic symptoms in terms of malfunctions in pattern-processing control. Control variables are necessary for flexibility in a module's response to different, sometimes conflicting, processing requirements. For the most part they can be regarded as gain control variables, because they modulate the gain on various signals. Gain control is ubiquitous throughout the nervous system (Prochazka, 1989), but its role in conscious processing at the cortical level has not been systematically addressed before now.

As indicated schematically in Figure 6.5, gain control variables can be classified broadly into two types: controls on (1) internal processing, and on (2) external information flow. Now we can provide plausible explanations for major psychotic symptoms as breakdowns in the control of specific pattern-processing capabilities identified in the preceding section.

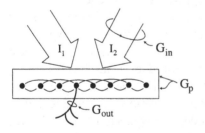

Fig. 6.5 Attentional control variables G_{in} and G_{out} regulate the gains of inputs and outputs. Processing within the module is regulated by a processing control variable G_P, of which there may be several kinds.

Thought disorder

The thought disorder that often appears in acute mania can be understood as a breakdown in the control of competitive pattern selection, with particular symptoms depending on the module(s) in which the breakdown occurs. Thus, instabilities in the selection of plans for speech output (encoded in activity patterns) can produce frequent, sudden switches in subject, even in midsentence. Moreover, when the influence of intended meaning on the selection of words and phrases is weakened, the selection will fall under the control of over-learned and low-level coding, resulting in punning, rhyming and stereotyped associations. Alternatively, perceptual confusion will result from inability to decide among multiple interpretations of sensory stimuli.

A typical module has a multitude of incompatible input patterns from other modules that compete for control of the module output. Regulation of the competition is essential to meet varying processing needs. One way to do this is by gain control of lateral interactions within the module. High gain biases the competition in favor of the presently active output pattern and so reduces the possibility of pattern switching. This is one mechanism for selective attention. On the other hand, low gain greatly increases the tendency for pattern switching activated by subliminal patterns. Therefore, the search of associative memory for new possibilities can be enhanced by lowering the gain. When the gain is too low, however, switching is excessive and stability of pattern formation is lost, resulting in thought disorder.

Thought disorder also occurs in schizophrenia, but with different characteristics from those just described for mania. Hoffman (1987) and Shenton, Solovay and Holzman (1987) review the literature on 'manic-like' and 'schizophrenic-like' thought disorders derived from analysis of psychotic speech. The primary difference is that manics exhibit the ability to organize a coherent discourse plan to express a single message or gestalt, though its execution is disrupted by unregulated switches, as described above; whereas, schizophenic discourse plans are incoherent patchworks of disparate gestalts that are comparatively stable (without the frequent switching apparent in manic discourse). Manic speech also tends to be extravagant, loosely structured and often inappropriately flippant, unlike schizophrenic speech.

Hoffman employs a simple Hopfield network to simulate disordered thought and so explain it by a network mechanism. His network is able to simulate the sudden switches characteristic of manic-like disorder, but his mechanism for producing switches is quite different from the breakdown of competitive pattern selection described above, and it is much too simple to explain the extravagance and playfulness in manic speech or the response to drug treatment, described below.

Hallucinations

We have seen that perception involves a superposition (or fusion) of 'bottom-up' sensory inputs with 'top-down' expectations. Separate control of the gains on these two inputs confers powerful processing capabilities, including cognitive abilities such as spatial visualization. There is now substantial evidence that visual mental imagery involves activation of the same modules activated in visual perception, with the major difference that primary visual cortex is coactivated only in the latter case (Farah, 1989). Evoked mental images can serve as 'expectations' priming primary visual cortex for the detection of objects. Evidently, if the top-down gain is too strong and is not shut off by the matching process, it can produce percepts of objects not presented in the sensory input. This is a plausible explanation for visual hallucinations. During dreaming, sensory input is shut off and perception is dominated by internally generated expectations, though it has often been noted that some sensory inputs, such as sounds, are automatically integrated into the dream.

The explanation for auditory hallucinations is somewhat different, as is to be expected because they commonly occur in schizophrenia without visual hallucinations, whereas the opposite is common in manic–depressive illness. Frith (1992) argues for a common mechanism underlying auditory hallucinations and delusions. A gain control version of that mechanism is considered next.

Reality check

ART tells us that, in some modules, input from two different brain loci must be compared for consistency. This pattern-matching process can be interpreted broadly as a reality check, but its specific psychological interpretation will depend on the module. For example, in a sensory module a top-down expectation may be compared with a bottom-up sensory input, or in a motor module an intended plan of action may be compared with an executed plan. In every case, theory suggests that gain control is needed to regulate the degree of mismatch allowed.

A number of mental disorders appear to be explicable as consequences of reality check failure due to a malfunction of matching gain control. According to ART, competitive pattern selection in one module (M_2 in Figs. 6.3 and 6.4) is governed by a reality check in another module (M_1). From the viewpoint of network theory, obsessive–compulsive disorder (OCD) is evidently a malfunction of the competitive pattern-selection mechanism, with inappropriate patterns repeatedly winning the competition for expression as thoughts and/or behaviors. This could be realized, for example, in a network where the nodes in M_2 activate behavioral plans or intentions while the activity patterns of 'context nodes' in M_1' encode contextual conditions for the release of those plans. Failure of matching gain control in this case would allow activation of behavior unrelated to context. Alternatively, reality check could fail because certain context nodes are preferentially activated and overwhelm the contribution from other contextual factors. The result is perseveration in the choice of behavioral plans dominated by a single contextual factor. This kind of failure in plan selection can arise from malfunction in the biasing of the context nodes. Such biasing is needed to adjust sensitivity to various contextual factors. This issue is addressed in the next section.

The gain control malfunction just described can account for obsessive activation of certain thoughts or the compulsive activation of certain behaviors, depending on the module in which it occurs. The fact that 'behavior unrelated to context' and perseveration are also important features of psychotic disorders suggests that this malfunction occurs in mania and schizophrenia as well as in OCD. Reality check failures in other modules may well account for other mental disorders.

In a cogent analysis, Frith (1992) argues that all positive symptoms of schizophrenia, such as delusions and auditory hallucinations, can be explained as a breakdown in self-monitoring of thoughts and behavior. He notes that self-monitoring in the sensorimotor system is necessary to distinguish perceptual changes due to body movement from those due to external causes. Mechanisms for doing that have been most thoroughly studied, both experimentally and theoretically, in the case of eye–head movements. In that case, an intended movement is encoded in a corollary discharge and compared 'downstream' with sensory input on the actual movement. A detailed network model of all this which does justice to empirical data has been worked out by Grossberg and Kuperstein (1989). Though Frith is unaware of this theoretical work, he notes that empirical evidence indicates that voluntary eye movement is initiated in the frontal eye fields (within frontal cortex) along with a corollary discharge. Frith speculates that every willed (voluntary) movement is initiated in frontal cortex along with a corollary discharge, and, further, that 'positive symptoms (of schizophrenia) occur because the brain structures for willed actions send corollary discharges to the posterior parts of the brain concerned with perception ... In consequence, self-generated changes in perception are misinterpreted as having an external cause.' Thus, for example, subvocal speech may be misperceived as having an external source – an auditory hallucination. Obviously, comparison of an intended movement (corollary discharge) with sensory input is a kind of reality check on available information before the construction of a conscious percept. Failure of the reality check may be due to structural damage to the necessary connections or, as has been noted, to gain control malfunction.

Disorders of attention and short-term memory

The cardinal principles enable us to extend the concepts of attention and attentional control to the information processed by an individual module. Gain controls on input and output channels can be regarded as attentional controls because they bias the module's response to information from those channels. The relative gain in a channel is therefore a measure of attention allocated to information from that channel. Of course, this 'network concept of attention' should not be confused with any of the various 'psychological concepts of attention.' The network concept certainly has implications for attentional behavior, and it may well provide the ultimate foundation for grounding psychological concepts of attention in neuropsychology. At the same time, the network concept is much broader, for it embraces biases on internal signals in such psychological tasks as discrimination. It has the potential, therefore, of demonstrating deep similarities among such different behaviors as attention and discrimination.

To make fine discriminations among different inputs to a module, there must be separate gain control for each channel or even for the input to each node of the module. Let us refer to the cell populations that produce such gain control signals as bias nodes. Bias nodes lie outside the module, but each one projects to a specific target within the module. This determines a (more-or-less) topographic mapping between the locus of bias nodes and the module – an important anatomical clue to identifying bias nodes in the brain, as shall be seen later. As noted in the preceding section, malfunctions of input gain control may lead to such mental disorders as OCD.

In contrast to the topographically specific structure of input gain control, output gain control is nonspecific – which is to say that the same gain control signal is sent to all nodes of the module. This type of gain control can serve at least two important functions:

1. Selective attention to the current state. Increased output gain strengthens the competitive advantage of active nodes over inactive nodes. This enhances the currently active pattern, momentarily stabilizing it against erosion by new inputs that upset the competitive balance.
2. Learning of complex associations among activities in many different modules can be controlled by a nonspecific signal that enhances and stabilizes their currently active patterns simultaneously, thereby driving transfer of associations between them into LTM by Hebbian learning.

From this, we may expect that malfunctions of output gain control will produce deficits in attending to significant stimuli and learning complex associations.

Central brain state control

Our objective now is to make plausible identifications of the several gain control variables described in the last section with known neurotransmitter systems in the brain. This will help us identify the loci of specific brain malfunctions that may be responsible for mental disorders attributed to gain control failures. Moreover, additional information about neural circuitry supports a more elaborate analysis of brain mechanisms implicated in mental disorders.

For many years anatomical, physiological and behavioral research (which cannot be reviewed here) has been converging toward the conclusion that cortical activity is modulated by inputs from at least four nuclei: the locus coeruleus in the brainstem, the raphé dorsalis and ventral tegmentum in the midbrain, and the nucleus basalis in the basal forebrain. As shown schematically in Figure 6.6, each of these nuclei has extensive projections to the cerebral cortex, although differences in the structure of these projections are major clues about their functions. The projections can be described as 'chemically coded' because each of them transmits at its synapses a different neuromodulator: noradrenalin from the locus

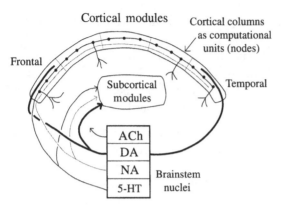

Fig. 6.6 Central brain state control system, output component. Activity in cortical modules is regulated by inputs from four subcortical nuclei with extensive chemically coded projections to cortex (see text). ACh, acetycholine; DA, dopamine; NA, noradrenalin; 5-HT, 5-hydroxytryptamine.

coeruleus, serotonin or 5-hydroxytryptamine (5-HT) from the raphé dorsalis, dopamine from the ventral tegmentum, acetylcholine (ACh) from the nucleus basalis. The term 'neuromodulator' has been used here to differentiate their modulatory functions from the functions of other neurotransmitters, such as glutamate and GABA, which are directly engaged in pattern processing and information transfer. For the latter functions, synaptic transmission must be *fast* (of the order of milliseconds), whereas for modulatory functions transmission is comparatively *slow* (on the order of 100 ms to minutes). Actually, ACh transmission can be either fast (for nicotinic receptors) or slow (for muscarinic receptors).

Besides transmission speed, another clue to the identification of some transmitters as modulators is the circuitry and topography of projections. Diffuse projections, for example, are inherently unable to transmit structured information, so they are strong indicators of modulatory function. Unfortunately, many published neural circuits fail to make the essential distinction between connections that are modulatory and those that transmit information. They fail to note that the very different information-processing functions of these two kinds of connections are reflected in very different topologies of circuit loops involving them (Percheron et al., 1989).

Owing to uncertainties about local circuitry and neural interactions, fully satisfactory explanations of neuromodulator actions are not available. However, we can evaluate functional descriptions of neuromodulation from indirect evidence, and this should eventually be helpful in making sense of local circuitry. It is suggested here that the four kinds of neuro-modulators are gain control variables with the functions already examined.

Vigilance control

To ascertain the functions of the four-tract control system schematized in Figure 6.6, an enormous number of pharmacological and lesion experi-ments have beeen performed on animals. The results have been confus-ing, more or less implicating each of the variables in nearly every aspect of learning and behavior. Koella (1982, 1984) argues that the four tracts are output components of a vigilance control network that regulates all behavioral states from alert wakefulness to paradoxical sleep. Other com-ponents of the network have been difficult to identify because they are not localized in a well-defined region of the brain.

In behavioral terms, the vigilance of an animal is a state of readiness to respond to particular stimuli. Koella has noted that the behavioral con-cept can be reduced to a more precise concept of network vigilance. We can define this concept more precisely still as network gain control, which has already been differentiated into several types. We have seen, though, that the various gain control functions embrace much more than is sug-gested by the term vigilance.

The term vigilance applies best to the function of the locus coeruleus/noradrenalin tract, though the term arousal is more widely used in the literature. However, empirical evidence supports the stronger claim that the locus coeruleus/noradrenalin tract modulates ouput gain of the entire neocortex. Relevant facts include: (1) the tract projects nonspecifically to all cortical modules; (2) the tract enhances cortical outputs in response to novel or stressful stimuli; and (3) lesions of the tract in animals impair their ability to learn complex tasks. This supports the conclusion that *through the locus coeruleus tract, noradrenalin modulates selective atten-tion and distributed associative memory in the neocortex.*

This conclusion helps explain the facts about Korsakoff's disease, for which there is anatomical evidence of damage to the noradrenalin system, typically preceded by alcohol abuse. Korsakoff patients can learn simple tasks but performance of complex tasks, such as discrimintion learning, is dramatically impaired; they have anteriograde amnesia back to (but not before) the onset of the disease; they have a variety of perceptual deficits consistent with impaired attention, including longer discrimination times and smaller orienting responses that habituate less quickly. Overall, Korsakoff patients have a limited ability to compare and integrate successive stimulus items.

The information-processing functions of selective attention and memory consolidation attributed to locus coeruleus/noradrenalin activity certainly do not exhaust the functions of noradrenalin in the brain. Disorders of noradrenalin activity are implicated in major depressive illness, but they most likely occur in the subcortical ventral noradrenalin bundle, which projects heavily to the hypothalamus, the major organ for internal body state regulation.

Behavior control and bipolar disorder

Cortical projections of the four nuclei in Figure 6.6 are especially relevant to psychiatry because they are most likely to be directly involved in the regulation of conscious processes and therefore of psychotic symptoms. It has already been noted that explanations for some psychotic symptoms and mental deficits can be achieved by identifying the cortical actions of the four tracts with particular kinds of gain control. The tracts also have subcortical projections regulating subconscious processing in modules that may be primary loci for some mental disorders. Indeed, the projection of a single nucleus to both cortical and noncortical targets is a strong clue that activity of the targets is coordinated by inputs from the nucleus. This is especially clear in the case of dopamine projections from the ventral tegmentum and the substantia nigra shown in Figure 6.7. Dopamine is clearly involved in the regulation of motor output. For that reason, Koella refers to dopamine as motor vigilance.

Figure 6.7 shows four nuclei that modulate the flow of information through two major pathways in the brain, named here as the Plan Selection Pathway and the Plan Execution Pathway. The first pathway is concerned with the organization and selection of behavioral plans. The latter is concerned with motivational and volitional control over plan selection. The pathways converge at the pallidum, the motor output module of the basal ganglia.

Without reviewing supporting empirical evidence (Hestenes, 1992), we can now describe how the primary symptom of *manic–depressive illness can be explained as a breakdown of gain control in the nucleus accumbens*, which functions as a gate through which the limbic system influences behavioral output. Dopamine input from the ventral tegmentum facilitates passage of limbic signals through the nucleus accumbens. In other

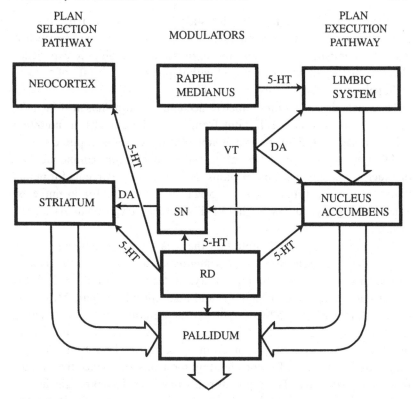

Fig. 6.7 Behavior control system schematic, showing principal components and connections. The system has two major pathways, one for the organization and selection of behavioral plans, the other for motivational/volitional control over plan execution. Activity in both pathways is modulated by dense, distributed dopamine (DA) and 5-hydroxytryptamine (5-HT) inputs. Many details including all feedback loops, have been omitted. VT, ventral tegmentum; SN, substantia nigra; RD, raphé dorsalis. (Adapted from Hestenes, 1992.)

words, dopamine input is a gain control variable that opens and closes the gate.

This nucleus accumbens gating model explains enhanced motor activity induced by amphetamines and other dopamine agonists as due to increased dopamine gain in the nucleus accumbens, which facilitates the execution of 'impulses' or 'urges' generated by the limbic system. Likewise, the pressured speech and impulsive behavior characteristic of mania are attributed to excess dopamine gain.

On the other hand, when dopamine gain in the nucleus accumbens is too low, an individual has difficulty initiating motivated behaviors and expressing interest or emotion. This state of depressed activity (or psychomotor retardation) is sometimes labeled as 'anhedonic,' because it may be accompanied by a subjective impression of inability to experience pleasure. It should not be confused with depression as a state of sadness or hopelessness, which must have a different origin.

Thus far, this discussion of nucleus accumbens gating has neglected the powerful influence of 5-HT input from the raphé dorsalis in inhibiting behavior. By a mechanism that is not well understood, raphé dorsalis/5-HT input opposes the action of ventral tegmentum/dopamine input to the nucleus accumbens. This explains the success of treatments for mania that increase the transmission of 5-HT in the brain, for example by administering high doses of the 5-HT precursor tryptophan (Hestenes, 1992).

Returning to Figure 6.7, note that the striatum is positioned to play a gating role in the selection pathway analogous to the role of the nucleus accumbens in the execution pathway. Indeed, the striatum and the nucleus accumbens are contiguous and anatomically similar. Moreover, the substantia nigra modulates gain in the striatum, just as the ventral tegmentum modulates gain in the nucleus accumbens, although the symmetry is broken by a projection from the latter to the substantia nigra that provides a means for coordinating the gains and hence the outputs from both pathways. The raphé dorsalis regulates flow through the two pathways in two ways: indirectly through its projections to the ventral tegmentum and the substantia nigra, and directly through its projections to the nucleus accumbens and striatum. One likely mode of behavior control is this: the locus coerulens signals the presence of stressful stimuli to cortex and inhibits the raphé dorsalis, which in turn disinhibits that nucleus accumbens and substantia nigra in preparation for vigorous behavioral response.

The anatomical contiguity and similarity of the nucleus accumbens and striatum suggest that they employ common physiological mechanisms, so they should have comparable malfunctions and responses to drugs. Indeed, low dopamine gain in the striatum produces Parkinsonian symptoms comparable to the anhedonia due to low dopamine gain in the nucleus accumbens. Moreover, the excess dopamine/nucleus accumbens gain in mania corresponds to excess striatal gain (or malfunction with equivalent effect) in Huntington's disease and Tourette's syndrome. In Tourette's syndrome the excess gain (or network defect) is probably localized in the striatum, where it can produce the spontaneous release of some stereotyped action.

Since the raphé dorsalis has 'the last word,' so to speak, in governing the release of behavioral plans, it may be that its malfunction is a common cause of bipolar disorder. The fact that mania is often accompanied by psychotic symptoms such as paranoia, thought disorder and, less frequently, hallucinations suggests that gain disregulation is not necessarily confined to the nucleus accumbens, but can spread to other modules sharing a common gain control nucleus. There are only two candidates to consider: the ventral tegmentum and the raphé dorsalis. Now, neuroleptics that reduce dopamine transmission are effective in bringing manic behavior rapidly under control; however, they do not concurrently eliminate psychotic symptoms, which typically take a considerably longer period to dissipate. This implicates raphé dorsalis gain malfunction as the cause of psychotic symptoms accompanying mania. It also suggests that mania without psychotic symptoms is due to ventral tegmentum gain malfunction.

More support for the view that 5-HT rather than dopamine is responsible for psychotic symptoms in mania comes from the literature on psychomimetic effects of drugs. The drugs inducing psychological states most similar to clinical psychosis are LSD and amphetamine, the principal representatives of two families of drugs with such effects. With sufficient doses, both drugs can produce delusions and hallucinations within a setting of clear consciousness, that is, without the thought disorder and disorientation that accompany the psychomimetic effects of other drugs, although thought disorder can be induced by higher doses. The mechanism of LSD action is believed to be a reduction of raphé dorsalis/5-HT transmission. On the other hand, the euphoric effects of amphetamine (speed) are attributed to increased dopamine transmission. With increasing doses, amphetamine induces stages similar to hypomania, mania and, ultimately in some people, paranoid psychosis. For this reason, it has been supposed that psychosis involves dopamine malfunction. One problem with this conclusion is the fact that neuroleptics, which are known to reduce dopamine activity, suppress but do not eliminate psychotic symptoms. Another is the fact that the onset of amphetamine psychosis occurs much later than the reduction in dopamine transmission. All this can be explained by the fact that amphetamine also reduces 5-HT activity. Though this effect is smaller than the dopamine reduction, it is cumulative with each dose, and the net reduction is between 40 and 70 percent over ten days. Furthermore, the onset and offset of behavioral effects (model psychosis) in cats correlate perfectly with large changes in 5-HT transmission. To this is added the fact that raphé dorsalis/5-HT transmission is turned off in REM sleep, when dreaming occurs. We conclude, therefore, that *reduced cortical 5-HT activity is the major factor, and possibly a sufficient factor in all model psychoses*, including dreaming. Surely it must be a major factor in clinical psychoses, though that remains to be demonstrated.

The problem remains to identify mechanisms that can explain the role of 5-HT in psychoses. Comparison with our previous gain control explanations for hallucinations and delusions suggests that *raphé dorsalis/5-HT regulates gain on top-down inputs and pattern matching in cortical modules.*

Executive control

Prefrontal cortex (less precisely, frontal cortex or frontal lobes) is sometimes described as 'the executive of the brain.' In this capacity it is believed to evaluate information about the state of the body and the environment and apply it to the selection and pursuit of goals. In brief, frontal cortex organizes and controls goal-directed behavior.

Frontal cortex is the 'Chief Executive Officer' for the behavioral control system (BCS) schematized in Figure 6.7. Our knowledge about the interaction of frontal cortex with the (rest of the) BCS is very patchy, but it does supply significant clues and constraints on the theoretical possibilities that we consider. Feedback from the BCS to frontal cortex is not shown in Figure 6.7, but Figure 6.6 does indicate densely distributed ventral tegmentum/dopamine innervation, which most probably modulates inputs to frontal cortex. Evidently, the two BCS pathways in Figure 6.7 implement the two major components of goal-directed behavior. Thus, we surmise that the execution pathway determines and maintains a goal while the selection pathway organizes motor plans to reach the goal. Much can be learned about the role of frontal cortex in behavioral control by examining what happens when it is impaired.

Damage to frontal cortex produces at least three characteristic symptoms: distractibility, lack of foresight, and situationally inappropriate behavior. The same symptoms appear in mania and schizophrenia, so they suggest a malfunction in frontal cortex. Cohen and Servan-Schreiber (1992) argue that all three symptoms can be attributed to a single functional deficit: *a disturbance in the internal representation of context*. They observe that goal-oriented behavior requires the construction and maintenance of an internal representation of context. More specifically, such a representation is essential for selective attention, which they define as the influence of context on the selection of task-appropriate information for processing.

The previous discussion about the roles of the nucleus accumbens and striatum (Fig. 6.7) in behavioral control suggests now that they provide a representation of contextual constraints controlling behavior – an operational representation of context. Thus, the nucleus accumbens integrates inputs from the limbic system (about the internal state of the body) and from sensory systems (about its external state); this is combined in the striatum with inputs from prefrontal cortex (about its intended state). When the prefrontal contribution is cut off, the operational context is determined solely by immediate sensory stimuli and limbic 'urges.' The result is distractible behavior. To explain less immediate symptoms of frontal dysfunction, it is necessary to consider how contextual representations are formed and maintained.

Cohen and Servan-Schreiber construct connectionist models to describe maintenance and control of contextual information by the frontal lobes, and to explain some symptoms of schizophrenia as gain control failures in the models when dopamine is identified as the control variable. A theoretically richer mathematical model of frontal lobe function has been developed by Levine, Leven and Prueitt (1992). This model simulates both normal and impaired performance on the Wisconsin Card Sorting Task (WCST), which is often used clinically to evaluate frontal lobe damage. Dehaene and Changeux (1991) have constructed a more specialized connectionist model to simulate WCST performance.

The Levine model employs an extended ART model, so it is entirely in the spirit of our approach, and we can use it to extend and strengthen our theory of mental disorders. By minor reinterpretations of components in the Levine model, we can incorporate the insights of Cohen and Servan-Schreiber along with some of our own.

Consider an ART model with two components, M_2 and M_1 as in Figures 6.3 and 6.4. Levine refers to the nodes in M_2 as 'category nodes' and in M_1 as 'feature nodes.' Instead, we interpret the nodes in M_2 as motor intentions and those in M_1 as context nodes. The idea is that an activation pattern in M_1 represents context, and an adaptive resonance selects a motor intention in M_2 which, through another channel, sends an 'executive order' to the BCS. This suggests that M_2 be identified with prefrontal cortex while M_1 represents a collection of other cortical modules where suitable contextual information can be stored. At least some of these modules must be sensory modules where the adaptive resonance activates a preparatory set or expectation that biases their response toward 'contextually relevant' features in sensory input. In other words, *resonant feedback from frontal cortex supports selective attention in sensory modules.* We can guess that more abstract representations of context are maintained in submodules of M_1 located in temporal cortex, for example.

The Levine model does, in fact, divide M_1 into submodules processing different 'contextual features.' It extends ART by introducing bias nodes to control the input gain on signals from each M_1 submodule into M_2. This gives the system control over the relative weights in the contextual input representation to M_2. It is an example of attentional input gain control described earlier. Extending the model further by introducing a mechanism for adjusting the weights in response to outcomes of motor acts competitively selected in M_2, we have a system capable of modifying its behavioral plans in response to experience. Levine and coworkers show that such a model can successfully simulate the performance of normal people on the WCST – in particular, the ability of normals to switch behavioral plans (or 'contextual set') in response to outcomes of behavior. Moreover, they show how such a model can explain paradoxical effects of frontal damage, namely, perseveration in the choice of unsuccessful behaviors on the one hand, and attraction to novel stimuli on the other.

With the interpretation of M_2 as prefrontal cortex, there is also a natural interpretation for the bias nodes on the Levine model as components of the nucleus basalis. The nucleus basalis has the kind of detailed topographic mapping onto the prefrontal cortex that we have already seen is needed for local attentional control of inputs. It has been noted that ACh is the neurotransmitter for the nucleus basalis projections. It is also of interest that there are similar cholinergic projections to the rest of cortex from other subcortical nuclei. If we are correct in guessing that these projections exert local gain control on cortical inputs, then we expect them to have a major role in regulating cognitive function. This view is supported by evidence that the progressive deterioration of cognitive abilities in Alzheimer's disease is due to deterioration of the cortical cholinergic system.

There is evidence that bias node activity in frontal cortex is modulated in at least two ways. Tonic 5-HT transmission is a powerful suppressor of ACh activity throughout the cortex. This may explain why dreaming occurs during REM sleep – for raphé dorsalis/5-HT transmission is shut off at that time, and this is accompanied by a sudden release of massive cholinergic activity (Hobson, 1988). In frontal cortex, ACh activity is also strongly affected by ventral tegmentum/dopamine transmission (Robinson, 1984). There is some evidence that the ventral tegmentum projections have the topological specificity needed for local control of ACh activity. The suggestion here is that there are theoretical reasons, consistent with empirical evidence, to believe that *dopamine (and 5-HT) modulates ACh bias control of input to the frontal lobes from other cortical modules*. It may be some time before empirical evidence is sufficient to evaluate this suggestion conclusively. In the meantime, it will be worthwhile to explore other possible means for frontal cortex input gain control.

The essential point is that the Levine model provides plausible mechanisms for maintaining 'contextual set' (input bias in frontal cortex) and for revising that set in response to experience. It has already been noted that three major symptoms of mania and schizophrenia can be explained as failures in the maintenance of contextual set. The identification of dopamine and 5-HT as regulators of contextual set in frontal cortex helps to pinpoint an anatomical locus for the disorders and to explain the action of antipsychotic drugs. Evidence supporting a role for dopamine gain control failure in schizophrenia is discussed at some length by Cohen and Servan-Schreiber. It should be noted, though, that they do not consider a role for 5-HT gain control. Also, it is quite possible that the muting of schizophrenic symptoms by reducing dopamine transmission with neuroleptics is merely compensating for other defects, and is not necessarily indicative of a dopamine gain control malfunction in schizophrenia. The evidence that manic–depressive illness is essentially due to gain control malfunction is much stronger, in particular, because 'gain control' drug therapy is generally more effective (Hestenes, 1992).

This completes our adaptation of the Levine model of frontal lobe function to account for a wider range of data on mental illness and neurology. The model can be applied to organize and interpret an enormous body of data from psychiatry, psychology, and neuroscience that cannot be addressed here. For example, it can be applied to elaborate the analysis of schizophrenic language deficits by Cohen and Servan-Schreiber. No doubt the model will have to be modified and extended to account for new data – that is in the nature of the 'modeling game' (Hestenes, 1987). The model itself suggests where to look for significant change. Thus, it suggests that a cognitive component of contextual set is determined by biasing cortical modules with cholinergic input through some unknown mechanism, while this set is modulated by the monoamines to account for the immediate (external and internal) environment.

It is interesting to speculate that the cholinergic system controls the formation of contextual representations from 'cognitive habits' such as stereotypes and prejudices.

Though this description of the BCS is quite fragmentary, it is sufficient for making sense of an immense body of information in the literature. Of course, details of the two major BCS pathways (see Fig. 6.7) need to be filled in. This will clarify additional mechanisms in mental disorders. For example, evidence suggests that OCD is caused by defective communication of frontal cortex with the striatum, possibly due to a dysfunction of 5-HT modulation (Hestenes, 1992). Along another line, there is much to be said about the role of the limbic system in behavioral control. Thus, it seems likely that paranoid delusions may be explained by excessive weighting of contextual set by 'fear processing' in the limbic system, perhaps because of dopamine or 5-HT dysfunction. The dopamine inputs to frontal cortex might be a means for expressing that, though a different role for dopamine inputs has been suggested above.

It hardly matters that our model may be seriously deficient or even completely wrong on some details. The important point is that it provides a framework for asking significant theoretical and empirical questions – a framework for organizing what we know and guiding research.

Clinical implications

A theoretical framework has been presented to explain essential roles of modulatory mechanisms in central control of information processing by the brain. This has enabled us to identify (tentatively, at least) specific gain control functions for the neuromodulators dopamine, noradrenalin, 5-HT, and ACh, and to account for a variety of mental disorders as breakdowns of control by these variables. Thereby, we can explain the psychiatric effects of various drugs by their biochemical effects on gain control. The clinical implications are many, but let us concentrate on claims about manic–depressive illness suggested by the theory.

Our main claim about mania is that it is due to a breakdown of gain control on the release of behavioral plans in the nucleus accumbens. Sometimes this is accompanied by secondary symptoms, such as thought disorder, when the gain control breakdown spreads to other modules. Neuroleptics can eliminate mania by re-establishing dopamine gain control, but, as explained below, they do not directly influence some secondary symptoms. Thought disorder in schizophrenia is different from that in mania and is probably not due to a gain control malfunction, though it can be modulated by using neuroleptics to reduce dopamine gain. Thus, a schizophrenic's alien voices can be muted by neuroleptics but not eliminated altogether. The symptoms of mania can be eliminated completely with suitable drug treatment precisely because they originate from gain control dysfunction. Evidently, the same drugs are less effective with schizophrenia because they merely compensate for some other kind of dysfunction.

A second claim about mania is that there are at least two subtypes, one originating in dopamine dysfunction, the other in 5-HT dysfunction. They correspond to two different clinical syndromes, sometimes referred to as pure mania and mixed mania. Pure mania is characterized as elevated mood and extravagant behavior without depression, anger or other symptoms. This is the classic case of poorly regulated behavioral activation due to excessive dopamine gain. It can be brought under control by neuroleptics that reduce dopamine activity.

In mixed mania, the mania is accompanied by some combination of depression, anger, fear or delusions. Neuroleptics can control the mania, but they cannot eliminate the secondary symptoms that do not originate from dopamine dysfunction. The analysis in the body of this chapter suggests, instead, that the whole syndrome arises from 5-HT dysfunction. It has been seen how this may explain secondary symptoms depending on the brain modules involved. Moreover, reduction of 5-HT gain control in the nucleus accumbens may allow dopamine activity to increase unchecked and so produce mania. All this suggests that mixed mania is best treated with drugs that enhance 5-HT activity.

Some support for this analysis of mania comes from the careful and extensive research on mood disorders by van Praag. He has concluded that there is a subgroup (possibly as large as 40 percent) of depressives in which 5-HT functioning is demonstrably disturbed (van Praag et al., 1990). In this group, anxiety and/or aggression dysregulation are the primary psychopathological features, while mood lowering is secondary. Treatment with drugs that enhance 5-HT activity is indicated. Van Praag has systematically investigated treatment with the 5-HT precursors L-tryptophan and 5-hydroxytryptophan (5-HTP). He found that 5-HTP is much more effective than L-tryptophan for treating depression and has traced the difference to the fact that 5-HTP also enhances noradrenalin activity whereas L-tryptophan does not. This explains paradoxical results in the literature on the use of L-tryptophan as an antidepressant. Van Praag has confirmed his explanation by demonstrating effective treatment of depression by L-tryptophan in combination with the noradrenalin precursor tyrosine. This work provides strong evidence for a coupling of noradrenalin/5-HT neuromodulatory controls analogous to the dopamine/5-HT coupling noted earlier.

The treatment of depression and other disorders with the monoamine precursors L-tryptophan/tyrosine deserves to be more widely investigated, including combinations with other drugs. Since the amino acids L-tryptophan/tyrosine are basic ingredients of food, their use as drugs might be expected to be especially safe, though the biochemistry is complex (Sandyk, 1992; Hestenes, 1992). However, in the United States the unrestricted sale of L-tryptophan was banned by the Federal Drug Administration (FDA) in 1990 because L-tryptophan ingestion was implicated in an outbreak of the debilitating eosinophilia–myalgia syndrome. The ban is still in place, though the case has been traced to a contaminant or an alteration in batches of L-tryptophan produced by a single company (Slutsker et al, 1990). Considering the broad usefulness of L-tryptophan (Sandyk, 1992), there seems to be no justification for continuing the ban other than commercial advantage to drug companies.

The purported role of 5-HT in mixed mania suggests commonality with van Praag's group of '5-HT depressives.' According to our theory, 5-HT constrains dopamine activity in the nucleus accumbens, so release of that constraint will increase the possibility of dopamine dysfunction and mania but will not necessarily cause it. Indeed, pure mania is supposed to be due to dopamine dysfunction despite the 5-HT constraint, though it might be allowed by an inherent weakness in that constraint. All this suggests a common mechanism of 5-HT dysfunction in mixed mania and 5-HT depression. It follows that a common treatment strategy is in order, especially, the use of monoamine precursors.

Hestenes (1992) reviews the literature on monoamine treatment of mania and presents detailed case histories of two sisters suffering from recurrent mixed mania. These cases are noteworthy for the use of gain control concepts to analyze symptoms and treatment. This is an opportunity to update those case histories and review the conclusions about monoamine treatment.

In both cases, L-tryptophan was used as a prophylactic against mania until 1990, when the FDA ban on the sale of L-tryptophan took effect. The younger sister has remained stable for six years since then without the support of lithium or any other drugs. One conclusion from her prior treatment for mania deserves to be reiterated because it is strongly supported by van Praag's (1991) evidence. A common result of neuroleptic treatment for acute mania or schizophrenia over many days is that the patient appears depressed, so antidepressants are introduced, sometimes creating unfortunate complications. However, there is good reason to believe that, in most cases, this so-called depression is simply due to depletion of catecholamine (dopamine and noradrenalin) stores by the neuroleptics. The most straightforward way to correct this condition, therefore, is to restock the depleted stores by administering the catecholamine precursor tyrosine. Hestenes (1992) gives details of one such successful treatment with 7 g tyrosine/day for two weeks. This tactic deserves to be more thoroughly studied. It may be that a tyrosine follow-up to acute neuroleptic treatment should be standard practice.

The case of the older sister is noteworthy because it is the longest and most thoroughly documented example of successful mania treatment and prophylaxis with L-tryptophan. After two severe manic episodes within two years, she was successfully stabilized on L-tryptophan for ten years until the ban in 1990. Thereafter, she went without any kind of treatment, but her sleep pattern, which had been fairly well controlled by L-tryptophan, became more erratic. After four years she had a severe manic episode and was put on a maintenance dose of lithium, but her adjustment was not as satisfactory as previously on L-tryptophan. Within a year she had another episode, including a suicide attempt. After acute treatment for the episode she was continued on lithium, but not without complaints. Recently she was able to secure L-tryptophan again. Here are some of her observations as she has switched gradually from lithium back to L-tryptophan maintenance. Throughout, her typical L-tryptophan dose has been 2 g/day, and her initial lithium dose was 1125 mg/day.

On lithium alone, her sleep is fragile and her circadian rhythm is not entrained, so she gets to sleep about two hours later each day, and her sleep time precesses around the clock. This is a major reason why she has not held a steady job for many years. Attempts to impose a conventional sleep schedule have been very stressful and ultimately unsuccessful. However, taking the daily L-tryptophan dose a half hour before bedtime not only reduces sleep latency and prevents sleep time precession, it even enables her to sleep an hour earlier if desired – something she could never do otherwise. She reports a pronounced difference in her subjective experience on taking L-tryptophan with and without lithium. Taking L-tryptophan without lithium, she feels a flood of beautiful imagery sweeping her into a dream, and she feels 'more alive' during the day. Taking L-tryptophan with lithium, she feels a fragile, slowly descending drowsiness with increasing sleep latency on successive nights.

Her original plan was to augment lithium treatment with L-tryptophan, as there is some reason to believe that they will act synergistically. However, she feels that the combination slows down her intellect, her reading comprehension and her reaction time. (Of course, the latter could actually be measured.) It makes her feel weak and clumsy and gives her a kind of drowsiness throughout the day.

Her report that L-tryptophan completely eliminates her anxiety is especially significant, as van Praag has emphasized anxiety as a sign of 5-HT dysfunction. As commonly reported by others, under lithium treatment her emotions are blunted. As the lithium dose was reduced, her normal ebullience returned. She now plans to eliminate lithium altogether, but would return to it if necessary. She has reconfirmed her belief that life with L-tryptophan is better for her.

The lesson to be learned from this is that monoamine precursors should probably play a greater role in psychiatric treatment, especially for mixed mania and 5-HT depression.

Summary

This chapter describes a robust theoretical framework for understanding the role of neuromodulators in brain state control. The framework provides the foundation for a new approach to psychiatric diagnosis and a guide for research into neurobiological mechanisms in mental illness. Clinical implications for manic–depressive illness and treatment with L-tryptophan are also discussed.

Note

The deepest theoretical ideas in this chapter come from the work of Stephen Grossberg, where they are extensively discussed, analyzed, and applied. However, several factors conspire to make entry into Grossberg's work difficult, even for accomplished scientists. Its mathematical sophistication is a barrier for some. Its extensive references to diverse branches of psychology and neuroscience are a barrier for others. Most of all, considerable time and effort are required to become conversant with Grossberg's conceptual framework, specialized vocabulary and analytical style. To soften the entry, Hestenes (1987) gives an introduction that amplifies the discussion of pattern-processing principles and mechanisms in this chapter. Levine (1991) gives a wide-ranging introduction to neural network with minimal mathematics that compares

Grossberg's approach to major alternatives. From Grossberg's own pro-
digious output the collection of his papers most relevant to the present
concerns is Grossberg (1982).

References

Banquet, J., Smith, M. & Guenther, W. (1992). Top-down processes, attention,
and motivation in cognitive tasks. In *Motivation, Emotion and Goal
Direction in Neural Networks*, ed. D. Levine & S. Leven, pp. 169–208.
Hillsdale, NJ: Lawrence Erlbaum.

Cohen, J. & Servan-Schreiber, D. (1992). Context, cortex and dopamine: a
connectionist approach to behavior and biology in schizophrenia.
Psychological Review, **99**, 45–77.

Dehaene, S. & Changeux, J-P. (1991). The Wisconsin Card Sorting Test:
theoretical analysis and modeling in a neuronal network. *Cerebral Cortex*,
1, 62–79.

Farah, M. (1989). The neural basis of mental imagery. *Trends in Neurosciences*,
12, 395–9.

Frith, C. (1992). *The Cognitive Neuropsychology of Schizophrenia*. Hillsdale,
NJ: Lawrence Erlbaum.

Grossberg, S. (1982). *Studies of Mind and Brain*. Dordrecht: D. Reidel.

Grossberg, S. & Kuperstein, M. (1989). *Neural Dynamics of Adaptive Sensory-
Motor Control*. New York: Pergamon.

Hestenes, D. (1987). How the brain works: the next great scientific revolution.
In *Maximum-entropy and Bayesian Spectral Analysis and Estimation
Problems*, ed. G. Smith & G. Erickson, pp. 173–205. Dordrecht/Boston:
D. Reidel.

Hestenes, D. (1992). A neural network theory of manic–depressive illness. In
Motivation, Emotion and Goal Direction in Neural Networks, ed. D. Levine
& S. Leven, pp. 209–59. Hillsdale, NJ: Lawrence Erlbaum.

Hobson, A. (1988). *The Dreaming Brain*. New York: Basic Books.

Hoffman, R. (1987). Computer simulations of neural information processing
and the schizophrenia–mania dichotomy. *Archives of General Psychiatry*,
44, 178–88.

Koella, W. (1982). A modern neurobiological concept of vigilance. *Experientia*,
38, 1426–37.

Koella, W. (1984). The organization and regulation of sleep. *Experentia*, **40**,
309–408.

Levine, D. (1991). *Introduction to Neural and Cognitive Modeling*. Hillsdale, NJ:
Lawrence Erlbaum.

Levine, D., Leven, S. & Prueitt, P. (1992). Integration, disintegration, and the
frontal lobes. In *Motivation, Emotion and Goal Direction in Neural
Networks*, ed. D. Levine & S. Leven, pp. 301–35. Hillsdale, NJ: Lawrence
Erlbaum.

Percheron, G., Francois, C., Yelnik, J. & Fenelon, G. (1989). The primate
nigro-striatal-pallido-nigral system. Not a mere loop. In *Neural
Mechanisms in Disorders of Movement*, ed. A. Crossman & M. Sambrook,
pp. 103–09. London: John Libby.

Pinker, S. (1994). *The Language Instinct*. Harmondsworth: Penguin.

Prochazka, A. (1989). Sensorimotor gain control: A basic strategy of motor systems? *Progress in Neurobiology*, **33**, 281–307.

Robinson, S. (1984). Serotonergic control of central cholinergic neurons. In *Dynamics of Neurotransmitter Function*, ed. I. Hanin, pp. 91–9. New York: Raven Press.

Sandyk, R. (1992). L-Tryptophan in neuropsychiatric disorders: a review. *International Journal of Neuroscience*, **67**, 127–44.

Shenton, M., Solovay, M. & Holzman, P. (1987). Comparative studies of thought disorders. *Archives of General Psychiatry*, **44**, 13–20, 21–30.

Slutsker, L., Hoesly, F., Miller, L., Williams, L. & Watson, J. (1990). Eosinophilia–myalgia syndrome associated with exposure to tryptophan from a single manufacturer. *Journal of the American Medical Association*, **246**, 213–17.

Smolensky, P. (1989). Connectionist modeling: neural computation/mental connections. In *Neural Connections, Mental Computation*, ed. L. Nadel, L. Cooper, P. Culicover & R. Harnish, pp. 49–67. Cambridge, MA: MIT Press.

van Praag, H. (1991). The monoamine hypothesis of depression. In *The Role of Serotonin in Psychiatric Disorders*, ed. S-L. Brown & H.M. van Praag. New York: Brunner/Mazel.

van Praag, H., Asnis, G., Kahn, R. et al. (1990). Monoamines and abnormal behavior, a multi-aminergic perspective. *British Journal of Psychiatry*, **157**, 723–34.

Part two

Clinical disorders

7

The nature of delusions: a hierarchical neural network approach

ERIC Y. H. CHEN and
GERMAN E. BERRIOS

For more than 300 years, delusions have been defined as 'pathological *beliefs*' (Berrios, 1996; Spitzer, 1990; see Table 7.1 for clinical examples). During the first half of the nineteenth century, Baillarger reinforced this view by suggesting that 'form' be distinguished from 'content' (Berrios, 1994). Analysis of *content* (i.e. of the semantics of 'belief') has since then generated clinical subtypes (e.g. depressive versus schizophrenic delusions) (Sérieux and Capgras, 1909; Jaspers, 1963; Moor and Tucker, 1979; Sims, 1988), supported psychoanalytical interest in symbols, and (more recently) encouraged correlational research, for example with biographical data, particularly amongst those interested in attribution theory (Bentall, 1994). The 'pathological belief' view has, in general, been less useful to the neurobiological study of delusions (Berrios, 1991; Fuentenebro and Berrios, 1995). Analysis of the *form* of delusions has also been useful in some cases. For example, it has led to stable diagnostic categories (Schneider, 1959; Jaspers, 1963), and to multidimensional approaches, whose main consequence has been the erosion of the old, categorical, 'all-or-none' view. Whether from the perspective of content or of form, most research has been cross-sectional and hence uninformative on how delusions actually change with time. Notable exceptions to this approach have been the work of Kendler, Glazer and Morgenstern (1983) and Garety and Hemsley (1994).

The multidimensional approach is not free from problems. For example, some dimensions of delusions such as 'bizarreness' remain ambiguous (Monti and Stanghellini, 1993). Borrowed from Kurt Schneider (Goldman et al., 1992), the term originally meant 'absurd', 'impossible' or 'contrary to common knowledge' (e.g. as in DSM-III-R: APA, 1987). Currently, however, 'bizarre' is used to mean 'improbable' and this shift in meaning has made the term more dependent upon subjective decision

Table 7.1. *Clinical examples of different types of delusions.*

Type of delusion	Clinical examples
Secondary delusion	A 34-year-old woman experienced voices scolding her and attributed this to a man having implanted a device in her denture which generated these voices
Non-bizzare delusion	A 54-year-old man believed that, since the day he was in a public toilet in which a young boy was also present, he had been under surveillance from the police and his movements had been videotaped because of the suspicion that he had committed indecent sexual behaviour towards the boy
Bizarre delusion	A 48-year-old man believed that he was controlled by insects which infested his body and had taken over his bodily function. These insects (which he called 'nits') were believed to be related to a galactic empire which had also been sending commands through stereo to instruct him to attend an intergalactic meeting on behalf of planet earth
Mood congruent non-bizarre delusion	A 68-year-old depressed woman was convinced that her husband was going to abandon her because she was unworthy of his commitment and had committed many minor mistakes in the past. When in this mental state, she was very distressed and was totally unable to be reassured by her husband
Mood congruent bizarre delusion	A 24-year-old elated man believed that he was a famous late Japanese admiral (killed in World War II) and marched naked in the street while thinking that he was in naval uniform

and context: not surprisingly, 'bizarreness' fails to achieve good inter-rater reliability (Flaum, Arndt and Andreasen, 1991; Goldman, et al., 1992) and hence its clinical usefulness has been called into question (Flaum et al., 1991). The authors believe that this is not a good reason to jettison this dimension and that further conceptual exploration should render it stable (Spitzer et al., 1993). However, such analysis cannot be undertaken unless the notion of delusion itself is examined afresh.

Conceptual analysis of delusion

The clinical phenomenon called 'delusion' remains opaque, and it is important to know whether this opaqueness is a fiendish intrinsic feature or is 'man-made', i.e. results from conceptual confusion. Four aspects of delusions will be explored to determine where earlier conceptual stipulations might have gone awry.

The raw datum of delusions

What is raw datum out of which the concept of delusion is constructed? By convention, it is a type of utterance which, in Anglo-Saxon descriptive psychopathology (DP), is reckoned always to contain a 'pathological belief'. At this stage, the process of conceptualizing delusions may fail, depending on: (a) what type of behaviour is made to count as raw datum, and (b) whether it is assumed that such datum provides sufficient information to categorize the utterance as a delusion (i.e. there is no need to resort to any contextual information).

With regard to (a) above, it is important to ascertain whether all delusions pertain to propositional attitudes (i.e. beliefs, thoughts, etc.) and never refer to emotions or acts for the idea of a delusional memory or volition would constitute a clinical non-sense. Anglo-Saxon psychiatry entertains such a narrow view, partially caused by the etymology of the English word 'delusion' (that defines it as an idea, and not as an emotion or act: *The Oxford English Dictionary*, 1994). In contrast to this, the French term *délire* is found to have a wider compass. Coined during the late sixteenth century, the word is a direct descendant from the agricultural Latin *deliratio*: 'a going out of the furrow, in ploughing' (Bloch and Wartburg, 1950). Metaphorical usage soon made the term refer to generic forms of behaviour such as 'giddiness, silliness, folly, dotage, madness' (Lewis and Short, 1879). When the term was rendered into the French vernacular *délire*, all these meanings came with it, and hence notions such as delusional 'emotions or acts' are clinically intelligible within French psychiatry. For example, Littré (1877) gives as its second definition: le délire de l'ésprit, de l'imagination, des passions. Porter la passion jusqu'au délire. (p. 1037).

A consequence of exclusively defining delusion as a pathological or wrong belief has been that aetiological accounts can only be pitched at the level of 'form and content' (e.g. the current cognitive approach). Furthermore, because the 'essence' of the phenomenon is considered as linguistic, there has been a tendency for it to be treated 'psychologically' rather than neurobiologically. The authors believe that the view that any human thought, emotion or act could, in principle, be 'delusional' is more heuristic in that it encourages a search for convergent brain mechanisms.

Content and form of delusions

A second area concerns the analysis of the content of the 'delusional' utterance. As mentioned above, delusions have conventionally been considered as beliefs that happen to be wrong, unshakeable, incorrigible, etc. The 'belief model' has proven useful in that it makes delusions unproblematic from the structural (form) point of view, paving the way for simplistic definitions in terms of 'wrongness' and/or evidential status of content. By assuming a continuity between 'normal' beliefs and delusions, it also opens the gate to the application of psychoanalysis and attributional theory to the 'study' of delusions.

In spite of the fact that the 'belief model' is no more than a hypothesis, it has been treated as a fact and its value has never been fully tested. For, however implausible it may sound, it could be asked why it is that delusions are not just verbal tics (like, say, the coprolalia of Tourette's syndrome), directly generated by some brain dysfunction? Why is it that their content is not just an aleatory (i.e. randomly acquired) foreign body trapped at the very moment when the delusion is formed and which has little association with whatever systems control belief formation?

The following counterclaims might be marshalled: (a) that in clinical practice delusions are just like beliefs – in both the way in which they are expressed and respond to treatment, and (b) that their content is bound to convey information connected in some way with the utterer or at least express his cultural codes. There is little force in these points. Indeed, the fact that some delusions may become degraded in response to cognitive therapy, for example, cannot be taken as evidence that the cognitive model of such delusions is correct. In general, human movements are particularly susceptible to semantic interpretation (even those of animals, like favourite pets, often are). For example, it is not long ago that spasmodic torticollis was considered as a 'looking away' from an anxiety-creating stimulus, and the tremor of Parkinson's disease as a 'shaking in anger'. In the case of utterances, the bias towards a semantic interpretation is even more marked. The point here is that such a bias is likely to act as a spurious reinforcer of the belief model, and thereby exaggerate the importance of content.

An intermediate position between the verbal tic and the just-a-belief hypotheses is to view delusions as beliefs manqué, i.e. utterances that only mimic or are just bad copies of beliefs. Such an approach would force the researcher to look at delusions as *sui generis* behavioural phenomena (utterances conveying aleatory ideas or images, pseudo-emotions and driven actions), which for yet unknown reasons are generated by brain loci in distress, and which in the moment of their manifestation, because they are channelled out along very narrow expressional systems, acquire certain similarities with behaviours that are normally recognized as beliefs, etc.

Informational value and loci

A third area in which error can be easily generated involves the type, amount, quality and loci of the information that delusions are supposed to convey. Since the central function of symptom-descriptions in psychiatry is to capture sufficient information to ascertain diagnosis and locate its neurobiological basis, one must ask what type of information is included in the form and content of a delusion? Is this information about brain loci, the utterer, or his or her cultural context? If all three, what conveys what? For example, does form tell one more about brain sites (i.e. are delusions isomorphic with or mappable upon a some brain system)? Does content tell one more about the patient's biography, personal cognitive capabilities and cultural background? Should content be taken (as it often is) prima facie? For example, can a persecutory delusional content foretell that the bearer of the delusion has a 'paranoid personality'? A model (far more complex than those available) is needed to deal with these questions. Firstly, it must be decided whether all delusions have the same structure and whether the latter is mappable onto (a) putative neurobiological addresses, and/or (b) linguistic mechanisms.

Delusion formation

A fourth area that might generate errors concerns that of models for delusion formation. Once again, the 'belief model' solves this problem by assuming that delusions are generated by the same cognitive mechanisms responsible for normal beliefs. The logic of this view suggests that delusional emotions or acts (were they to be countenanced by English-speaking psychiatry) are prepared in the same cauldrons as normal emotions and acts, respectively. But then, what would these three 'types' of delusions have in common?

Most theories of delusion formation (Arthur, 1964) are unrepentantly 'cognitive' in nature. Traditional psychology has adopted a 'sequential' paradigm according to which cognitive events issue seriatim out of a cascade of processes. This approach is unlikely to offer a satisfactory description of all aspects of cognition (Martindale, 1991). It can be argued, for example, that each single synaptic event requires a considerable amount of time (in the order of 10 ms) in relation to the latency of

172   *Eric Y. H. Chen and German E. Berrios*

cognitive events (in the order of several hundredths of a ms). The number
of steps that could be accommodated in a sequence (in the order of up to
100) is usually too small for any realistic sequential modelling of even
simple cognitive processes. (A simple serial computer program typically
contains computation in the region of several thousand individual steps
when iterative calculation is involved.) So, moving away from a purely
cognitive view of delusions should free the researcher to seek for other
models of delusion formation.

The role of parallel models

Several parallel models for psychoses have been proposed (see Chapter 8)
but none deals exclusively with delusions. A comprehensive model for the
latter should incorporate both parallel and sequential aspects of cognitive
processing (Callaway and Naghdi, 1982). Because mental symptoms are
structurally heterogeneous (Marková and Berrios, 1995), delusions are
likely to require a different model from, say, formal thought disorder.
This chapter proposes a preliminary model of delusion formation integrating both parallel and sequential aspects of cognitive processing. One
of the conspicuous conclusions of the model is that different dimensions
of delusional experience map onto different abnormalities in the parallel
or the sequential aspects of processing.

Existing models of delusion

All current models of delusion make assumptions about the nature of
normal cognition, and hence all theories of delusions are closely related
to prevalent views on cognition (Berrios, 1991). Hence, whether delusions
are explained in terms of other symptoms, or cognitive processes, or
neurobiological systems, will depend on what historical period one is
dealing with (Arthur, 1964).

Earlier models

At least since the seventeenth century, the view has been entertained that
delusions are related to low intelligence and/or inadequate powers of
reasoning and judgement (Berrios, 1994). During the nineteenth century,
some delusions were also conceived of as secondary to interpretations of
primary pathology affecting perception (e.g. hallucinations), emotions,
personality, and social interactions (for a review, see McKenna, 1994).

It has also been proposed (Bleuler, 1950) that delusions might arise from formal thought disorder, i.e. a combination of loose associations and faulty logical reasoning. When generalized, this approach suffers from the clinical observation that delusions may be the only symptom present (Munro, 1988; Chapman and Chapman, 1988).

Recent cognitive models

More recently, use has been made of cognitive psychology to explain delusions. For example, some theories consider delusions as secondary to putative abnormalities of attention, memory, etc. One such explanation has been offered by Maher and Ross (1984) who proposed that a spurious 'free floating sense of significance' may lead, through 'mistaken attributions', to 'delusions of reference'. Another theory (related to the defective sensory filter view) (e.g. Frith, 1979) proposes that delusions arise from a failure to 'limit the content of consciousness'; this view was later elaborated to incorporate 'faulty feedback monitoring' of actions and intentions (Frith, 1987). This view appears best suited for an account of delusions and thought possession (passivity), where symptoms arise from an apparent dissociation between intention and action. Hemsley and Garety (1986) have offered a further explanation focusing on deficits in the cognitive stages of the belief system: for example, deluded patients seem more likely to arrive at a conclusion based on (statistically) insufficient information, and are more prone to hold on to delusion in face of contradictory evidence (Huq, Garety and Hemsley, 1988). These models have in common the view that cognitive processing occurs in discrete stages (an assumption inherent in the so-called information-processing approach). In general, the above models fail to address the crucial feature of 'bizarreness'.

Parallel models or sequential models?

The parallel models described above are based exclusively on parallel algorithms. From anatomical studies it is clear, however, that the cerebral cortex involves sequential (output of particular cortical area forwarded as input to another area) as well as parallel organization (large number of neurons richly interconnected within one cortical area) (Nieuwenhuys, Voogd and van Huijzen, 1988; Anderson and Hinton, 1989; Kohonen, Oja and Lehtio, 1989; Shepherd, 1990; Braitenberg and Schuz, 1991). This means that parallel models cannot capture well cognitive functions such as symbolic processing and logical reasoning; on the other hand, sequential models (similar to those in a digital computer) cannot capture functions such as ability to retrieve memory from partial cues (content-addressable memory) or resistance to minor focal damage (graceful degradation). It would appear appropriate, therefore, that a new model of delusions should combine both parallel and sequential aspects of processing.

A hierarchical network model of cognitive processing

Cognitive information processing is conceptualized here as a sequence of 'pattern recognition tasks' (Fig. 7.1), with the nature of 'representation' becoming progressively more abstract and complex (or 'higher level'). At each stage, processing involves the mapping of 'information patterns' (in the form of 'input vectors') onto 'interpretative patterns' (i.e. vectors in the output space). For example, at a perceptual level, a collection of features such as colour, shape, surface texture etc. (information space) maps onto the identification of an object, e.g. a teapot (interpretation space). At a higher level, a collection of objects, e.g. teapot, dining table, waiter, menu (information space), maps onto the interpretation of a restaurant scenario (interpretation space). At an even higher level, the

SEQUENTIAL INFORMATION FLOW BETWEEN NETWORKS

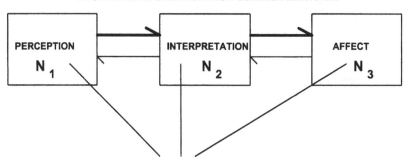

PARALLEL PROCESSING WITHIN EACH NETWORK

Fig. 7.1 Information processing is represented by three networks connected in sequence. Information primarily flows from the lower level 'perceptual' network (N_1) to the higher level 'affect' network (N_3). At each level of processing, information is processed in a parallel distributed fashion by a neural network, which essentially carries out pattern recognition tasks at the relevant level. From higher level networks, priming influence could be exerted over lower level networks.

combined data of a restaurant scenario and an attractive companion (information space) map onto romantic, positive affects (interpretation space). At each of these stages, the nature of processing is essentially similar: the simultaneous (i.e. parallel) consideration of a large number of informational features in relation to past experience and the arrival at an interpretation consistent with both past knowledge and current information.

In the model proposed here, cognitive processing is represented by three neural networks arranged one after another in a hierarchy of processing levels (the exact number of networks is of no consequence to the basic arguments) (Figure 7.1). The first network (N_1) represents processing of 'perceptual information'; the second network (N_2) represents 'high-order cognitive interpretation'; and the third network (N_3) represents 'affective states'. Each network forwards its outputs to the next network and in turn receives top-down 'priming' (see below) from a higher level network (Fig. 7.2). The model incorporates parallel processing within each network and sequential processing between different networks.

Processing within each network

Processing within each network can be considered as a pattern-recognition task that is 'parallel' in nature (Fig. 7.2). The pattern is represented by an array of activity distributed across units in the network, each unit encoding a 'micro-feature' of the input pattern. Processing involves each unit computing information simultaneously (i.e. in parallel) and communicating the result to all other units at each time step. This process goes on until a steady state is arrived at. Processing of input information patterns is partly determined by past correlations ('memories') encoded by weights of each connection in the network, and partly by global parameters of the network (such as the degree of 'noise', see below) (Hopfield, 1982; Amit, 1989; Muller and Reinhardt, 1991). This final steady pattern of activity across the network maximally satisfies external information (input pattern) and internal constraints (encoded as connection weights) and represents the outcome of processing (i.e. 'the interpretation' of the input information) (Rumelhart et al., 1986). Such constraint-satisfaction processes have been used to model the retrieval of content-addressable memory based on 'partial' or 'noisy' cues (Amit, 1989; Muller and Reinhardt, 1991). Description of computational details can be found in Chen (1994; 1995).

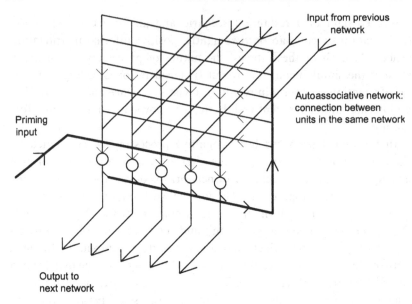

Fig. 7.2 In this detailed figure of one component network in the system, five units are represented by circles. Connections are represented by straight lines, with arrows indicating direction of information flow. Each unit receives input from three sources: (1) from a lower level network; (2) priming input from a higher level network; and (3) input from other units in the same level network. Outputs of each units are also directed: (1) to the next higher level network; (2) to prime a lower level network; and (3) to other units in the same level (this connection is omitted in the figure for the sake of clarity). The connections between a unit and all other units at the same level characterize an 'autoassociative' network. Each of these connections carries a weight which determines how much information should flow through it. The weights are specified via a learning process involving exposure to patterns. The activation of each unit is determined as a function of all its inputs. The activation level then determines the information transmitted to the output lines. Information is represented by patterns of activity across a large number of units.

Basin of attraction and spurious attractors

When an input pattern is presented to a network, the network evolves into a state corresponding to one of the previously stored patterns. The set of initial input patterns that eventually leads to retrieval of a particular stored pattern is called its 'basin of attraction' (Amit, 1989). With a larger basin of attraction, a larger set of inputs (that may initially have only modest resemblance to the target pattern) may eventually lead to retrieval of the target (stored) pattern.

In the situation of 'memory overload' (where there is an attempt to store a larger number of patterns than that permitted by the capacity of the network), 'spurious attractors' arise (Amit, 1989; Muller and Reinhardt, 1991). 'Spurious attractors' are 'alien' stable patterns that do not correspond to any of the previously learned patterns. The combination of micro-features in a spurious attractor does not correspond to previously encountered regularities in the environment.

Processing across different networks

Within a series of networks (see Fig. 7.1), information flows predominantly in one direction (from low level to high level). However, information from a high-level network could influence the processing of a low-level network by a 'priming' effect (which corresponds to the 'top-down' effects proposed in cognitive psychology) (Callaway and Naghdi, 1982).

Priming

The influence by activity in a higher level network of processing in a lower level network corresponds to the cognitive process of 'priming'. Priming enhances the probability for a network to settle into the primed pattern. This process is implemented by selectively contributing to the subthreshold activation of a set of units corresponding to the primed pattern in such a way that a smaller amount of subsequent activation will be required to prompt the network towards retrieval of the primed pattern (for details, see Berrios and Chen, 1993).

Modelling delusions

Abnormal interpretations (delusions) are modelled here as failures in mapping input patterns to appropriate sets of interpretations. Such distortions of mapping from the representational space to the interpretation space may result from a variety of mechanisms. The model proposes that different types of mapping failure lead to different structural characteristics in delusions (Fig. 7.3; Table 7.2).

Spurious attractors and bizarre (impossible) delusions

Intrinsic problems affecting a single network responsible for high-level interpretation (N_2) lead to the formation of spurious attractors in that

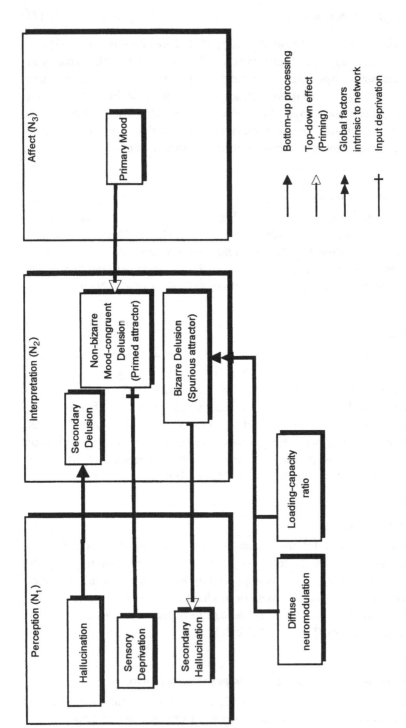

Fig. 7.3 Different mechanisms leading to delusions according to the network model.

Table 7.2. *Relationship between network states, cognition and clinical symptom.*

Clinical symptom	Perception network (N1)	Interpretation network (N2)	Affect network (N3)	Response to treatment (prediction from model)
Secondary delusions	*Neural model* Abnormal processing	Normal	Normal	
	Cognitive events Threatening voices	Persecutory ideas secondary to threatening noises	Fear secondary to persecutory ideas	Responsive as long as primary symptom controlled
Primary bizarre delusion	*Neural model* Normal	Abnormal spurious attractors	Normal	
	Cognitive events Normal	Fixed interpretation irrespective of input and incongruous with general knowledge	Normal	Treatment response less satisfactory or questionable
Mood-congruent delusions	*Neural model* Normal	Primed to, e.g., depressive interpretation	Fixed at, e.g., depression	
	Cognitive events Normal	Negative interpretation that is non-bizarre	Depressed mood	Good response as long as mood improves
Mood-congruent bizarre delusion	*Neural model* Normal	Spurious attractor	Fixed, at, e.g., depression	
	Cognitive events Normal	Fixed interpretation irrespective of input and incongruous with general knowledge	Depressed mood	Poor response even if mood improves; anti-psychotic medication may be necessary

network (Fig. 7.3). Spurious attractors may arise as a result of a number of different network conditions. Factors implicated in the precipitation of psychotic illnesses could be meaningfully represented by some of these network conditions in the model. For example, a reduction in network size or in the number of connections may correspond to reduced global neural resources (which could be due to genetic, neurodevelopmental, or acquired factors). A change in the noise level in the system may also correspond to altered neuromodulation by monoamines (Chen, 1994).

It is important to note that spurious attractors emerge as a result of abnormal processing within a network. Spurious attractors in the 'interpretation' network (N_2) result in alien patterns in the interpretation space that bear no resemblance to previous experience and are characterized by an absurd clustering of features that are incongruous with one another. The resulting pattern therefore defies general knowledge (i.e. disregards encoded correlation between environmental features).

Spurious attractors usually have a large 'basin of attraction', which means that a broad range of different input patterns will map onto the spurious interpretation. This model therefore addresses the formal characteristics of bizarre delusions. It depicts the latter as unshakeable interpretations (trapped at basin of attraction of a spurious attractor) that are absurd, internally incongruous (violation of encoded correlations), and are inferred from apparently unrelated observations in a manner not understandable by others (expansion of basin of attraction).

Effects of pathological priming and non-bizarre delusions

In the 'interpretation' network (N_2), a normal output pattern may become excessively and persistently primed by pathology at a higher level network, i.e. a fixed state of activity in the 'affective' network (N_3) (see Fig. 7.3). This leads to a persistently biased interpretation of any input into the 'interpretation' network (N_2) in favour of the primed pattern. For example, if processing at the level of affect is fixed (due to a primary mood pathology) at a state of 'depression', feedback priming at the level of interpretation (N_3 to N_2) will be in favour of a 'negative' interpretative pattern. The 'negative patterns' will become a dominant output of the 'interpretation' network (N_2) regardless of what the inputs are. Even normal and neutral inputs from the 'perception' network (N_1 to N_2) might lead to a predominantly negative set of interpretations. This effect would be further enhanced by a decrease in the level of noise (which corresponds to impaired monoamine modulation), thus reducing the chances of a spontaneous 'jump' out of that state.

In contrast to spurious attractors, primed patterns are pre-existing patterns with pathologically enlarged 'basins of attraction'. There is no intrinsic abnormality within the patterns themselves, which are coherent clusters of interpretative features. The abnormality lies in the pathologically enlarged set of informational input that maps onto a particular interpretation. Examples of this type of biased misinterpretation are mood-congruent delusions, e.g. delusion of worthlessness in affective disorder, and non-bizarre delusions in delusional disorders (e.g. delusion of jealousy).

Global factors

Relative weight of internal and external information

A further mechanism for delusion formation in our model involves changes in the relative emphasis given to external input and internal constraints in the retrieval of a pattern. Biases towards internal weights result in a system that is less responsive to incoming data and therefore more susceptible to the generation of internal patterns (memories). This corresponds clinically to situations in which a decrease in the intensity of external information (e.g. in sensory deprivation, sensory impairment, or in delirium) leads to a relative dominance of internal information and predisposes to delusion formation (see Fig. 7.3).

Global noise level and cognitive inflexibility

The 'noise' parameter in a neural network refers to the extent to which the computation rule is probabilistic rather than deterministic (Amit, 1989; Muller and Reinhardt, 1991). In a more deterministic network, the unfolding network pattern evolves by alteration in the activity of a small number of units at a time. The output pattern is arrived at by incremental revisions of the previous pattern and therefore its trajectory is more likely to be 'trapped' in an interpretative pattern which, although more satisfactory than the preceding ones, does not necessarily attain the overall best fit to external data and internal constraints (local minima). 'Noise' in a network allows a certain possibility of jumping out from such states, so that there is a better chance of settling in a globally optimized (overall best-fit) solution (Amit, 1989). This computational phenomenon corresponds closely to the cognitive flexibility in a changing mental set, i.e. capacity to reconsider all information and to come to an alternative interpretation that may differ considerably from an earlier one.

Empirical evidence suggests that the modulatory role of diffuse catecholamine projection systems (including the dopamine system) may act to suppress random background firing of target cortical neurons (therefore reducing noise) (Reader et al., 1979; Godbout et al., 1991). Although this may have the effect of increasing the 'signal-to-noise' ratio in information transmission (Keeler, Picher and Ross, 1989; Cohen and Servan-Schreiber, 1992, 1993), excessive suppression of neural noise results in a rigid and deterministic neural system more likely to be trapped by locally stable states. At a cognitive level, this situation manifests as fixation on a particular interpretation with an impaired ability to switch to alternatives (cognitive inflexibility).

Therefore, under normal circumstances, interpretative cognitive function requires the neural noise level to be within an optimal range. Too much noise interferes with signal transmission; too little noise reduces cognitive flexibility. Reduction in cognitive flexibility implies that once an abnormal interpretation is arrived at, there is little possibility of revision. In this way it closely resembles the dimension of 'incorrigibility' of delusional experiences. The same mechanism may be related to the finding of perseverative errors shown by schizophrenic patients in the Wisconsin Card Sorting Test (Scarone, Abbruzzese and Gambini, 1994). It is also consistent with the observations of Huq et al. (1988) that patients tended to arrive earlier at a (statistically unwarranted) conclusion and to maintain that conclusion despite contrary evidence.

Classical secondary delusions

Yet another mechanism could explain the generation of delusions secondary to hallucinations: pathology at the lower level perceptual network (N_1) (i.e. hallucination) leads to abnormal input patterns correctly processed by the interpretation network (N_2) to produce an interpretation consistent with the pathological perception (see Fig. 7.3).

Priming effect on the perceptual network

Finally, a fixed pattern at the interpretation network (N_2) also primes the perceptual network (N_1) in favour of perception consistent with a particular interpretation of the environment (see Fig. 7.3). For example, the interpretation of being watched and criticised by others (delusion of reference) leads to a priming in perception so that irrelevant overheard conversations are experienced as voices talking about oneself (i.e. a hallucinatory experience secondary to a delusion). 'Top-down' influence on hallucination has also been suggested by Bentall (1990).

Discussion

Based on a neural network framework, different types of processing dysfunction are suggested to explain a variety of abnormal interpretations (summarized in Table 7.2). Spurious attractors lead to 'odd' interpretations that are internally inconsistent and at variance with general knowledge (defined as absurd clusters of semantic features incongruous with one another and resulting in a construct that defies general knowledge). Priming from 'upstream' pathology leads to 'mistaken' interpretations, i.e. an unlikely, unjustified but potentially conceivable interpretation.

This model also offers a unique theoretical basis for the re-definition and differentiation between bizarre (impossible) and non-bizarre delusions. This more restrictive conceptualization of bizarreness efficiently addresses the subset of delusions that conventionally have been described as 'bizarre'. Whilst 'bizarreness' may reflect abnormalities inherent at the same level of processing (horizontal dimension), top-down or bottom-up processes constitute an independent dimension (vertical). Thus 'mood congruity' of a delusion, for example, may evidence a top-down priming influence. Tracing of a delusion to a primary perceptual disorder evidences, in turn, a bottom-up influence. On the other hand, the dimension of 'incorrigibility' is related to a global cognitive factor represented in the model by the extent to which processing is subjected to deterministic rather than probabilistic rules (which in turn maps biologically to levels of noise in cortical neuronal activity).

Albeit speculative, this model provides a framework for empirical research. For example, because it considers the 'horizontal' and 'vertical' dimensions of delusion as independent, it can predict that in clinical practice delusions should show varied permutations of mood congruity and bizarreness (suggesting that pathology affects the two mechanisms) independently. Further predictions may also be made: for example, the extent to which 'bizarreness' and 'mood congruity' are 'orthogonal' could be empirically determined by using a multidimensional rating scale. Similarly, the model offers a specific prediction in situations in which a delusion results from factors extrinsic to the interpretation network, namely that removal or cessation of the primary cause should result in degradation of the delusion. (However, the correlation between the dynamics of the delusion and that of the primary pathology need not be linear.) For example, if mood-congruent delusions are assumed to be produced by top-down priming from the level of affect (as evident by being typically non-bizarre), resolution of the mood disorder should result in softening of the delusion. On the other hand, the model predicts that mood-congruent delusions linked to spurious attractor properties (i.e. bizarreness) should show a course less dependent upon an improvement in affect (see Table 7.2). This prediction could be tested by longitudinal comparison between bizarre and non-bizarre mood-congruous delusions. Other parameters from the model are also accessible to measurement. For example, cognitive flexibility can be reflected in executive function tests such as perseverative errors in the Wisconsin Card Sorting Test.

We are aware of the fact that caution must be exercised in the mapping of model components to brain structures. Anatomical studies show that organization in the cortex is complex and defies macroscopic lobar boundaries. Each level of processing (function) may correspond to a (structural) system of richly interconnected cortical areas (of similar architectonic status) that transcend lobar or cortical–subcortical boundaries (Barbas and Pandya, 1991; Fuster, 1995). For example, the interpretative network may correspond to a connected system involving specific parts of the temporal cortex, frontal cortex as well as subcortical structures. Other strengths and limitations of mapping neural network models onto brain structures have already been extensively discussed (Crick and Asanuma, 1986; Churchland and Sejnowski, 1992).

Conclusions

The first stage in the development of a concept of delusion appropriate for empirical research must be a conceptual analysis to determine the locus of opacity in delusions. As shown in this chapter, the 'received view' has resulted from stipulations that are now an obstacle to understanding. Dictated by history, social power and fashion, these stipulations are rarely reviewed, and hence research into delusions remains a prisoner of the past. One way out of this trap is by boldly making use of different conceptual frames. One such conceptual frame has been a structural or multidimensional view of delusions; another is neural network models. Simple neural network models, however, are limited in their capacity to represent complex cognitive events. A hierarchical neural network model based on current understanding of cognitive processes is proposed here which incorporates both parallel and sequential aspects of information processing.

It is also suggested that disruption of specific parameters in this model leads to processing abnormalities that are similar in form to subtypes of delusions, for example bizarre and non-bizarre delusions, mood-congruent and mood-incongruent delusions, and 'secondary' delusions. Thus, bizarre delusions arise from disturbed intrinsic processing within the same hierarchical level; mood congruity from dysfunction in network interaction across different hierarchical levels.

The role of cognitive inflexibility and sensory deprivation is also discussed in relation to our model. This chapter also proposes a new theoretical basis for the differentiation between bizarre delusions (odd belief systems) and non-bizarre delusions (wrong interpretations), and makes a number of specific predictions about the clinical course (and empirical ascertainment) of different types of delusions.

References

Amit, D.J. (1989). *Modelling Brain Function: The World of Attractor Neural Networks*. Cambridge: Cambridge University Press.

Anderson, J.A. & Hinton, G.E. (1989). Models of information processing in the brain. In *Parallel Models of Associative Memory*, ed. G.E Hinton & J.A. Anderson, pp. 23–64. Hillsdale, NJ: Lawrence Erlbaum.

APA (1987). *Diagnostic and Statistical Manual of Mental Disorders*, 3rd edn, revised. Washington DC: American Psychiatric Association.

Arthur, A.Z. (1964). Theories and explanations of delusions: a review. *The American Journal of Psychiatry*, **121**, 105–15.

Barbas, H. & Pandya, D.N. (1991). Patterns of connections of the prefrontal cortex in the rhesus monkey associated with cortical architecture. In *Frontal Lobe Function and Dysfunction*, ed. H.S. Levin, H.M. Eisenberg & A.L. Benton, pp. 35–58. Oxford: Oxford University Press.

Bentall, R.P. (1990). The illusion of reality: a review and integration of psychological research on hallucinations. *Psychological Bulletin*, **107**, 82–95.

Bentall, R.P. (1994). Cognitive biases and abnormal beliefs: towards a model of persecutory delusions. In *The Neuropsychology of Schizophrenia*, ed. A.S. David & J.C. Cutting, pp. 334–57. Hillsdale, NJ: Lawrence Erlbaum.

Berrios, G.E. (1991). Delusions as 'wrong beliefs': a conceptual history. *British Journal of Psychiatry*. **159** (Suppl. 14), 6–13.

Berrios, G.E. (1994). Delusions: selected historical and clinical aspects. In *The Neurological Boundaries of Reality*, ed. E.M.R. Critchley, pp. 251–67. London: Farrand Press.

Berrios, G.E. (1996). *The History of Mental Symptoms. Descriptive Psychopathology since the 19th century.* Cambridge: Cambridge University Press.

Berrios, G.E. & Chen, E.Y.H. (1993). Recognising psychiatric symptoms: relevance to the diagnostic process. *British Journal of Psychiatry*, **163**, 308–14.

Bleuler, E. (1950). *Dementia Praecox or the Group of Schizophrenias*, translated by J. Zinkin. New York: International University Press.

Bloch, O. & Wartburg, W. (1950). *Dictionnaire Etymologique de la Langue Française.* Paris: Presses Universitaires de France.

Braitenberg, V. & Schuz, A. (1991). *Anatomy of the Cortex.* Berlin: Springer-Verlag.

Callaway, E. & Naghdi, S. (1982). An information processing model for schizophrenia. *Archives of General Psychiatry*, **39**, 339–47.

Chapman, L.J. & Chapman, J.P. (1988). The genesis of delusions. In *Delusional Beliefs*, ed. T.F. Oltmans & B.A. Maher, pp. 167–83. New York: Wiley.

Chen, E.Y.H. (1994). A neural network model of cortical information processing in schizophrenia 1: interaction between biological and social factors in symptom formation. *Canadian Journal of Psychiatry*, **39**, 362–7.

Chen, E.Y.H. (1995). A neural network model of cortical information processing in schizophrenia 2: role of hippocampal–cortical interaction: a review and a model. *Canadian Journal of Psychiatry*, **40**, 21–6.

Churchland, P.S. & Sejnowski, T.J. (1992). *The Computational Brain.* Cambridge, MA: MIT Press.

Cohen, J.D. & Servan-Schreiber, D. (1992). Context, cortex, and dopamine: a connectionist approach to behaviour and biology in schizophrenia. *Psychological Review*, **99**, 45–77.

Cohen, J.D. & Servan-Schreiber, D. (1993). A theory of dopamine function and its role in cognitive deficits in schizophrenia. *Schizophrenia Bulletin*, **19**, 85–104.

Crick, F.H.C. & Asanuma, C. (1986). Certain aspects of the anatomy and physiology of the cerebral cortex. In *Parallel Distributed Processing: Explorations in the Microstructure of Cognition*, Vol. 2: *Psychological and Biological Models*, ed. J.L. McClelland & D.E. Rumelhart, pp. 333–71. Cambridge, MA: MIT Press.

Flaum, M., Arndt, S. & Andreasen, N. (1991). The reliability of 'bizarre' delusions. *Comprehensive Psychiatry*, **32**, 59–65.

Frith, C.D. (1979). Consciousness, information processing and schizophrenia. *British Journal of Psychiatry*, **134**, 225–35.

Frith, C.D. (1987). The positive and negative symptoms of schizophrenia reflect impairments in the perception and initiation of action. *Psychological Medicine*, **17**, 631–48.

Fuentenebro, F. & Berrios, G.E. (1995). The predelusional state: a conceptual history. *Comprehensive Psychiatry*, **36**, 251–9.

Fuster, J. (1995). *Memory in the Cerebral Cortex: An Empirical Approach to Neural Networks in the Human and Non-human Primate.* Cambridge, MA: MIT Press.

Garety, P.A. & Hemsley, D.R. (1994). *Delusions: Investigations into the Psychology of Delusional Reasoning.* Oxford: Oxford University Press.

Godbout, R., Mantz, J., Pirot, S., Glowinski, J. & Thierry, A. (1991). Inhibitory influence of the mesocortical dopaminergic neurons on their target cells: electrophysiological and pharmacological characterization. *Journal of Pharmacology and Experimental Therapeutics*, **258**(2), 728–38.

Goldman, D., Hien, D.A., Haas, G.L., Sweeney, J.A. & Frances, A.J. (1992). Bizarre delusions and DSM-III-R schizophrenia. *American Journal of Psychiatry*, **149**(4), 494–9.

Hemsley, D.R. & Garety, P.A.. (1986). The formation and maintenance of delusions: a Bayesian analysis. *British Journal of Psychiatry*, **149**, 51–6.

Hopfield, J.J. (1982). Neural networks and physical systems with emergent collective computational abilities. *Proceedings of the National Academy of Science of the USA*, **79**, 2554–8.

Huq, S.F., Garety, P.A. & Hemsley, D.R. (1988). Probabilistic judgements in deluded and non-deluded subjects. *Quarterly Journal of Experimental Psychology*, **40A**, 801–12.

Jaspers, K. (1963). *General Psychopathology*, translated by J. Hoenig & M.W. Hamilton. Manchester: Manchester University Press.

Keeler, J.D., Picher, E.E. & Ross, J. (1989). Noise in neural networks: thresholds, hysteresis, and neuromodulation of signal-to-noise. *Proceedings of the National Academy of Science of the USA*, **86**, 1712–16.

Kendler, K.S., Glazer, W.M. & Morgenstern, H. (1983). Dimensions of delusional experience. *American Journal of Psychiatry*, **140**(4), 466–9.

Kohonen, T., Oja, E. & Lehtio, P. (1989). Storage and processing of information in distributed associative memory systems. In *Parallel Models of Associative Memory*, ed. G.E. Hinton & J.A. Anderson, pp. 129–70. Hillsdale, NJ: Lawrence Erlbaum.

Lewis, C.T. & Short C. (1879). *A Latin Dictionary*. Oxford: Clarendon Press.

Littré, É. (1877). *Dictionnaire de la Langue Française*. Paris: Hachette.

Maher, B. & Ross, J.S. (1984). Delusions. In *Comprehensive Textbook of Psychopathology*, ed. H.E. Adams & P. Sutker, pp. 383–409. New York: Plenum Press.

Marková, I.S. & Berrios, G.E. (1995). Mental symptoms: are they similar phenomena? The problem of symptom heterogeneity. *Psychopathology*, **28**, 147–57.

Martindale, C. (1991). *Cognitive Psychology: a Neural-Network Approach*. Belmont, CA: Brooks/Cole.

McKenna, P.J. (1994). *Schizophrenia and Related Syndromes*. Oxford: Oxford University Press.

Monti, M.R. & Stanghellini, G. (1993). Influencing and being influenced: the other side of 'bizarre delusions' 1. Analysis of the concept. *Psychopathology*, **26**, 159–64.

Moor, J.H. & Tucker, G.J. (1979). Delusions: analysis and criteria. *Comprehensive Psychiatry*, **20**(4), 388–93.

Muller, B. & Reinhardt, J. (1991). *Neural Networks: An Introduction*. Berlin: Springer-Verlag.

Munro, A. (1988). Delusional (paranoid) disorders. *Canadian Journal of Psychiatry*, **33**, 399–404.

Nieuwenhuys, R., Voogd, J. & van Huijzen, C. (1988). *The Human Central Nervous System: A Synopsis and Atlas*. Berlin: Springer-Verlag.

Reader, T.A., Ferron, A. Descarres, l. & Jasper, H.H. (1979). Modulatory role for biogenic amines in the cerebral cortex: microiontophoretic studies. *Brain Research*. **160**, 217–29.

Rumelhart, D.E., Smolensky, P., McClelland, J.L. & Hinton, G.E. (1986). Schemata and sequential thought processes in parallel distributed

188   *Eric Y. H. Chen and German E. Berrios*

processing models. In *Parallel Distributed Processing: Explorations in the Microstructure of Cognition:* Vol. 2: *Psychological and Biological Models,* ed. J.L. McClelland & D.E. Rumelhart, pp. 7–57. Cambridge, MA: MIT Press.

Scarone, S., Abbruzzese, M. & Gambini, O. (1994). The Wisconsin Card Sorting Test discriminates schizophrenic patients and their siblings. *Schizophrenia Research,* **10**(2), 103–7.

Schneider, K. (1959). *Clinical Psychopathology.* New York: Grune and Stratton.

Sérieux, P. & Capgras, J. (1909). *Les Folies Raisonnantes.* Paris: Alcan.

Shepherd, G.M. (1990). *The Synaptic Organization of the Brain.* Oxford: Oxford University Press.

Sims, A. (1988). *Symptoms in the Mind.* London: Baillière.

Spitzer, M. (1990). On defining delusions. *Comprehensive Psychiatry,* **31**(5), 377–91.

Spitzer, R.L., First, M.B., Kendler, K.S. & Stein, D.J. (1993). The reliability of three definitions of bizarre delusions. *American Journal of Psychiatry,* **150**, 880–4.

The Oxford English Dictionary (1994). Oxford: Oxford University Press.

8

'Produced by either God or Satan': neural network approaches to delusional thinking

SOPHIA VINOGRADOV, JOHN H. POOLE and
JASON WILLIS-SHORE

A schizophrenic man is convinced that the CIA performed cardiac surgery on him on the army and gave him a lizard's heart; now his blood pumps through only three chambers, which means any medication he takes is going to be very dangerous for him.

A lonely erotomanic woman tells an elaborate story of how California politician, Jerry Brown, secretly fell in love with her when she wrote him a fan letter 20 years ago; Brown still signals his passion to her whenever he is photographed in profile.

Most of us would agree that these are examples of delusional thinking, one of 'the main psychiatric phenomena' encountered by clinicians in everyday practice (Brockington, 1991). In keeping with Jaspers' classic description of half a century ago (1946), these examples show the hallmark characteristics of subjective certainty, incorrigibility, and impossible (or improbable) content. Until now, clinical psychiatry has been preoccupied with only one of these features, namely the *content* – and thus we focus on whether a patient's delusion is bizarre, on whether it is well systematized, on whether it is paranoid or somatic or grandiose. Yet any experienced clinician also knows two other perplexing things about delusions. The first is that 'however sharply they may be defined logically, they are not sharply demarcated from normal thinking' (Brockington, 1991, p. 42). The second is that delusional thinking is more than the sum of its contents. As Sedler (1995, p. 259) notes (italics added):

Whereas . . . delusions may or may not invoke the whole of psychic life to explain their specific contents, it is the *form* in which these contents appear, the delusional structure that sustains them, which must command our attention.

189

(For) although the strange, outlandish, or incomprehensible content of delusions is the feature that superficially engages one's attention, and indeed has dominated clinical theory, it is clear that these features alone are insufficient to understand what makes a delusion.

So what exactly *does* make a delusion, this tenacious belief that the patient clings to despite all of the contradictory evidence of everyday reality? How different is it from the range of thinking processes we all engage in? More recent descriptions have emphasized these formal properties of delusional thinking (e.g. Berrios, 1991; Vinogradov, King and Huberman, 1992a; Spitzer, 1995; Sedler, 1995) in order to make sense of the apparently illogical way some patients have of experiencing the world. A formal approach to delusions ignores the details of content and focuses instead on the thinking processes or cognitive operations of the delusional patient. The authors propose that such an approach is ultimately the most useful and valid way to understand delusional thinking from a neurobiological point of view – and, therefore, from a clinical point of view as well.

As is shown in this chapter, neural network models may be able to explain, at least in part, how disordered information processing in the brain can give rise to delusional thinking in all its myriad clinical manifestations. Why is an understanding of this approach crucial for those who are interested in psychopathology? The authors argue that it is only such an approach that allows us to grasp *in a neurobiologically sound manner* the way in which cerebral pathophysiology interacts with environmental stressors and individual psychodynamics to give rise to one of the most classic signs of mental illness (see Brockington, 1991).

Let us return, as our starting point, to the examples about the lizard heart and Jerry Brown's secret passion. Putting aside the content (interesting as it is), what can we hypothesize about the structure of the patients' thinking processes in these two examples? How would we characterize their cognitive operations?

Delusions appear to involve *both* the personal, narrative-based episodic memory system ('This is what happened to me, I remember it – I had secret cardiac surgery/Jerry Brown fell in love with me') *and* the knowledge, belief, or generic (semantic) memory system ('This is factual, I know this to be true – the CIA always puts lizard hearts into people/people convey secret messages in photographs'). As such, delusional thinking spreads beyond memory of one's personal past. It has a life of its own in the present and it influences ongoing perceptions, thoughts, and actions. It also connects or binds together many different aspects of a person's experience. Nowhere is this more evident than when a patient develops ideas of reference and is on the cusp of assigning meaning to the experience:

At first it was as if parts of my brain 'awoke' which had been dormant and I became interested in a wide assortment of people, events, places, and ideas which normally would make no impression on me . . . (I felt) there was some overwhelming significance in all this, produced by either God or Satan, and I felt I was duty-bound to ponder on each of these new interests, and the more I pondered the worse it became. The walk of a stranger on the street could be a sign to me which I must interpret, every face in the window of a passing streetcar would be engraved on my mind, all of them concentrating on me and trying to pass me some sort of message.
(MacDonald (1964) as cited in Benioff, 1995.)

Delusions are a person's attempt to explain his or her overwhelmingly significant experience; they represent the creation of a personal narrative. This narrative – this self-generated explanation of events – becomes integrated into the individual's episodic memory. When these memory records are later activated, the delusional person can no longer discern that they were internally generated explanations for a whole set of experiences. Instead, the individual has become certain that the explanations are part of something that really happened, part of the real, external world. The delusional explanations have become part of the person's generic, background knowledge (semantic memory), and like all knowledge, will influence the person's ongoing experience of events.

Delusional thinking must, therefore, at its most fundamental level, be related to aberrant long-term memory formation and retrieval, probably both in the episodic and in the generic memory systems, with subsequent effects on perception and interpretation of incoming stimuli. (Although cognitive psychologists tend to distinguish between the two aspects of long-term memory, evidence strongly suggests that they are highly interrelated at both a neuroanatomic and functional level – Fuster, 1995.) Over the past 20 years, connectionist models of information processing in the brain have made great strides in exploring various aspects of normal memory functioning in humans (e.g., Collins and Loftus, 1975; Anderson, 1983; McClelland and Rumelhart, 1985). The logical next step is to use connectionist models to understand some of the *abnormal* memory information processing that occurs in psychiatric disorders characterized by delusions.

This chapter discusses such a neural network information-processing approach to delusional thinking in three sections:

a brief review of the literature on cognitive aspects of delusional thinking

a presentation of neurological, neuropsychological, and experimental data that support a neural network model of delusional syndromes

an overview of current connectionist models that are relevant to this approach.

No attempt is made to present a complete neural network model of delusional thinking. The empirical data base on the cognitive and neuro-psychological aspects of delusion formation in clinical populations is still scanty. Furthermore, connectionist modeling continues to struggle to develop cogent schemas for relatively simple memory phenomena; it is not yet able to account for all of the rich and complex attentional, con-textual, and affective inputs that must influence the formation and retrie-val of abnormal memories in susceptible individuals. Rather, the usefulness of the connectionist approach to understanding what we observe clinically and to planning future research is illustrated.

Cognitive aspects of delusional thinking

I got caught speeding once, about ten years ago, near LA. The cop stopped me and gave me a ticket. I realized last summer who the cop was: it was Mark Fuhrman from the OJ Simpson case. Then I suddenly realized that he gave me another ticket once when I was speeding near Las Vegas, about six years ago. I'm not sure how he got there. Maybe LA police sometimes work in other places, too. For substitution or restitution and promotion. And then I knew they would want me to be a witness in the OJ Simpson trial. They'd want me to say whether or not Fuhrman was an honest cop. And I knew they were following me, because of the OJ case. They're rich, they can follow me anywhere. The doctor I saw yesterday looked like one of their lawyers.
LK, a 40-year-old Caucasian male with delusional disorder.

Maher (1974, 1988) has proposed that delusions are the result of normal cognitive processes applied to unusual or faulty perceptual data. Humans tend to see causality in covariation or coincidence; scientific researchers do it all the time, and it is adaptive from an evolutionary point of view. A painting on a cave wall is followed by a good hunt, a certain clump of marsh grass hides some edible tubers – humans will make a link between events, which can (sometimes) enhance their survival. Likewise, when we are presented with distorted or troubling incoming sensory data, we attempt to make sense of it, to assign meaning to it. For example, if someone has a neurologic disease that causes auditory hallucinations, then his or her brain will work very hard to come up with an explanation for those voices – perhaps it is God, telling him or her to have faith and be healed.

The vignette above illustrates that there is something more to delusional thinking than just this, however. Certainly, Mr. K. has distorted perceptions that are 'explained away' by his delusion: his uneasy sense of being followed is due to his important role in the OJ Simpson case. But it goes the other way, too: his conviction about his role itself distorts his perceptions of current and past events. Also, there is a certain vagueness, a tangentiality, even some unusual word use, as he describes his experiences – what Chapman, Edell and Chapman (1980) have noted as cognitive slippage during description of symptoms.

Indeed, Chapman and Chapman (1988) have pointed out that schizophrenics show striking cognitive slippage when they discuss their delusional topics; schizophrenics also show a selection bias in that they focus more often on stimuli that are strong or prominent, and they neglect weaker stimuli, resulting in a 'constriction of the evidence considered.' These investigators propose that delusions, anomalous perceptual experience, and thought disorder are independent phenomena that can augment each other, but that none of the three uniformly occurs first in a causal sequence.

Faulty cognitive operations are involved in delusional thinking

Several lines of experimental evidence suggest that delusional thinking is not simply the result of anomalous perceptions, but that it involves some specific faulty cognitive operations. Deluded subjects make more external attributions for negative events and more internal attributions for positive events; they also tend to see coincidences as significant (Kaney and Bentall, 1992). Deluded subjects request less information before reaching a decision on a probabilistic inference task (Huq, Garety and Hemsley, 1988) and they show a reasoning bias when they perform such tasks (Garety, Hemsley and Wessely, 1991). Johnson (1988) has proposed that, in patients with delusional thinking, there is a loss of control over thoughts. This produces a paucity of reflective, cognitive–operations information, and so the thoughts become particularly easy to confuse with external stimuli.

The experimental work in schizophrenia, a clinical disorder characterized by delusions, is also suggestive. Here, the cognitive deficits relevant to delusional thinking appear to involve problems with specific aspects of memory function. Symptom severity, which includes positive symptom profiles and therefore the presence of delusions, is a significant predictor of impaired memory (Sullivan et al., 1994). Schizophrenic patients show compromised episodic memory (Gold et al., 1992), but preservation of procedural memory, implicit memory, and some aspects of primary short-term memory (Clare et al., 1993). Interestingly, semantic memory is also anomalous in schizophrenia (Manschreck et al., 1988; Kwapil et al., 1990; Spitzer et al., 1993, 1994; Chen et al., 1994) – especially in the realm of controlled processing (i.e. attention-based and effort-based aspects) (Henik, Priel and Umansky, 1992; Henik et al., 1995; Vinogradov, Ober and Shenaut, 1992b; Ober, Vinogradov and Shenaut, 1995, 1996).

Of particular relevance to delusions, schizophrenics show defects in their memory for the *source* of information (Harvey, Earle-Boyer and Levinson, 1988; Harvey et al., 1990; Bentall, Baker and Havers, 1991; Vinogradov et al., 1997. When schizophrenics are asked to recall the source of information ('make up a word' *vs* 'read the word') after a long delay, they often misattribute self-generated items to the experimenter (Vinogradov et al., 1997). Source monitoring is conceptualized as a meta-memory function that, while dependent on intact encoding, storage, and retrieval, also requires monitoring and regulation of contextual information. Thus, some researchers have concluded that delusions, such as experiences of alien control in schizophrenia, probably reflect a disorder in central error correction (Malenka et al., 1987) and in central monitoring of perception, memory, and action (Frith and Done, 1989; Bentall et al., 1991).

The various faulty cognitive operations reviewed thus far suggest, among other things, that delusional patients have problems with reasoning, attentional processes, and central monitoring, all aspects of the executive functions of the prefrontal cortex. In addition, there is a poorly defined ensemble of memory deficits. Taken together, these information-processing defects undoubtedly play a role in establishing cognitively biased but tenaciously held explanatory schemata – based on faulty executive monitoring of records in episodic and/or semantic memory. Manifestation of frankly delusional beliefs may also require that these information-processing deficits are superimposed on a predisposition to specific cognitive biases – a kind of stickiness or viscosity of cognition – due to distressing life events, negative emotional states, absence of disconfirming feedback, and the like. Thus, a person's delusional interpretation of events would reflect both predisposing biases and impaired executive functions.

We know that normal subjects tend to interpret unexplained states of physiologic arousal negatively, and that subjects who report negative feelings will almost always provide an explanation for them (Maslach, 1979). Psychiatric patients who experience physiologic arousal as part of their illness will also attempt to explain the arousal, and will show a bias towards various negative kinds of explanations. For example, the patient with panic attacks becomes convinced they are caused by the crowds in a shopping mall and develops agoraphobia; the hypervigilant veteran with post-traumatic stress disorder decides that being around Vietnamese immigrants is dangerous; the obsessive–compulsive patient becomes convinced that her intense anxiety is caused by failure to return home to check whether the door is locked, even though she has already done so repeatedly. Yet – despite the negative bias to their explanatory systems – not all of these patients develop true delusional thinking (i.e., imperviousness to logical analysis and disconfirming evidence).

It seems likely that an unpleasant state of anxious arousal is necessary, but not sufficient, to develop delusions. In other words, problems in memory processing (which themselves must be quite anxiety producing) both result in and are superimposed upon heightened arousal, strongly negative emotional tone, memories of previous experiences, and motivation to find explanations. This in turn reinforces underlying cognitive biases in the affected individual. Longitudinal research certainly indicates that premorbid interests and preoccupations color the content of delusions in schizophrenia when an individual finally develops an acute psychotic episode (Harrow, Rattenbury and Stoll, 1988; Chapman and Chapman, 1988).

In our clinical research, we have also observed the contrasting phenomenon. We have interacted with higher-functioning schizophrenia spectrum patients (DSM-IV residual schizophrenia or schizotypal personality disorder). These patients had brief psychotic episodes in the past and continue to demonstrate mild forms of the cognitive anomalies of schizophrenia, but have never developed detailed, well-systematized, overarching delusions. Instead, they move through life focused on vague mystical or religious experiences, or are preoccupied with their memories of difficulties faced in late adolescence (such as a hostile social clique or an aggressive boyfriend). Clinically, these patients seem to lack the exaggeration of cognitive biases, and thus appear to be protected from elaborating complicated delusional explanations for their experiences.

The role of cognitive bias in delusional thinking

Let us examine this concept of cognitive bias more closely. It has already been suggested that delusional thinking occurs because some part of long-term memory processing is not working very well. What is interesting about cognitive bias is that it actually suggests that some part of cognition is working *too well*. Shapiro has described this most eloquently:

A suspicious person is a person who has something on his mind. He looks at the world with fixed and preoccupying expectations, and he searches repetitively, and only, for confirmation of it . . .
Suspicious people are not simply people who are apprehensive and 'imagine things.' They are, in actual fact, extremely keen and often penetrating observers. *(Shapiro, 1965.)*

Paranoid subjects show better nonverbal receiving ability than normals when asked to identify correctly videotapes of people's facial expressions (LaRusso, 1978). Paranoid schizophrenics, who by definition are preoccupied by one or more delusions (and/or hallucinations), are more ready to impute the presence of stimuli and to draw inferences more liberally from presenting stimulation, despite processing it less adequately than controls (Broga and Neufeld, 1981). They also report illusory correlations between randomly correlated pairs of words, particularly when they are of a paranoid content (Brennan and Hemsley, 1984).

Magaro (1981) reviewed the experimental information-processing literature contrasting nonparanoid schizophrenics and paranoid individuals and concluded that paranoids have preconceived and idiosyncratic cognitive sets that interfere with their ability to respond to tasks requiring attentional mechanisms. Stroop task experiments by Carter et al. (1993) demonstrated that paranoid schizophrenics showed a greater than normal interference effect (as compared to disorganized schizophrenics who showed a greater than normal facilitation effect). In a pilot study, evidence was found that paranoid schizophrenics show more inhibition dominance than nonparanoids on a semantic priming task (unpublished data); in a recent experiment, it was demonstrated that paranoid schizophrenics showed nonsignificant priming on a lexical detection task, consistent with interference in automatic spread of activation in semantic memory (Ober et al., 1996).

Schizophrenics with systematized delusions show better verbal ability and verbal memory than those without, as well as a greater discrepancy between premorbid verbal ability and current attentional functioning (Kremen et al., 1994). Paranoid schizophrenics are not vulnerable to distraction on a digit span task in the same manner as nonparanoid schizophrenics (Rund, 1982), and do not make as many perseverative errors on the WCST (Rosse et al., 1991). They process complex information more efficiently (Langell, Purisch and Golden, 1987) and show evidence of increased inhibitory processes on the P300 AERP task (Louza and Maurer, 1989). Thus, certain aspects of cognitive bias suggest that something in the brain is functioning too well, rather than not well enough. As Shapiro describes it:

On the one hand, the paranoid person searches intensely for confirmation of his anticipations. On the other hand, those same rigid anticipations of what he will find allow him to feel entitled to discredit and disregard apparent contradictions . . . In this process, intellectual capacity, keenness, and acuteness of attention become . . . instruments of bias. This keenness enables suspicious people to make, as they often do, brilliantly perceptive mistakes. *(Shapiro, 1965.)*

What aspects of brain function might account for this keen anticipation, this tendency to make brilliantly perceptive mistakes? We can only propose a tentative and partial answer. The data we have briefly reviewed suggest 'interference effects,' as if the set of memory associations that is brought to bear on a task is too rigid, too strong, too tightly connected, so that it interferes with the subject's ability to evaluate and respond flexibly to the task at hand. Indeed, it is as if incoming percepts are evaluated only in terms of certain rigid sets of associations, and the percepts themselves become connected to (and absorbed by) this rigid set of associations. These observations imply dysfunction in cortical association areas responsible for the generation of context or expectations, areas which are, by definition, involved in the 'storage' of memories. At the same time, the data suggest that there are domains of relatively intact prefrontal cortical functioning.

Baer (1979, cited in Strauss, 1988) has pointed out that patients with complex partial seizures (temporal lobe epilepsy), who can show hyper-religiosity, hypergraphia, and interpersonal 'stickiness,' often also have a propensity to impute particular significance to trivial stimuli; a feature that may be related to sensory-limbic hyperconnectiveness. In schizophrenia, Saykin et al. (1991) found a selective impairment in memory and learning consistent with temporo-limbic dysfunction, while Gur et al. (1994) from the same laboratory found that severity of delusional thinking was correlated with problems in left midtemporal lobe function (on functional neuroimaging) as well as deficits in verbal memory. In a comparison of schizophrenic subjects with bipolars and normals, Wood and Flowers (1990) found that a focal suppression of left hemispheric peri-Sylvian activation during memory task performance uniquely characterized schizophrenia, as did a deficit in narrative prose memory. These clinical research data hint at a relationship between cognitive bias and posterior brain areas involved in memory storage and retrieval.

Some preliminary conclusions

Based on a brief review of the cognitive aspects of delusional thinking, the following preliminary conclusions are suggested.

Delusional thinking is associated with problems in long-term memory processing with a concomitant misattribution of sources of information. There is evidence of both episodic and generic memory anomalies (especially in the realm of controlled, attentional processing), as well as defects in reasoning and central monitoring or meta-memory operations. In other words, there are *deficits* in the brain systems that are responsible for the organization and encoding of memories – and for the monitoring of associated contextual information (consistent with executive dysfunction in prefrontal cortex).

Delusional thinking is associated with cognitive bias, which is the inadequate processing of all relevant information combined with the 'overprocessing' of certain other types of information. There is suggestive evidence of involvement of language systems and of temporal lobe function, including sensory–limbic hyperconnectivity. In other words, there is *overdrive* in the brain systems that are responsible for the set of expectations that are brought to tasks involving perception as well as the set of associations that is formed during perception.

Given these preliminary conclusions, let us turn now to the neurological and neuropsychological data pointing to the brain systems that might be involved in delusional thinking.

Delusional thinking is associated with disconnection of reciprocally innervated brain systems

Clinical research over the past 15 years indicates that a number of delusional syndromes are caused by dysfunction of specific brain systems important for the formation of general schemata and the utilization of specific memories. Several neuropathological conditions that point to the neural bases of delusions are examined first. Then evidence is considered for cerebral impairment in two psychiatric disorders that involve severe reality distortion: the obsessive–compulsive and schizophrenia spectrum disorders. Taken together, this body of work supports a neural network model of delusional syndromes based on disconnection of reciprocally innervated brain systems – particularly those involved in the retrieval and inhibition of sensorimotor schemata.

The neuropathology of delusional syndromes

Acute-onset delusional syndromes

Even patients with no prior tendency for psychosis may develop delusional symptoms following cerebral impairment. For example, studies of senile dementia patients who have no prior history of psychiatric disturbance (Cummings and Victoroff, 1990; Mendez et al., 1990) indicate that delusions occur in 40 percent of cases. In progressive dementias, these symptoms occur in the early and middle stages of the illness and cease as cognitive functions continue to decline (Drevets and Rubin, 1989). This suggests that, for delusions to manifest, no only must there be defective cerebral functioning, but also certain subsystems must be *preserved*. Thus, two questions arise: (1) which subsystems have failed? and (2) what is the effect of this failure on still-functioning modules?

Delusions of imperfection

Strong evidence for neurologic etiology comes from several delusional syndromes, which have in common the belief that something has gone wrong with familiar objects or people, i.e., reduplicative and dysmorphic delusions (Malloy and Duffy, 1994). Reduplicative delusions involve the fixed belief that imperfect doubles have replaced familiar places (reduplicative paramnesia), important people in one's life (Capgras delusion), or even oneself (doppelganger delusion). Dysmorphic delusions involve the fixed belief that one's own body is disfigured (body dysmorphic delusion), diseased (hypchondriasis), infested by bacteria or parasites (Ekbom delusion), or dead (Cotard delusion). These delusions can occur in the absence of neurodiagnostic findings. However, a large proportion of cases are accompanied by neurologic signs (Malloy, Cimino and Westlake, 1992) or may result from neurologic disorders acquired in adulthood (e.g. toxic metabolic conditions, traumatic brain injury, dementia).

Several reviews of the neurological evidence in adult-onset cases with these syndromes point to involvement of the frontal lobes in virtually all cases (e.g., Ruff and Volpe, 1981; Hakim, Verma and Greiffenstein, 1988). Associated behavioral features are also characteristic of frontal dysfunction, and include amnesia with confabulation, poor insight into consequences of actions, and lack of concern regarding one's illness. Furthermore, impairment of right frontal functioning may be a prerequisite for the development of delusional thinking, in that most studies point to either right or bilateral frontal damage.

Beyond this rather nonspecific requirement, the content of reduplicative and dysmorphic delusions appears to be influenced both by personality factors (pre-illness biases in the system) and by the exact location of additional nonfrontal damage – most frequently in the perceptual association areas of the right temporal or parietal lobes (Malloy and Duffy, 1994). For example, specific areas in the inferior temporal cortex are dedicated to recognition of familiar faces, and lesions in this region are associated with the impression that familiar pepole have been imperfectly replicated (Alexander, Stuss and Benson, 1979; Malloy et al., 1992). In contrast, the posterior temporo-parietal area specializes in identifying objects, and impairments in this region can produce the sensation that familiar objects or places have been replaced by dilapidated surrogates (Benson, Gardner and Meadows, 1976). Finally, the anterior parietal region contains a schematic map of the body, and lesions here can produce impressions of bodily distortion or dysfunction.

Anorexia nervosa, a disorder involving not only severe disruption of eating behaviors but also marked body-image distortion, may exemplify the confluence of premorbid cognitive biases with neurocognitive dysfunction. A large volume of research has documented that anorexia is associated with specific predisposing psychosocial factors, such as culture-specific and subculture-specific models of beauty, socioeconomic level, and family members' reactions to adolescent body changes. Evidence (reviewed by Braun and Chouinard, 1992) has also accumulated that this disorder tends to be associated with neuropsychological and/or electrophysiological disturbances in the right temporo-parietal cortex, possibly accompanied by frontal metabolic disturbances. Many patients with anorexia nervosa have beliefs of delusional intensity that they are grossly overweight (despite clear evidence to the contrary), and that losing even more weight will yield feelings of success and social acceptance. This appears to result both from premorbid cognitive and emotional biases as well as from a breakdown in self-monitoring and regulation.

All of the above delusions involve the erroneous conviction that something is seriously wrong with oneself or one's world. The contrary conviction – that nothing is wrong – can also be triggered by neurologic deficits, particularly when associated with the perceptual deficit, anosognosia.

Anosognosia

When brain trauma causes an acute loss of sensory, motor, or language abilities, patients' capacity accurately to appraise their own functions may or may not be spared. This ability depends primarily upon specific multisensory perceptual and cognitive functions, based in a cortical region at the confluence of temporal, parietal, and occipital lobes. In the right hemisphere, this region is involved in judging whether one's own body is functioning properly, while in the left hemisphere it evaluates the progress and effectiveness of verbal communications. Anosognosia, the inability to perceive dysfunction in oneself, is a common consequence of lesions in this region. When damage is in the *right* temporo-parieto-occipital area, patients often cannot recognize even complete loss of limb function, such as left hemiplegia or anesthesia. When such patients are confronted with evidence of their dysfunction (such as an immobile left arm), they often respond with confabulations that can reach delusional proportions ('That's someone else's arm'). Similarly, when the *left* temporo-parietal area is damaged, patients frequently cannot recognize even severe disruption in their semantic language functions, such as an inability to name objects or comprehend language, and their production of fluent but empty speech (Wernicke's aphasia). This combination of incomprehensible language with an inability to see the deficit in oneself often leads to agitated, paranoid states, which can easily be misdiagnosed as schizophrenia.

The role of central monitoring and control functions

Given that delusional symptoms are related to dysfunction in posterior association areas, why would frontal dysfunction also be an essential component of these syndromes? The prefrontal cortex is the final common convergence for perceptual information collated by posterior association areas. The process of monitoring one's internal and external environment involves intensive reciprocal communication between the posterior heteromodal sensory association area and the prefrontal heteromodal association cortex (Mesulam, 1985). Indeed, 85 percent of pathways to the prefrontal cortex that convey environmental information originate in the posterior association areas – 60 percent from tertiary association cortex, and 25 percent from secondary association areas (Strub and Black, 1988). In this role, the prefrontal cortex coordinates diverse brain functions that are involved in shifting and focusing attention. It also provides the central *control* function of maintaining adaptive concepts and responses while suppressing irrelevant concepts and responses (Goldman-Rakic, 1987a, 1987b). Thus, if the frontal lobes and their reciprocal connections with the posterior cortex are intact, irrelevant, maladaptive percepts from the posterior cortex, despite their alarming nature, may eventually be ignored or even suppressed. Conversely, if frontally based monitoring and control functions are disrupted, then any perceptual defects, prexisting temperamental tendencies – or even the subtle perceptual biases that are normal features of human perception – may take on a degree of autonomy that severely distorts thinking and behavior.

Automatisms

The converse occurrence – loss of frontal regulatory functions while perceptual and motor systems remain intact – further highlights the role of frontal dysfunction in delusional states. For example, the supplementary motor area regulates exploration of the environment by alternately allowing or suppressing basic searching behaviors initiated by limbic motivational centers. Damage to this area can release automated behaviors from control, resulting in 'alien hand syndrome,' in which the patient's hand persistently manipulates objects without conscious initiation or control. The uncanny sensation of a seemingly autonomous limb frequently causes patients to believe they have been possessed or are controlled by an outside force (Goldberg, Mayer and Toglia, 1981).

Temporal lobe epilepsy

Temporal lobe epilepsy is a disorder involving partial seizures (not generalized to the entire brain) originating in cortical or limbic structures of the temporal lobe. Temporal lobe epilepsy has been of considerable theoretical interest due to apparent associations with altered behavior and personality. Temporo-limbic ictal phenomena (occurring at or near the time of seizure) are highly diverse, potentially including intense perceptual, motor, mnestic, autonomic, and emotional manifestations (Bigler,

1988). This suggests that stimulation of temporo-limbic circuitry can activate templates for a wide variety of phenomena – in short, almost any experience that the brain is capable of producing (Spiers et al., 1985).

Interictal manifestations (occurring between seizures) are thought to result primarily from chronic irritation of brain systems near the epileptic focus. (This is a topic with some disagreement, as attempts are made to distinguish specific neurologic effects from general 'psychological' reactions to seizures, medication effects, etc.) While no interictal behaviors are inevitably associated with temporal lobe epilepsy, most studies have found specific personality traits, including: heightened emotionality, dependency, obsessionality, paranoia, and reduced sexuality (Hermann and Riel, 1981; Brandt, Seidman and Kohl, 1985; Fedio, 1986). In addition, circumstantiality (verbosity with poor closure), hypergraphia (incessant impulse to write), intense philosophical interest or religiosity, and sense of personal destiny are also frequently observed (Hermann and Riel, 1981; Rao et al., 1992; Sanders and Mathews, 1994).

The temporo-limbic system specializes in collating sensory input with internally stored perceptual and emotional templates, in interpreting their relevance, and in encoding this for later retrieval. Temporal lobe epilepsy research suggests that repeated, uncontrolled discharges in this system can result in a heightened drive to ascribe meaning to details, in activation of emotions, and in difficulty perceiving pragmatic cues that guide social interactions. Baer (1979) proposed that these are due to sensory-limbic hyperconnectivity, which results in the overinvestiture of emotions in the details of perception and ideation.

The interictal manifestations of temporal lobe epilepsy are reminiscent of the behavioral distortions and cognitive biases of psychoses (i.e., circumstantiality, paranoia, heightened sense of meaningfulnes, poor social pragmatics). However, these tendencies typically do not take on psychotic proportions, and patients with temporal lobe epilepsy are not generally considered to have an elevated risk for psychosis. As discussed for right temporo-parietal lesions, this may be due to the presence of intact prefrontal systems that are able to monitor, regulate, and to some degree override posterior perceptual systems and therefore to maintain adaptive functioning. Nonetheless, when one examines psychiatric populations, left temporal lobe epilepsy is over-represented in schizophreniform disorders (Sherwin, 1982; Flor-Henry, 1983). In such cases, the temporal lobe epilepsy tends to be associated with diffuse cerebral pathology (Hermann and Whitman, 1984) and, thus, a reduced capacity to compensate for biases in temporo-limbic functioning.

Synthesis: a neuropsychological model of delusional syndromes

Memories and perceptual maps of one's world are mainly stored in the *primary* association areas of the cerebral cortex, located between the primary sensory and motor areas (Markowitsch, 1985; Damasio, Tranel and Damasio, 1990; Killackey, 1990). Modality-specific memories and schemata (e.g., of sights, melodies, tactile impressions, motoric sequences) are typically stored in the *secondary* association areas, immediately adjacent to the primary sensory or motor area of the same modality. The integration of multiple, 'heteromodal' sensorimotor features of experience occurs in two *tertiary* association areas: the temporal-occipital-parietal juncture, and the prefrontal cortex (Strub and Black, 1988). Finally, each of these regions is intimately connected with subcortical structures (the limbic system, basal ganglia, and thalamic nuclei) responsible for the encoding and retrieval of memories along with their associated emotional relevance.

These association areas are storage sites for fundamental schemata – internal maps of the world that guide our perceptual, cognitive, and metacognitive processes. As discussed below, the posterior associative and limbic structures contain perceptual templates by which sensory input is recognized, logically interpreted, and imbued with emotional color. Likewise, frontal associative and subcortical structures contain regulatory schemata for cognition and action, and include such processes as: generating and choosing among options, monitoring and correcting errors, assessing emotional motivation of actions, and imposing self-control.

The posteriorly located temporal-occipital-parietal-limbic (TOPL) circuits are most directly responsible for the formation and storage of perceptual schemata. They provide the framework within which sensory percepts are recognized, interpreted, evaluated, and imbued with emotional valence. In these circuits, lateralized hemispheric specialization is a salient organizing principal. The language-dominant (usually left) TOPL specializes in verbal, sequential, and detail-oriented schemata for evaluating self and environment. For example, it monitors the linguistic sensibility of speech (by oneself and others), and provides the internal labels for explaining events, evaluating the accuracy and significance of minute perceptual details, and analyzing cause–effect sequences. In short, it generates a verbally encoded associative network for sequentially analyzing the minutiae of experience.

In a complementary manner, the right TOPL specializes in visuospatial schemata for evaluation of self and environment, using mainly nonverbal, globally organized, simultaneous processing of patterns. It provides internal templates against which complex perceptual configurations can be compared, thereby differentiating the familiar from the alien, the functional from the dysfunctional, the beautiful from the discordant. In sum, it generates a configurally encoded associative network for synthetically interpreting the 'rightness or wrongness' of objects, organisms, and their functions. When they function normally together, the perceptual–memory circuits of the left and right TOPL generate and store a complex associative network in which narrative, sequential analyses of perceptual details are meshed with a visuospatial map of the overall pattern of perceptions, and the whole is then colored with emotional significance.

The frontal–basal ganglia-limbic-thalamic (FBGLT) circuits are the primary regulators of 'action' in the physical and cognitive realms. In contrast to the schema-generating and storage function of the TOPL circuits, the FBGLT circuits are involved in the regulatory integration, monitoring, and control of existing schemata. FBGLT circuits are involved in such processes as the organization of learning, the retrieval of memories, the generation of multiple behavioral options, the ability to make context-appropriate choices, the formation of expectancies, the sustained execution of plans, and the suppression of inappropriate responses. Furthermore, the prefrontal cortex is the final common pathway for metacognitive processes such as self-monitoring, self-regulation, and self-consciousness (Stuss and Benson, 1987; Perecman, 1987).

The FBGLT circuits manifest lateralized differences similar to the posterior areas – including left frontal regulation of verbal, sequential, detail-oriented behavior, and right frontal regulation of configural, simultaneous, pattern-oriented processing. In addition, there is a striking functional divergence along the dorsal–ventral axis, with the dorsolateral prefrontal circuit and the ventrally located orbitomedial circuit enacting complementary roles of elaboration and inhibition over thoughts, emotions, and behavior (Mesulam, 1985; Cummings, 1993; Malloy and Richardson, 1994).

Clinical and experimental research suggests that a wide variety of delusional syndromes involve disruption of the ciruits which connect three basic modules:

the posterior perceptual-association and limbic circuits involved in interpreting the world;

the anterior motor-association, basal ganglia, and limbic structures involved in initiating and maintaining actions;

the prefrontal association areas involved in monitoring and controlling behaviors.

Specifically, structural or functional disconnection results in the excessive autonomy of functional units, with an oversimplification and perseveration of their functions. This results in their unmodulated domination over surrounding processes. For example, if impaired posterior TOPL circuits begin to free-run, unconstrained by prefrontal regulation, then surrounding circuits will be dominated by irrelevant schemata that prompt the false recognition of threat, alienness, or damage. Similarly, if anterior motor or speech-generating circuits are isolated from prefrontal regulation, one may become convinced that one's actions or verbally encoded thoughts are under external control or come from an alien source.

Application of the neuropsychological model to two psychiatric disorders

We will apply this neuropsychological model of delusional thinking to two common and debilitating psychopathological conditions, obsessive–compulsive disorder (OCD) and schizophrenia.

Obsessive–compulsive disorder

Let us consider OCD briefly insofar as it contributes to our understanding of delusional mechanisms (see Chapter 9 for in-depth discussion of neural network approaches to OCD). OCD is characterized by relentless, obsessional thoughts that one's world is full of specific dangers or contaminations. Patients cannot suppress these thoughts, which are associated with severe anxiety and which prompt either constant cleaning (of hands, objects, etc.) or endless compulsive checking (that the door is locked, that the gas is turned off). Neuropsychological, neuroimaging, and evoked potential studies consistently indicate that OCD involves dysfunction within a circuit linking the temporal pole of the limbic system (an area involved in anxious ideation), basal ganglia (especially the caudate nucleus, responsible for initiation of actions), and the orbitofrontal cortex (involved in suppressing nonadaptive responses) (Abbruzzese et al., 1995; Baxter et al., 1987, 1988; Malloy et al., 1989). The latter two areas are typically *hyper*metabolic in OCD, which suggests that the problem is not loss of function within these areas. Rather, there appears to be inadequate serotonergic activity within inhibitory projections connecting these three structures, resulting in inadequate negative feedback – a situation that can be pharmacologically ameliorated (Benkelfat et al., 1990; Insel and Winslow, 1992).

Thus, OCD illustrates the consequences of functionally disconnecting the temporo-limbic and basal ganglia structures known to be responsible for the recognition of danger, narrative elaboration, anxiety, and initiation of behavior, from the frontal areas responsible for suppressing inappropriate responses. Patients develop a stereotyped, anxiety-charged narrative that takes on a 'free-running' quality and cannot be inhibited. In many cases, the affected person realizes that the incessant thoughts are irrational; in some patients, however, the symptoms attain delusional proportions, resisting all attempts at factual demonstration and logic. As discussed previously, the model presented here makes the testable prediction that these two groups differ primarily in the intactness of frontal circuitry involved in the monitoring and evaluation of experience.

Schizophrenia: a pervasive reality distortion syndrome

This section summarizes some of the neurocognitive anomalies consistent with our model that may contribute to the formation of delusional beliefs in schizophrenia. Schizophrenia involves one or more episodes of sustained psychosis (delusions, hallucinations, severely disorganized behavior) with a significant loss of adaptive functioning. As every clinician knows, however, beyond this basic definition, patients with schizophrenia manifest a heterogeneous mix of possible symptoms and deficits, with no single lesion or dysfunction occurring in all cases of the disorder. Any truly integrative model of schizophrenia must therefore define its common biological substrate as a *pattern of functional (dis)organization* in the brain, one that allows for divergence among subjects in the details of impairment. In light of this consideration, it is fascinating that both neural network *hypo*connectivity and *hyper*connectivity have been proposed as central to the deficits of schizophrenia (David, 1994; Hemsley, 1994).

A first possible approach to defining neurocognitive impairment in schizophrenia emphasizes failures in automatic regulatory processes. For example, the P50 auditory event-related potential, which typically is inhibited when stimuli are repeated in close succession, has been used as an index of 'sensory gating,' or filtering of redundant stimuli. Many schizophrenics fail to inhibit this response to repeated stimuli, suggesting a failure of filtering that may lead to information overload and interference with selective attention (Freedman et al., 1987). Recent studies have found that absence of P50 gating is associated with altered semantic information processing, namely hyperpriming on a mainly automatic priming task (Vinogradov et al., 1996). This suggests that a failure of inhibitory controls over sensory perception may be coupled to overly productive, automatic associative processes in semantic memory.

A second approach focuses on regulatory failures in schizophrenia, but at the level of controlled (effort-based) processes, using tasks mediated by different regions of the frontal lobes and their projections. Such studies provide evidence of hypometabolism in the dorsolateral prefrontal cortex when schizophrenics engage in tasks requiring flexible problem-solving strategies, such as the Wisconsin Card Sort (WCS; Weinberger, Berman and Zec, 1986), and in the premotor, sensorimotor, and mesial frontal lobes during complex motor tasks (Guenther et al., 1994). Individuals affected by schizophrenia, however, do not show a uniform pattern of deficits affecting all aspects of prefrontal cortical function, and various measures of frontal integrity do not necessarily correlate highly with one another (Goldberg and Weinberger, 1988). This suggests considerable heterogeneity of the 'frontal syndrome' even within schizophrenia. For example, while Seidman et al. (1995) found schizophrenics to be severely impaired on the WCS and on two tasks thought to be sensitive to orbitofrontal integrity, Abbruzzese et al. (1995) only found WCS performance to be impaired.

To integrate these studies, Poole et al. (1996b) administered a battery of frontally related tasks to schizophrenics and normal controls, along with a computer-administered semantic priming procedure under conditions requiring either automatic or controlled information processing. The schizophrenics showed impairment on three, relatively independent, factor-derived indices: cognitive inflexibility, motor incoordination, and inhibitory failures. Inhibitory failures were associated with hyperpriming on an automatic semantic priming task. Cognitive inflexibility was associated with absence of priming on a mainly controlled semantic priming task. Motor incoordination was unrelated to both automatic and controlled semantic information processing. Individuals exhibited varying combinations of these deficits. Taken together, these studies suggest that, while impairment of FBGLT circuits is common in schizophrenia, individuals differ widely in terms of the exact structural and functional domains affected. Three affected sites are suggested: dorsolateral prefrontal with impaired formation of strategic sets, orbitofrontal with impaired inhibition of nonadaptive responses and 'hyperassociations,' and basal ganglia with impaired motor sequencing.

A third domain of neurocognitive analysis of schizophrenia is that of memory functions. These studies (e.g., Gold et al., 1992; Paulsen et al., 1995) typically find that the majority of memory difficulties in schizophrenia involve suboptimal organization of storage and retrieval processes, not true amnesia (i.e., failure to encode or maintain a stable memory trace). While simple recognition memory is typically intact, certain aspects of metarecognition, such as source monitoring and recall, are typically impaired (Harvey et al., 1988, 1990; Bentall et al., 1991). Source monitoring is that aspect of memory which involves tracking the origin of experiences and memories. Vinogradov et al. (1997) studied source monitoring in schizophrenia, using a task that required recall of whether words were generated by the subject, the experimenter, or were new. Schizophrenics had two types of source-monitoring anomalies: a failure to recognize items that were self-generated, and a response bias towards identifying items as experimenter generated. The net result was a tendency to say that self-generated items had an external source.

These findings of a projective, externalizing tendency in schizophrenics' memory processes parallel what is seen when causal expectancies are examined. Bentall (1994) found that delusional schizophrenics show an enhancement of the self-serving bias typically seen in normals, i.e., an exaggerated tendency to attribute negative outcomes to external causes and to attribute positive outcomes to one's own effort. These findings from memory and attribution studies suggest that in some schizophrenics, delusional beliefs may be rooted in an exaggeration of the normal cognitive biases towards projective externalization. In the study by Vinogradov et al. (1997), subjects with the worst source-monitoring performance had significantly higher ratings of unusual thought content, disorganized behavior, and motor incoordination – suggesting that these cognitive biases reflect a breakdown in self-regulation of thoughts and behavior. Liddle (1995) has proposed that the symptoms of schizophrenia reflect disorder of the supervisory mental processes responsible for initiation, selection, and monitoring of self-generated mental activity, and that the underlying neuropathology entails disordered functional connectivity within the neural networks of multimodal association cortex.

A fourth domain of cognitive analysis in schizophrenia focuses on perceptual accuracy. For example, impaired recognition of emotional cues (facial expression and vocal prosody) has been repeatedly documented in schizophrenia, with a severity comparable to that produced by right-hemispheric lesions (Borod et al., 1990, 1993). In a study that controlled for general cognitive level (IQ) and nonemotional perceptual abilities (facial and vocal discrimination), Poole et al. (1996a) found that inaccurate affect recognition was associated with the severity of schizophrenics' reality distortion (delusions, hallucinations), disorganization (loose associations, bizarre appearance/behavior), and cognitive symptoms (distractibility, stereotyped thinking). These findings suggest that some schizophrenics have a core disturbance of affect recognition, which may be differentiated from less-specific deficits, and is associated with psychotic symptoms, stereotyped thinking, and loss of attentional control.

Thus, depending on the subject sample – indeed, on the individual examined – schizophrenics show impairments in any of several relatively automatic perceptual/associative processes (sensory gating, semantic associations, affect recognition), as well as any of several relatively controlled monitoring/regulatory processes (organization of memory, source monitoring, strategy formation, response sequencing, response inhibition). We propose that no single one of these impairments is necessary or sufficient for schizophrenia, but that these diverse deficits reflect a single meta-organizational pattern: functional disconnection between the perceptual and the regulatory domains, resulting in stimulus-driven responses and autonomous, stereotyped mental productions.

Delusional thinking and neural network models

The discussion has so far been focused on the clinical and empirical evidence that supports a neural network approach to delusional thinking. However, several investigators have developed specific computational models that can be applied to the cognitive processes involved in delusional thinking. These models will be examined briefly and their salient features highlighted. Interestingly, the themes already discussed from a phenomenological, cognitive psychological, and neuropsychological/ neuroanatomical point of view – that is, functional disconnections between domains of information processing combined with hyperassociations within domains – resurface now in these various connectionist models.

Hoffman's model of positive symptoms in schizophrenia (1989/1993)

Hoffman and colleagues have developed a neural network model in which a disruption of communication between cortical areas leads to the characteristic symptoms of schizophrenia, including auditory hallucinations, experiences of thought broadcasting, delusions, and the paranoid state (Hoffman and Dobscha, 1989; Hoffman and McGlashan, 1993). They argue that diminished frontal metabolism in schizophrenic patients reflects a normal developmental process of axonal pruning gone awry. Citing evidence of dramatic reductions in synaptic density over the course of normal adolescence (Huttenlocher, 1979; Phelps and Chugani, 1986), Hoffman and his colleagues suggest that the 'hypofrontality' of schizophrenia results from a breakdown in the pruning shut-off mechanism that normally kicks in at around 16 years of age. This pathological and excessive neuronal pruning is the cornerstone of their neural network model of schizophrenia (Hoffman and McGlashan, 1994).

Hoffman and Dobscha's computer simulations of brain information processing use a Hopfield-type network in which each 'neuron' receives synaptic input from all other neurons. The authors explain that 'the behavior of a Hopfield network can be intuitively thought of as a physical system that tends to orient itself in certain stable "crystalline" structures . . . These structures correspond to specific, reproducible patterns of activation . . . [which] can be thought of as memories of the system' (Hoffman and Dobscha, 1989, p. 480). The connection weights are initially set from exemplar patterns (which function as attractors), so that a set of associations is encoded in the equilibrium state. The initializing input pattern serves as a 'seed.' Weights then remain fixed and only sequential updating of activation values takes place. Finally, the network is systematically pruned, i.e., network connections are functionally eliminated.

The results of the simulation show that when this network is over-pruned, patches of output activation patterns tend to fall into fixed, autonomous states that are inappropriate given the input. Additionally, these pathological outputs do not resemble any particular encoded memory and they repeatedly interfere with the overall flow of information in the system. Hoffman calls these pervasive and pathological outputs 'parasitic foci.'

According to this model, the emergence of parasitic foci within human cortical pathways contributes to the formation of positive symptoms in schizophrenia (Hoffman and McGlashan, 1993, 1994). For instance, a parasitic focus arising in cortical circuits responsible for speech perception will lead to 'factitious speech percepts' (p. 126), which might be experienced as verbal hallucinations (Hoffman and McGlashan, 1993). A parasitic focus falling in the communication pathways between speech production and speech perception areas could subtly influence or shape one's own *inner* thoughts and could simultaneously contort *external* auditory and verbal perceptions into the same mold (Hoffman et al., 1994). Experientially, one would (mis)perceive people as saying the same things one was thinking, which could result in symptoms of thought broadcasting or mind reading (Hoffman et al., 1994).

Hoffman and McGlashan carry this model a step further to illustrate how a parasitic focus in cortical association areas related to narrative memory might precipitate paranoid delusions. Specifically, they hypothesize that story memories would become dominated by a fixed, autonomous, and persistent associative activation pattern. Seemingly unrelated perceptions would easily trigger the parasitic focus which, given its observed tendency to dominate information flow, would consistently distort the schizophrenic patient's internal narrative. Due to the fixed nature of the parasitic focus, delusional beliefs would be resistant to disconfirming evidence.

In sum, this model relates reduced synaptic density caused by excessive axonal pruning in schizophrenia to a loss of control of narrative memory, which ultimately results in the formation of delusions. This model suggests that functional disconnection (excessive axonal pruning) between certain cortical circuits results in autonomous, hyperactive information flow within pathological and pervasive output patterns (parasitic foci).

Cohen and Servan-Schreiber's model of disturbances in the processing of context in schizophrenia (1992)

Cohen and Servan-Schreiber have constructed a neural network model that relates the neuromodulatory effects of dopamine in the prefrontal cortex to information processing deficits in schizophrenia. The authors point out that the cognitive impairments observed in schizophrenics on attentional and lexical disambiguation tasks commonly reflect a deficit in the processing of contextual information. They cite evidence that the prefrontal cortex plays an important role in the processing of contextual information (Goldman-Rakic, 1987a, 1987b; Diamond and Goldman-Rakic, 1989) and that the proper functioning of the prefrontal cortex is dependent on the neuromodulatory effects of mesocortical dopamine projections (Levin, 1984; Weinberger, Berman and Chase, 1988). Using a computer model, Cohen and Servan-Schreiber explain how reduced dopaminergic tone in the prefrontal cortex may directly influence the processing of contextual information.

The authors begin by constructing back-propagation network models that simulate normal human performance on attentional and lexical disambiguation tasks. Although the models require architectural modifications for each task, they share some common features, including a 'discourse module.' The discourse module is important as it holds a representation of general information about context. For instance, in the lexical disambiguation task, given the phrase 'without a pen . . . you can't sign a check' or the phrase 'without a pen . . . you can't keep chickens,' the subject must interpret the appropriate meaning of the ambiguous word 'pen' given the context in which it is used. While the semantic module processes the meaning of individual words, the discourse module processes or holds the meaning of the phrase. Network information cycles in and out of the semantic and discourse modules; the meaning of individual words (e.g., keep chickens or sign a check) influences the interpretation of a phrase and vice versa.

To simulate schizophrenics' performance on these tasks, the authors reduce their model's dopamine analogue: the gain parameter. The gain parameter functions as a multiplier for the effects of excitatory and inhibitory inputs to the unit, and thus is analogous to a neuromodulator. When the gain is reduced in the discourse module, presumably analogous to reduced mesocortical dopamine activity in the prefrontal cortex, the network's performance closely resembles that of schizophrenic patients. This occurs on all of the cognitive tasks, and only when the gain parameter in the discourse module of each model is reduced. Cohen and Servan-Schreiber interpret these results as support for their hypothesis that schizophrenic deficits in attention and language-processing tasks are a consequence of reduced dopaminergic activity in the prefrontal cortex. When gain is reduced, the effects of both excitatory and inhibitory inputs to cortical circuits are reduced, which in turn has an impact on information processing and memory functions, especially those related to the processing of context.

The authors do not specifically address how these cognitive deficits might lead to the clinical symptoms of schizophrenia. Nevertheless, they argue that their modeling approach provides a powerful and much-needed tool for exploring the complex connections between physiology and behavior. They postulate a decrease in the dopaminergic 'gain function' to the prefrontal cortex, which implies a functional hypoconnectivity between mesolimbic areas and their dopaminergic projections to prefrontal cortex. They also emphasize that this results in inadequate processing of contextual or discourse level information by the prefrontal cortex, a notion that echoes some of the metamemory (source-monitoring) deficits explored earlier in this chapter.

Vinogradov, King, and Huberman: spread of activation, phase transitions, and the paranoid process (1992a)

Vinogradov and her associates have proposed a spreading activation network model of the process of delusion formation with an emphasis on discrete phase transitions in the network. This process occurs along a phenomenological continuum that can be viewed in three overlapping stages. The first is that of the initial paranoid state, when the predisposed individual experiences a sense of connections or associations among temporally contiguous perceptions. In the second stage, the individual begins to assign meaning to these associations, and ultimately a self-generated schema is learned that allows the individual to explain his or her experience. Finally, by the third stage, with this explanatory schema in place, the delusion becomes crystalized and self-perpetuating. New perceptions and events not only become connected to a past set of associations, they serve to confirm the ever-more tenaciously held delusional beliefs and thus become integrated into the explanatory schema itself.

Vinogradov et al. suggest that the initial paranoid state, which is best characterized as one of overactivation or hyperconnectivity, can be described with a neural nework model of memory formation. This state results from the dynamic interplay among three model parameters: (1) the average number of links per node; (2) the weights for each link; and (3) the relaxation rate of an individual node. Abnormally large numbers of links between nodes, abnormally large link weightings, and/or an abnormally sluggish node relaxation rate could create an overactive, hyperassociative network state where temporally contiguous perceptions become pathologically 'connected' to one another, as is the case in the initial paranoid state.

Vinogradov et al. carry this model a step further to explain the process by which this initial paranoid state becomes crystalized into a fixed delusion. Changes in the network parameters (links per node, weights per link, or relaxation rate) will precipitate major changes in the behavior of networks, leading to abrupt phase transitions characterized by an explosive growth in the expansiveness of network activation (Shrager, Hogg and Huberman, 1987). The hyperassociative network state (the paranoid state) is already predisposed to form more connections among events or perceptions; as the number of these connections or links grows, computer simulations show that an abrupt phase transition occurs (Fig. 8.1). It is manifested by an explosion of network activation such that a single giant cluster of nodes becomes activated. The charac-

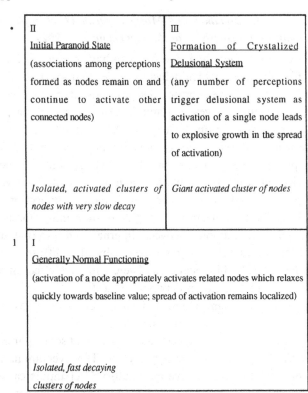

Fig. 8.1 Phase diagram for the characteristics of spreading activation networks as a function of the number of links per node, the weights per link, and the relaxaiton rate of network nodes. (Adapted from Vinogradov et al., 1992a.)

teristics of the spreading activation network in this phase are analogous to those that occur in the crystalization of the fixed delusion where any number of various perceptions, experiences, and thoughts can trigger expression of the entire delusional system.

This neural network model suggests that hyperconnectivity within a given cortical circuit, perhaps related to decreased inhibitory processes influencing the circuit, leads to the delusional patient's initial experience of associations between a variety of events. Hyperconnectivity within the memory network ultimately results in abrupt phase transitions and thus in the formation of a fixed, crystalized delusion.

Krieckhaus, Donahoe, and Morgan: paranoid schizophrenia and
dopamine hyperactivity in the hippocampus (1992)

Krieckhaus, Donahoe, and Morgan have presented a model of paranoid schizophrenia in which delusions arise from aberrations in the consolidation of declarative memory. They propose that this dysfunctional process results from changes in synaptic connections in the parietal-temporal-occipital association cortex (PTO). These changes in PTO connective networks are secondary to their modulatory inputs from dopamine D2 hypersensitive neurons in the CA1 region of the hippocampus. Krieckhaus et al. postulate that long-term, declarative memory stores are 'embodied' in the numerous synaptic connection strengths in the PTO. These connection strengths are normally modified as a result of complex interactions between internal and external inputs. They are further modified – or reinforced – by the diffuse modulatory inputs from the CA1 hippocampus. The cumulative effect of these reinforcing inputs is to strengthen network connections that are consistently paired. That is, these reinforcement signals strengthen the associations between perceptions that warrant association.

Krieckhaus et al. suggest that in paranoid schizophrenia, CA1 neurons of the hippocampus are hyperactive. The overstimulation of PTO networks by the hyperactive modulatory CA1 inputs causes inappropriate connections to be strengthened. As a result, unrelated and temporally contiguous perceptions are experienced as strongly associated and interconnected. This hyperassociative state ultimately leads to the formation of delusions. The model also explains the ameliorating effects of D2 dopamine antagonists (neuroleptics) on delusions: presumably, dopamine-hypersensitive CA1 hippocampal neurons are rendered less sensitive by these agents, which reduces the overstimulation of the PTO memory networks.

Like Cohen and Servan-Schreiber's work, this model examines the modulatory effect of dopaminergic tone on information-processing circuits, although here it is a case of increased gain on memory circuits in PTO, rather than reduced gain on discourse or context circuits in prefrontal cortex. Like Vinogradov et al.'s model, Krieckhaus and colleagues propose that unrelated and temporally contiguous perceptions are experienced as strongly related because of a hyperassociative state in memory circuits – and that this gives rise to paranoid delusions. Though not explicitly stated, one might infer that CA1 dopamine overactivity could be a result of impaired inhibitory input to this area from frontal afferents (as suggested in Weinberger's neurodevelopmental model of schizophrenia, 1987).

Chen's model of cortical information processing in schizophrenia (1994/1995)

Recently, Chen has developed a model similar to Hoffman's (Hoffman and Dobscha, 1989) in its design and function, but Chen considers the additional roles of dopaminergic modulation, of cognitive overload, and of hippocampal dysfunction in schizophrenia through treatment of different intrinsic parameters within the neural network (Chen, 1994, 1995; also see Chapter 3 by Chen and Berrios).

Chen observes that when the level of noise in his neural network model is reduced, a situation analogous to increased dopaminergic suppression of random firing in cortical neurons, 'spurious attractors' – the fixed and autonomous activation patterns that Hoffman calls parasitic foci – become prevalent throughout the network. These spurious attractors in turn lead to the formation of delusions, presumably through the same hypothetical mechanisms detailed by Hoffman (see the discussion of Hoffman's model above).

Chen also details the effects of bombarding the information-processing network with a high degree of input relative to processing capacity, analogous to high cognitive demands placed upon an individual under excessive stress. This high memory loading in the neural network results in parasitic foci dominating the network. Chen proposes that his model provides evidence for the interaction of both biological and social factors in the formation of psychotic symptoms. An increase in the dopamine-mediated suppression of the random firing of cortical neurons in biologically predisposed individuals, paired with stressful social factors such as those prevalent in early adulthood, may precipitate delusional thinking through aberrant information processing in memory systems.

Chen goes on to simulate the effects of dysfunctional hippocampal–cortical communication. Rolls (1989, cited in Chen, 1995) has argued that hippocampal processing of information serves to 'orthogonize' input such that overlapping or correlated incoming events (e.g., perceptions) are coded onto cortical output patterns that are separated from one another. Chen experiments with this process by presenting input patterns that have varying degrees of overlap to his neural network, modeling a possible aspect of hippocampal dysfunction in schizophrenia.

His results indicate that a failure in input orthogonization could lead to delusional thinking. Chen finds that the higher the degree of input pattern overlap, the more prevalent the same fixed and meaningless output patterns (parasitic foci) become. This occurs even under circumstances of relatively low cognitive load. Chen notes that such a failure in input orthogonization, i.e., a failure to separate input patterns, would result in the categorization difficulties that have been observed in schizophrenia (Chen, Wilkins and McKenna, 1994). Such deficits may play a role in establishing the cognitive biases that precipitate delusional thinking.

Like Vinogradov and Krieckhaus, Chen underscores the important role played by inputs becoming associated, though he uses different terminology. Similarly to Vinogradov, he infers that this hyperassociation plays a causative role in producing abnormally functioning memory circuits (for Krieckhaus, abnormal memory associations are the result of overactive dopamine input). Like Krieckhaus, Chen focuses on dopamine overactivity and its effects on cortical information processing; Krieckhaus and Chen also both assign a deficit to the hippocampus. However, as does Hoffman, Chen examines the role of lack of communication between cortical circuits (excessive pruning for Hoffman, decreased random firing or noise for Chen), which results in autonomously functioning cicuits or parasitic foci. Somewhat similarly to Cohen and Servan-Schreiber, Chen looks into the effect of cognitive overload on overall information processing in the system (Cohen and Servan-Schreiber would call it decreased dopamine to prefrontal cortex), and concludes that it impairs the ability of the system to engage in contextual processing – a sort of 'dopamine steal' syndrome.

Ruppin et al.'s attractor network model for positive psychotic symptoms in schizophrenia (1995)

Ruppin and colleagues (1995) have proposed a neural network model for delusions and hallucinations in schizophrenia in which synaptic degeneration in inputs is accompanied by an increase in local connections in the network (the analog of new synaptogenesis). In this attractor network, general memory retrieval was normal, but there was spontaneous activation on noncued memory patterns when either the noise in the system or the strength of internal connections increased beyond a certain threshold level. Like the positive symptoms of schizophrenia, the spontaneous retrieval bias of this network was both self-limiting and self-reinforcing; it is suggestive of the response biases seen in schizophrenic patients on source memory tasks (e.g., the response bias towards labeling internal events as externally generated – see Vinogradov et al., 1997). In addition, this model generated interesting predictions about the pathophysiology and psychopathology of schizophrenia: the notion of synaptic compensation for the degenerated inputs, the notion of increased spontaneous neural activity in these attractor networks, and the well-known clinical phenomenon of environmental cuing of delusional memory retrieval.

An integration of the neural network models

Let us now integrate these six models, with an emphasis on the features they share that are most pertinent to delusional thinking.

1. All of the models point, either explicitly or implicitly, to the important role played by a functional disconnection between domains of brain information processing. Decreased communication between cortical circuits and/or frontal–hippocampal circuits are most often emphasized (excessive pruning – Hoffman, Ruppin; reduced dopamine input to prefrontal cortex with impairment in discourse or contextual level processing – Cohen and Servan-Schreiber; decreased inhibitory processes to memory association circuits and/ or hippocampus – Vinogradov, Krieckhaus, Chen; decreased random firing in cortical neurons – Chen).

2. Nearly all of the models focus on hyperassociation within memory circuits with pathological and autonomously functioning output patterns (parasitic foci – Hoffman; increased connectivity with abrupt phase transitions in memory circuits – Vinogradov; increase in local connections with spontaneous activation of noncued memory patterns – Ruppin; hyperassociative state in PTO memory circuits – Krieckhaus; spurious attractors – Chen).

3. Several of the models either explicitly or implicitly acknowledge the general effect of cognitive overload, cognitive limitations, and/or excessive activation of limbic areas, i.e., emotional overload and stress (reduced functional capacity of prefrontal cortex – Cohen and Servan-Schreiber; tendency of the system to overload and move towards abnormal states of activation – Vinogradov, Chen, Ruppin).

4. Three of the models underscore the importance of integrating the role of dopamine neuromodulation into models of brain information processing, especially those involving context-processing or

monitoring functions and memory formation (Cohen and Servan-Schreiber, Krieckhaus, Chen).

Future directions

Convergent evidence from cognitive psychology, neuropsychology, and neural network modeling supports the idea that delusional thinking is the result of two fundamental aspects of brain function gone awry:

1. a disconnection that occurs between normally integrated domains of cortical information processing (overall central monitoring and/or inhibitory functions are disconnected from memory association/ schemata formation);
2. a form of 'free-running' overdrive or hyperconnectivity that occurs within given isolated regions of memory formation, expectations, association, and retrieval – with pathological outputs as the result.

This approach allows us to answer two questions about delusional thinking that have long perplexed psychopathologists. The first is the notion of severity. If brain pathology exists along a continuum of dysfunction, as it almost certainly does, then it makes sense that there may be milder or more severe forms of delusional thinking (improbable delusions *vs* impossible delusions), depending on a person's level of neurobiologic dysfunction. Second, a formal, cognitive approach allows those of us who are clinicians to move beyond the perplexing and often bizarre contents of our patients' delusions to reflect on the ways in which brain pathology interacts with environmental and intrapsychic stressors to give rise to the unique signs and symptoms of each individual.

As neural network models of psychopathology become more sophisticated, they will obviously need to address the important questions of variation. First, what is the effect on the overall information-processing system when one varies the relative contributions of the two domains of malfunction described above? Second, what is the effect of varying the extent and severity of the malfunctions, both independently and concomitantly? Third, might there be variations in the underlying causes of malfunction? We suggest that such variations in real brain systems account for the large clinical heterogeneity observed in patients with delusional thinking – from the almost-believable and well-circumscribed preoccupations of the erotomanic, to the disorganized, kaleidoscopic delusions of the schizophrenic, to the patently absurd 'stuck loop' of the severely obsessive–compulsive patient.

Finally, a major challenge for models of the future will be to integrate the contributions of the following.

1. Premorbid biases in the system. How do an individual's psychodynamics (prior memory records) influence the formation of delusions? At the same time, why, despite an almost infinite number of idosyncratic variations, is there so much thematic coherence to patients' delusional systems? As Sedler (1995) puts it: 'The frequency with which certain themes recur – jealousy, persecution, grandiose ideas, somatic ideas – long has provided a basis for subtyping delusions but this alone fails to tell us whether these themes are biographically pregnant or simply general categories of human interest gone awry' (p. 258).

2. Affective state and emotional valence. What are the contributions of emotional state to the initiation and sustenance of delusional thinking? How do certain delusions obtain a strong negative emotional valence, while others have a neutral or even more positive valence? How is the role of affect different in delusions associated with mood disorders from those associated with thinking disorders?

3. The subjective sense of 'relief' and the inherently rewarding properties of the delusional system. What accounts for the relief that delusions provide? Why is having an explanation experienced by the human brain so rewarding? Dopamine release is triggered by surprise or unmet expectations; does an explanatory system reduce anxiety-producing dopamine overdrive?

4. The role of certainty. Why do delusional individuals have such a high degree of conviction or certainty about their beliefs? How is the level of certainty signaled? Why is this certainty not open to feedback or evidence to the contrary? What is the role of dopaminergic (and/or serotonergic) overdrive in the development of pathological certainty?

5. Brain dopamine systems. What is the possible relationship between the formation of delusions and brain dopamine systems that mediate responses to novelty/unmet expectations? Are delusions a means the brain can use to change inputs that are experienced as unexpected/novel/surprising into inputs that are expected (and so decrease dopaminergic tone)?

6. Integration with current findings in laboratory neuroscience. Multiple unit recording in primates of cortical representations of auditory stimuli in primary auditory cortex is mappable,

manipulable, and subject to refinement (Recanzone, Schreiner and Merzenich, 1993). Multiple unit intracortical recording experiments in primates have also conclusively demonstrated that structuring the expectation for a particular visual stimulus will modify its representation in primary visual cortex (Desimone and Duncan, 1995). In other words, expectation results both in a widespread inhibition of extrinsic stimulus-driven responses within the cerebral cortex and in a positive and highly specific representation of the 'remembered' (expected) events (Desimone and Duncan, 1995). Expectancy signals are likely to be powerful, distributed inhibitory and excitatory effects from frontal cortex sources; the role of expectation as a factor in the accuracy of perceptual responses (representations in primary sensory cortex) is a new area of laboratory neuroscience investigation, one that will generate valuable empirical data in the coming years (Susan Smiga and Michael Merzenich, personal communication). Neural network models of normal brain function will need to account for the net balance between input signals, intrinsic cortico-cortical connections, and output variables in the maintenance of associational relationships between stimulus expectations and stimulus representations, yet allow for cognitive and perceptual flexibility. Models of psychopathology will have the far more daunting task of coherently describing breakdowns in one or another of this elaborate set of interrelated processes.

The implications of neural network approaches to delusional thinking are sure to be far reaching. As hinted at by this last factor, future research will touch not just upon the study of psychopathology, but upon our understanding of normal human brain function as well, including the complex associational relationships between expectations (cortical representations of remembered events) and ongoing perceptions (cortical representations of current stimuli). As we understand more clearly what makes a delusion, we will gain new insights into the power of rigid belief systems and extremist dogma in general, into their emotionally and cognitively rewarding aspects, and into our ability as human beings to see only what we want to see and to be seduced and manipulated by simplistic explanatory schemes.

References

Abbruzzese, M., Bellodi, L., Ferri, S., & Scarone, S. (1995). Frontal lobe dysfunction in schizophrenia and obsessive–compulsive disorder: a neuropsychological study. *Brain and Cognition*, **27**, 202–12.

Alexander, M., Stuss, D. T. & Benson, D. F. (1979). Capgras syndrome: a reduplicative phenomenon. *Neurology*, **29**, 334–9.

Anderson, J. R. (1983). *The Architecture of Cognition*. Cambridge, Mass: Harvard University Press.

Baer, D. (1979). Temporal lobe epilepsy: A syndrome of sensory-limbic hyperconnection. *Cortex*, **15**, 357–84.

Baxter, L. J., Thompson, J. M., Schwartz, J. M. et al. (1987). Trazodone treatment response in obsessive–compulsive disorder correlated with shifts in glucose metabolism in the caudate nuclei. *Psychopathology*, **20**, 114–22.

Baxter, L. J., Schwartz, J. M., Mazziotta, J. C. et al. (1988). Cerebral glucose metabolic rates in nondepressed patients with obsessive–compulsive disorder. *American Journal of Psychiatry*, **145**, 1560–3.

Benioff, L. (1995). What is it like to have schizophrenia? In *Treating Schizophrenia*, ed. S. Vinogradov, pp. 81–107. San Francisco: Jossey Bass.

Benkelfat, C., Nordahl, T. E., Semple, W. E. et al. (1990). Local cerebral glucose metabolic rates in obsessive–compulsive disorder: Patients treated with clomipramine. *Archives of General Psychiatry*, **47**, 840–8.

Benson, D. F., Gardner, H. & Meadows, J. C. (1976). Reduplicative paramnesia. *Neurology*, **26**, 147–61.

Bentall, R. P. (1994). Cognitive biases and abnormal beliefs: Towards a model of persecutory delusions. In *The Neuropsychology of Schizophrenia*, ed. A. S. David & J. C. Cutting. Hove, UK: Lawrence Erlbaum Associates.

Bentall, R. P., Baker, G. A. & Havers, S. (1991). Reality monitoring and psychotic hallucinations. *British Journal of Clinical Psychology*, **30**(Pt 3), 213–22.

Berrios, G. E. (1991). Delusions as 'wrong beliefs': a conceptual history. *British Journal of Psychiatry*, **159** Suppl., 6–13.

Bigler, E. D. (1988). *Diagnostic and Clinical Neuropsychology*. Austin: University of Texas Press.

Borod, J. C., Martin, C. C., Alpert, M., Brozgold, A. & Welkowitz, J. (1993). Perception of facial emotion in schizophrenic and right brain-damaged patients. *Journal of Nervous Mental Disease*, **181**, 494–502.

Borod, J. C., Welkowitz, J., Alpert, M. et al. (1990). Parameters of emotional processing in neuropsychiatric disorders: Conceptual issues and a battery of tests. *Journal of Communicable Diseases*, **23**, 247–71.

Brandt, J., Seidman, L. J. & Kohl, D. (1985). Personality characteristics of epileptic patients: a controlled study of generalized and temporal lobe cases. *Journal of Experimental and Clinical Neuropsychology*, **7**, 25–38.

Braun, C. M. & Chouinard, M. J. (1992). Is anorexia nervosa a neuropsychological disease? *Neuropsychology Review*, **3**, 171–212.

Brennan, J. H. & Hemsley, D. R. (1984). Illusory correlations in paranoid and non-paranoid schizophrenia. *British Journal of Clinical Psychology*, **23**, 225–6.

Brockington, I. (1991). Factors involved in delusion formation. *British Journal of Psychiatry*, **159** Suppl., 42–5.

Broga, M. I. & Neufeld, R. W. (1981). Multivariate cognitive performance levels and response styles among paranoid and nonparanoid schizophrenics. *Journal of Abnormal Psychology*, **90**, 495–509.

Carter, C. S., Robertson, L. C., Nordahl, T. E., O'Shora-Celaya, L. J. & Chaderjian, M. C. (1993). Abnormal processing of irrelevant information in schizophrenia: the role of illness subtype. *Psychiatry Research*, **48**, 17–26.

Chapman, L. J. & Chapman, J. P. (1988). The genesis of delusions. In *Delusional Belief*, ed. T. F. Oltmanns & B. A. Maher, pp. 167–83. New York: John Wiley and Sons.

Chapman, L. J., Edell, W. A. & Chapman, J. P. (1980). Physical anhedonia, perceptual aberration, and psychosis proneness. *Schizophrenia Bulletin*, **6**, 639–53.

Chen, E. Y. (1994). A neural network model of cortical information processing in schizophrenia. I: Interaction between biological and social factors in symptom formation. *Canadian Journal of Psychiatry*, **39**, 362–7.

Chen, E. Y. (1995). A neural network model of cortical information processing in schizophrenia. II: role of hippocampal–cortical interaction: a review and a model. *Canadian Journal of Psychiatry*, **40**, 21–6.

Chen, E. Y., Wilkins, A. J. & McKenna, P. J. (1994). Semantic memory is both impaired and anomalous in schizophrenia. *Psychological Medicine*, **24**, 193–202.

Clare, L., McKenna, P. J., Mortimer, A. M. & Baddeley, A. D. (1993). Memory in schizophrenia: what is impaired and what is preserved? *Neuropsychologia*, **31**, 1225–41.

Cohen, J. D. & Servan-Schreiber, D. (1992). Context, cortex, and dopamine: a connectionist approach to behavior and biology in schizophrenia. *Psychological Review*, **99**, 45–77.

Collins, A. M. & Loftus, E. F. (1975). A spreading-activation theory of semantic processing. *Psychological Review*, **82**, 407–28.

Cummings, J. L. (1993). Frontal–subcortical circuits and human behavior. *Archives of Neurology*, **50**, 873–80.

Cummings, J. L. & Victoroff, J. I. (1990). Noncognitive neuropsychiatric syndromes in Alzheimer's disease. *Neuropschiatry, Neuropsychology and Behavioral Neurology*, **3**, 140–58.

Damasio, A. R., Tranel, D. & Damasio, H. (1990). Face agnosia and the neural substrates of memory. *Annual Review of Neuroscience*, **13**, 89–109.

David, A. S. (1994). Dysmodularity: a neurocognitive model for schizophrenia. *Schizophrenia Bulletin*, **20**, 249–55.

Desimone, R. & Duncan, J. (1995). Neural mechanisms of selective visual attention. *Annual Review of Neuroscience*, **18**, 193–222.

Diamond, A. & Goldman-Rakic, P. S. (1989). Comparison of human infants and rhesus monkeys on Piaget's AB task: evidence for dependence on dorsolateral prefrontal cortex. *Experimental Brain Research*, **74**, 24–40.

Drevets, W. C. & Rubin, E. H. (1989). Psychotic symptoms and the longitudinal course of senile dementia of the Alzheimer's type. *Biological Psychiatry*, **25**, 39–40.

Fedio, P. (1986). Behavioral characteristics of patients with temporal lobe epilepsy. *Psychiatric Clinics of North America*, **9**, 267–81.

Flor-Henry, P. (1983). Hemisyndrome of temporal lobe epilepsy: Review of evidence relating psychopathological manifestations in epilepsy to right-

and left-sided epilepsy. In *Hemisyndromes: Psychobiology, Neurology, and Psychiatry*, ed. M. S. Myslobodsky, pp. 149–94. New York: Academic Press.

Freedman, R., Adler, L. E., Gerhardt, G. A. et al. (1987). Neurobiological studies of sensory gating in schizophrenia. *Schizophrenia Bulletin*, **13**, 669–78.

Frith, C. D. & Done, D. J. (1989). Experiences of alien control in schizophrenia reflect a disorder in the central monitoring of action. *Psychological Medicine*, **19**, 359–63.

Fuster, J. M. (1995). *Memory in the Cerebral Cortex: An Empirical Approach to Neural Networks in the Human and Nonhuman Primate*. Cambridge, MA: MIT Press.

Garety, P. A., Hemsley, D. R. & Wessely, S. (1991). Reasoning in deluded schizophrenic and paranoid patients. Biases in performance on a probabilistic inference task. *Journal of Nervous and Mental Diseases*, **179**, 194–201.

Globus, G. G. & Arpaia, J. P. (1994). Psychiatry and the new dynamics. *Biological Psychiatry*, **35**, 352–64.

Gold, J. M., Randolph, C., Carpenter, C. J., Goldberg, T. E. & Weinberger, D. R. (1992). Forms of memory failure in schizophrenia. *Journal of Abnormal Psychology*, **101**, 487–94.

Goldberg, G., Mayer, N. H. & Toglia, J. U. (1981). Medial frontal cortex infarction and the alien hand sign. *Archives of Neurology*, **38**, 683–6.

Goldberg, T. E. & Weinberger, D. R. (1988). Probing prefrontal function in schizophrenia with neuropsychological paradigms. *Schizophrenia Bulletin*, **14**, 179–83.

Goldman-Rakic, P. S. (1987a). Circuitry of primate prefrontal cortex and regulation of behavior by representational memory. In *Handbook of Physiology – The Nervous System*, ed. F. Plum & V. Mountcastle, pp. 373–417. Bethesda, MD: American Physiological Society.

Goldman-Rakic, P. S. (1987b). Circuitry of the frontal association cortex and its relevance to dementia. *Archives of Gerontology and Geriatrics*, **6**, 299–309.

Guenther, W., Brodie, J. D., Bartlett, E. J. et al. (1994). Diminished cerebral metabolic response to motor stimulatition in schizophrenics: A PET study. *European Archives of Psychiatry and Clincal Neuroscience*, **244**, 115–25.

Gur, R. E., Mozley, P. D., Shtasel, D. L. et al. (1994). Clinical subtypes of schizophrenia: differences in brain and CSF volume. *American Journal of Psychiatry*, **151**, 343–50.

Hakim, H., Verma, N. P. & Greiffenstein, M. F. (1988). Pathogenesis of reduplicative paramnesia. *Journal of Neurology, Neurosurgery, and Psychiatry*, **51**, 839–41.

Harrow, M., Rattenbury, F. & Stoll, F. (1988). Schizophrenic delusions: An analysis of their persistence, of related premorbid ideas, and of three major dimensions. In *Delusional Beliefs*, ed. T. F. Oltmanns & B. A. Maher, pp. 184–211. New York: John Wiley and Sons.

Harvey, P. D., Docherty, N. M., Serper, M. R. & Rasmussen, M. (1990). Cognitive deficits and thought disorder: II: An 8-month followup study. *Schizophrenia Bulletin*, **16**, 147–56.

Harvey, P. D., Earle-Boyer, E. a. & Levinson, J. C. (1988). Cognitive deficits and thought disorder: a retest study. *Schizophrenia Bulletin*, **14**, 57–66.

226   Sophia Vinogradov, John H. Poole and Jason Willis-Shore

Hemsley, D. R. (1994). A cognitive model for schizophrenia and its possible neural basis. *Acta Psychiatrica Scandinavica*, **384** (Suppl.), 80–6.

Henik, A., Nissimov, E., Priel, B. & Umansky, R. (1995). Effects of cognitive load on semantic priming in patients with schizophrenia. *Journal of Abnormal Psychology*, **104**, 576–84.

Henik, A., Priel, B. & Umanksy, R. (1992). Attention and automaticity in semantic processing of schizophrenic patients. *Neuropsychiatry, Neuropsychology, & Behavioral Neurology*, **5**, 161–9.

Hermann, B. P. & Riel, P. (1981). Interictal personality and behavioral traits in temporal lobe and generalized epilepsy. *Cortex*, **17**, 125–8.

Hermann, B. P. & Whitman, S. (1984). Behavioral and personality correlates of epilepsy: a review, methodological critique, and conceptual model. *Psychological Bulletin*, **95**, 451–97.

Hoffman, R. E. & Dobscha, S. K. (1989). Cortical pruning and the development of schizophrenia: a computer model. *Schizophrenia Bulletin*, **15**, 77–90.

Hoffman, R. E. & McGlashan, T. H. (1993). Parallel distributed processing and the emergence of schizophrenic symptoms. *Schizophrenia Bulletin*, **19**, 19–40.

Hoffman, R. E. & McGlashan, T. H. (1994). Corticocortical connectivity, autonomous networks, and schizophrenia [comment]. *Schizophrenia Bulletin*, **20**, 257–61.

Hoffman, R. E., Oates, E., Hafner, R. J., Hustig, H. H. & McGlashan, T. H. (1994). Semantic organization of hallucinated 'voices' in schizophrenia. *American Journal of Psychiatry*, **151**, 1229–30.

Huq, S. F., Garety, P. A. & Hemsley, D. R. (1988). Probabilistic judgements in deluded and non-deluded subjects. *Journal of Experimental Psychology*, **40**, 801–12.

Huttenlocher, P. R. (1979). Synaptic density in human frontal cortex – developmental changes and effects of aging. *Brain Research*, **163**, 195–205.

Insel, T. R. & Winslow, J. T. (1992). Neurobiology of obsessive compulsive disorder. *Psychiatry Clinics of North America*, **15**, 813–24.

Jaspers, K. (1946). *General Psychopathology*, transl. 1963, J. Hoenig & M. W. Hamilton. Manchester: Manchester University Press.

Jobe, T. H., Harrow, M., Martin, E. M., Whitfield, H. J. & Sands, J. R. (1994). Schizophrenic deficits: neuroleptics and the prefrontal cortex. *Schizophrenia Bulletin*, **20**, 413–6; discussion 417–21.

Johnson, M. K. (1988). Discriminating the origin of information. In *Delusional Beliefs*, ed. T. F. Oltmanns & B. A. Maher, pp. 34–65. New York: John Wiley and Sons.

Kaney, S. & Bentall, R. P. (1992). Persecutory delusions and the self-serving bias. Evidence from a contingency judgment task. *Journal of Nervous and Mental Diseases*, **180**, 773–80.

Killackey, H. P. (1990). The neocortex in memory storage. In *Brain Organization and Memory: Cells, Systems, and Circuits*, ed. J. L. McGaugh, N. M. Weinberger & G. Lynch, pp. 265–70. New York: Oxford University Press.

Kremen, W. S., Seidman, L. J., Goldstein, J. M., Faraone, S. V. & Tsuang, M. T. (1994). Systematized delusions and neuropsychological function in paranoid and nonparanoid schizophrenia. *Schizophrenia Research*, **12**, 223–36.

Krieckhaus, E. E., Donahoe, J. W. & Morgan, M. A. (1992). Paranoid schizophrenia may be caused by dopamine hyperactivity of CA1 hippocampus. *Biological Psychiatry*, **31**, 60–70.

Kwapil, T. R., Hegley, D. C., Chapman, L. J. & Chapman, J. P. (1990). Facilitation of word recognition by semantic priming in schizophrenia. *Journal of Abnormal Psychology*, **99**, 215–21.

Langell, M. E., Purisch, A. D. & Golden, C. J. (1987). Neuropsychological differences between paranoid and nonparanoid schizophrenics in the Luria–Nebraska Battery. *International Journal of Clinical Neuropsychology*, **9**, 88–95.

LaRusso, L. (1978). Sensitivity of paranoid patients to nonverbal cues. *Journal of Abnormal Psychology*, **87**, 463–71.

Levin, S. (1984). Frontal lobe dysfunctions in schizophrenia. II: Impairments of psychological and brain functions. *Journal of Psychiatry Research*, **18**, 7–72.

Liddle, P. F. (1995). Inner connections within domain of dementia praecox: role of supervisory mental processes in schizophrenia. *European Archives of Psychiatry and Clinical Neuroscience*, **245**(4–5), 210–15.

Louza, M. R. & Maurer, K. (1989). Differences between paranoid and nonparanoid schizophrenic patients on the somatosensory P300 event-related potential. *Neuropsychobiology*, **21**, 59–66.

Magaro, P. A. (1981). The paranoid and the schizophrenic: the case of distinct cognitive style. *Schizophrenia Bulletin*, **7**, 632–61.

Maher, B. A. (1974). Delusional thinking and perceptual disorder. *Journal of Individual Psychology*, **30**, 98–113.

Maher, B. A. (1988). Delusions as the product of normal cognition. In *Delusional Beliefs*, ed. T. F. Oltmanns & B. A. Maher, pp. 333–6. New York: John Wiley and Sons.

Malenka, R. C., Angel, R. W., Thiemann, S., Weitz, C. J. & Berger, P. A. (1987). Central error-correcting behavior in schizophrenia and depression. *Biological Psychiatry*, **21**, 263–73.

Malloy, P., Cimino, C. & Westlake, R. (1992). Differential diagnosis of primary and secondary Capgras delusions. *Neuropsychiatry, Neuropsychology, and Behavioral Neurology*, **5**, 83–96.

Malloy, P. & Duffy, (1994). The frontal lobes in neuropsychiatric disorders. In *Handbook of Neuropsychology*, Vol. 9, ed. F. Boller & J. Grafman, pp. 203–32. New York: Elsevier Science.

Malloy, P., Rassmussen, S., Braden, W. et al. (1989). Topographic evoked potential mapping in obsessive–compulsive disorder: evidence of frontal lobe dysfunction. *Psychiatry Research*, **28**, 63–71.

Malloy, P. F. & Richardson, E. D. (1994). Assessment of frontal lobe functions. *Journal of Neuropsychiatry*, **6**, 399–410.

Manschreck, T. C., Maher, B. A., Milavetz, J. J., Ames, D., Weisstein, C. C. & Schneyer, M. L. (1988). Semantic priming in thought disordered schizophrenic patients. *Schizophrenia Research*, **1**, 61–6.

Markowitsch, H. J. (1985). Hypotheses on mnemonic information processing in the brain. *International Journal of Neuroscience*, **27**, 191–227.

Maslach, C. (1979). Negative emotional biasing of unexplained arousal. *Journal of Personality and Social Psychology*, **37**, 953–69.

McClelland, J. L. & Rumelhart, D. E. (1985). Distributed memory and the representation of general and specific information. *Journal of Experimental Psychology, General*, **114**, 159–97.

Mendez, M. F., Martin, R. J. Smyth, K. A. & Whitehouse, P. J. (1990). Psychiatric symptoms associated with Alzheimer's disease. *Journal of Neuropsychiatry*, **2**, 28–33.

Mesulam, M. M. (1985). Patterns in behavioral neuroanatomy: Association areas, the limbic system, and hemispheric specialization. In *Principles of Behavioral Neurology*, ed. M. M. Mesulam, pp. 1–70. Philadelphia: F. A. Davis.

Ober, B. A., Vinogradov, S. & Shenaut, G. K. (1995). Semantic priming of category relations in schizophrenia. *Neuropsychology*, **9**, 220–8.

Ober, B. A., Vinogradov, S. & Shenaut, G. K. (1996). Automatic versus controlled semantic priming of lexical decision in schizophrenia. *Neuropsychology*, **11**, 506–13.

Paulsen, J. S., Heaton, R. K., Sadek, J. R. et al. (1995). The nature of learning and memory impairments in schizophrenia. *Journal of the International Neuropsychology Society*, **1**, 88–99.

Perecman, E. (1987). Consciousness and the meta-functions of the frontal lobes: Setting the stage. In *The Frontal Lobes Revisited*, ed. E. Perecman, pp. 1–10. New York: IRBN.

Phelps, M. E. & Chugani, J. C. (1986). Functional development of the human brain from 5 days to 20 years of age. *Journal of Nuclear Medicine*, **27**, 901.

Poole, J., Corwin, F. & Vinogradov, S. (1996a). Cognitive and clinical correlates of inaccurate affect perception in schizophrenia. Under review.

Poole, J. H., Vinogradov, S., Ober, B. A. & Shenaut, G. (1996b). Components and implications of frontal dysfunction in schizophrenia. Under review.

Rao, S. M., Devinsky, O., Grafman, J. et al. (1992). Viscosity and social cohesion in temporal lobe epilepsy. *Journal of Neurology, Neurosurgery, and Psychiatry*, **55**, 149–52.

Recanzone, G. H., Schreiner, C. E. & Merzenich, M. M. (1993). Plasticity in the frequency representation of primary auditory cortex following discrimination training in adult owl monkeys. *Journal of Neuroscience*, **13**, 87–103.

Rolls, E. T. (1989). Functions of neuronal networks in the hippocampus and neocortex in memory. In *Neural Models of Plasticity: Experimental and Theoretical Approaches*, ed. J. H. Byrne & W. O. Berry, pp. 240–65, San Diego, CA: Academic Press.

Rosse, R. B., Schwartz, B. L., Mastropaolo, J., Goldberg, R. L. & Deutsch, S. I. (1991). Subtype diagnosis in schizophrenia and its relation to neuropsychological and computerized tomography measures. *Biological Psychiatry*, **30**, 63–72.

Ruff, R. L. & Volpe, B. T. (1981). Environmental reduplication associated with right frontal and parietal lobe injury. *Journal of Neurology, Neurosurgery, and Psychiatry*, **44**, 382–6.

Rund, B. R. (1982). The effect of distraction on focal attention in paranoid and non-paranoid schizophrenic patients compared to normals and non-psychotic psychiatric patients. *Journal of Psychiatric Research*, **17**, 241–50.

Ruppin, E., Reggia, J. A. & Horne, D. (1995). A neural model of delusions and hallucinations in schizophrenia. In *Advances in Neural Information*

Processing Systems, Vol. 7, ed. G. Tesauro, D. Touretzky & T. Leen, pp. 149–56. Cambridge, Mass: MIT Press.

Sanders, R. D. & Mathews, T. A. (1994). Hypergraphia and secondary mania in temporal lobe epilepsy: Case reports and literature review. *Neuropsychiatry, Neuropsychology and Behavioral Neurology*, 7, 114–17.

Saykin, A. J., Gur, R. C., Mozley, P. D. et al. (1991). Neuropsychological function in schizophrenia: selective impairment in memory and learning. *Archives of General Psychiatry*, 48, 618–24.

Sedler, M. J. (1995). Understanding delusions. *Psychiatric Clinics of North America*, 18, 251–62.

Seidman, L. J., Kalinowski, A. G., Kremen, W. S. et al. (1995). Experimental and clinical neuropsychological measures of prefrontal dysfunction in schizophrenia. *Neuropsychology*, 9, 481–90.

Shapiro, D. (1965). *Neurotic Styles*. New York: Basic Books.

Sherwin, I. (1982). The effect of location of an epileptogenic lesion on the occurrence of psychosis in epilepsy. *Advances in Biological Psychiatry*, 8, 81–97.

Shrager, J., Hogg, T. & Huberman, B. A. (1987). Observation of phase transitions in spreading activation networks. *Science*, 236, 1092.

Spiers, P. A., Schomer, D. L., Blume, H. W. & Mesulam, M. M. (1985). Temporolimbic epilepsy and behavior. In *Principles of Behavioral Neurology*, ed. M. M. Mesulam, pp. 289–326. Philadelphia: F. A. Davis.

Spitzer, M. (1995). A neurocomputational approach to delusions. *Comprehensive Psychiatry*, 36, 83–105.

Spitzer, M., Braun, U., Hermle, L. & Maier, S. (1993). Associative semantic network dysfunction in thought-disordered schizophrenic patients: direct evidence from indirect semantic priming. *Biological Psychiatry*, 34, 864–77.

Spitzer, M., Weisker, I., Winter, M., Maier, S., Hermle, L. & Maher, B. A. (1994). Semantic and phonological priming in schizophrenia. *Journal of Abnormal Psychology*, 103, 485–94.

Strauss, M. E. (1988). On the experimental psychopathology of delusions. In *Delusional Beliefs*, ed. T. F. Oltmanns & B. A. Maher, pp. 157–63. New York: John Wiley and Sons.

Strub, R. L. & Black, F. W. (1988). *Neurobehavioral Disorders: A Clinical Approach*. Philadelphia: F. A. Davis.

Stuss, D. T., & Benson, D. F. (1987). The frontal lobes and control of cognition and memory. In *The Frontal Lobes Revisited*, ed. E. Perecman, pp. 141–58. New York: IRBN.

Sullivan, E. V., Shear, P. K., Sipursky, R. B., Sagar, H. J. & Pfefferbaum, A. (1994). A deficit profile of executive, memory, and motor functions in schizophrenia. *Biological Psychiatry*, 36, 641–53.

Vinogradov, S., Solomon, S., Ober, B. A., Biggins, C. A., Shenaut, G. K. & Fein, G. (1996). Do semantic priming effects correlate with sensory gating in schizophrenia? *Biological Psychiatry*, 39, 821–4.

Vinogradov, S., Willis-Shore, J., Poole, J. H., Marten, E., Shenaut, G. K. & Ober, B. A. (1997). Clinical and neurocognitive aspects of source monitoring in schizophrenia. *American Journal of Psychiatry*, 154, 1530–7.

Vinogradov, S., King, R. J. & Huberman, B. A. (1992a). An associationist model of the paranoid process: application of phase transitions in spreading activation networks. *Psychiatry*, 55, 79–94.

Vinogradov, S., Ober, B. A. & Shenaut, G. K. (1992b). Semantic priming of word pronunciation and lexical decision in schizophrenia. *Schizophrenia Research*, **8**, 171–81.

Weinberger, D. R. (1987). Implications of normal brain development for the pathogenesis of schizophrenia. *Archives of General Psychiatry*, **44**, 660–9.

Weinberger, D. R., Berman, K. F. & Chase, T. N. (1988). Mesocortical dopaminergic function and human cognition. *Annals of the New York Academy of Science*, **537**, 330–8.

Weinberger, D. R., Berman, K. F. & Zec, R. F. (1986). Physiologic dysfunction of dorsolateral prefrontal cortex in schizophrenia: I. Regional cerebral blood flow evidence. *Archives of General Psychiatry*, **43**, 114–24.

Wood, F. B. & Flowers, D. L. (1990). Hypofrontal vs. hypo-Sylvian blood flow in schizophrenia. *Schizophrenia Bulletin*, **16**, 413–24.

9

Neural network modelling of cognitive disinhibition and neurotransmitter dysfunction in obsessive–compulsive disorder

JACQUES LUDIK and DAN J. STEIN

In recent years there has been a dramatic revolution in our conceptualization of obsessive–compulsive disorder (OCD). OCD has long been considered a prototypical psychogenic condition, one that allowed an important window onto the workings of the unconscious mind. The disorder was thought to be relatively uncommon and refractory to treatment. In the last decade or so, however, advances in the neurobiology of OCD have led to a view that this disorder is best understood as one of the neuropsychiatric disorders, with specific brain dysfunction underlying complex behavioural symptoms. Furthermore, OCD is now recognized to be one of the most common psychiatric disorders (Karno et al., 1984; Weissman et al., 1994), and the introduction of novel pharmacotherapeutic and psychotherapeutic interventions has significantly improved its outcome (Baer and Minichiello, 1990; Jenike, 1992).

One of the most interesting aspects of current research on OCD is the new perspective that is being brought to questions about brain–behaviour relationships. Clearly, patients with OCD suffer from psychological symptoms, with anxiety-provoking intrusive thoughts (obsessions) leading to repetitive and ritualistic responses (compulsions). Functional imaging studies, however, demonstrate that these symptoms are mediated by specific dysfunctional brain circuits. Of significant interest is that both medication and psychotherapy lead to normalization of these circuits. Thus, while OCD may involve brain dysfunction, a comprehensive understanding of the condition also requires attention to brain-based emergent psychological structures and processes (Stein and Hollander, 1992).

In order to think about and further study this kind of integration of biological and behavioural data, clinicians and researchers may find it useful to draw on the theoretical constructs and empirical methods of cognitive science. Computational models seem to provide a sophisticated theoretical framework for incorporating both neuroscientific and psychological domains, and also for undertaking rigorous testing of integrative hypotheses. This chapter starts with an outline of recent advances in the neurobiology and neuropsychology of OCD, and continues with a neural network model of OCD, which, it is argued, allows a useful perspective on the intersection between these different approaches.

Neurochemistry of obsessive–compulsive disorder

A particularly important impetus was given to research on the neurobiology of OCD by the finding that the disorder responds to treatment with the serotonergic reuptake inhibitor (SRI), clomipramine, but not to the noradrenergic tricyclic antidepressant, desipramine (Zohar and Insel, 1987). This finding differentiates OCD from many other psychiatric disorders, such as depression and panic disorder, which respond to a range of antidepressants, and strongly suggests a specific role for serotonin in the mediation of OCD symptoms. More recently, clinical trials of serotonin selective reuptake inhibitors (SSRIs) have consistently demonstrated efficacy in the treatment of OCD (Greist et al., 1995; Stein, Spadaccini and Hollander, 1995).

Additional support for the hypothesis that serotonin plays an important role in OCD has been provided by a range of studies. Cerebrospinal fluid (CSF) concentrations of the serotonin metabolite 5-hydroxyindoleacetic acid (5-HIAA) may be raised in a subgroup of OCD patients, with these levels falling during clomipramine treatment (Thoren et al., 1980). Furthermore, in some studies, pharmacological challenges with the serotonin agonist m-chlorophenylpiperazine (m-CPP) resulted in exacerbation of OCD symptoms in a subgroup of OCD patients (Zohar et al., 1987; Hollander et al., 1992). These behavioural findings were no longer present after pharmacotherapy with SRIs.

Nevertheless, other patients with OCD do not appear to have elevated CSF 5-HIAA, show no symptom exacerbation after m-CPP, or do not respond to treatment with SRIs. While some of the these findings may reflect methodological limitations of the relevant research, another explanation of the data is that neurochemical systems in addition to serotonin also play a role in OCD. In particular, there is increasing evidence that dopamine is also important (Goodman et al., 1990). Dopamine is strongly implicated in the mediation of involuntary movements, and there are now data showing that tics are common in OCD and that OCD symptoms are frequent in tic disorders (Pauls and Leckman,

1986). Indeed, it has even been suggested that OCD and tic disorders are different phenotypic manifestations of an underlying genetic dysfunction (Pauls and Leckman, 1986).

Serotonin and dopamine are known to have significant functional interactions, and both preclinical and clinical findings provide support for the hypothesis that dopamine is also involved in OCD (Goodman et al., 1990). Administration of dopamine agonists may result in stereotypies in animals and in increased compulsive behaviours in humans (Frye and Arnold, 1981; Borcherding et al., 1990). Furthermore, patients with OCD and comorbid tics who fail to respond to a SRI may respond to the combination of a SRI and a dopamine blocker (McDougle et al., 1994). While additional neurochemical systems are also likely to be involved in OCD, current data therefore support a particular role for serotonin and dopamine.

Neuroanatomy of obsessive–compulsive disorder

While both serotonin and dopamine neurons have widespread connections, it is notable that they converge on the basal ganglia. Certainly, the basal ganglia are thought to play an important role in involuntary movement disorders, suggesting that these structures are also important in OCD. Indeed, some of the earliest evidence that OCD is mediated by specific neuroanatomical structures emerged after the influenza epidemic in the early 1900s. Patients who developed the sequela of encephalitis lethargica sometimes had both involuntary movements, presumably on the basis of basal ganglia pathology, and also obsessive–compulsive symptoms.

Several strands of more recent evidence support an important role for the basal ganglia in OCD. Patients with various neurologial conditions involving the basal ganglia, including Sydenham's chorea and Huntington's disease, may have comorbid OCD (Wise and Rapoport, 1989). Furthermore, patients with OCD may have increased neurological soft signs suggestive of basal ganglia pathology. Finally, both structural and functional brain imaging studies have implicated basal ganglia pathology in OCD. Thus, some computerized tomography (CT) (Luxenberg et al., 1988) and magnetic resonance imaging (MRI) (Robinson et al., 1995) studies have found decreased caudate volume in OCD patients, while functional imaging studies have found decreased activity in caudate after effective treatment of OCD (Baxter et al., 1992; Insel, 1992).

Occasionally, patients with frontal lobe lesions present with OCD symptoms, and OCD patients may show evidence of frontal lobe impairment on electrophysiological studies. An MRI study found subtle abnormalities in right frontal lobe, while some functional imaging studies have documented increased prefrontal or orbito-frontal activity before treatment, with normalization after treatment (Baxter et al., 1992; Insel, 1992). In addition, surgical lesions to cortical–basal ganglia pathways may result in improvement in OCD symptoms (Wise and Rapoport, 1989). Taken together, these various findings suggest that cortical–basal ganglia-thalamic-cortical circuits play a significant role in the mediation of OCD symptoms.

Indeed, it may be hypothesized that some sort of malfunctioning feedback or feedfoward circuit could explain the repetitive nature of OCD symptoms. The basal ganglia have been conceptualized as a repository for repetitive motor programmes, reminiscent of the repetitive behavioural sequences seen in OCD, which might then be released excessively as a result of basal ganglia pathology and dysfunctional gating of impulses (Wise and Rapoport, 1989). Increased orbito-frontal activity on functional imaging might then reflect the resistance that OCD patients describe in response to their symptoms. Alternatively, increased orbito-frontal activity may reflect a primary dysfunction in regulating internal cues, which manifests in dysregulation of goal-directed behaviours (Insel, 1992).

Neuropsychology of obsessive–compulsive disorder

What are the functional implications of brain neurotransmitter and cortical–basal ganglia abnormalities? An increasing range of work has documented that OCD is characterized by specific neuropsychological impairments (Stein, Hollander and Cohen, 1994). One of the most consistent neuropsychological findings has been impairment on tests of set-shifting (Head et al., 1989; Martinot et al., 1990; Hollander, Liebowitz and Rosen, 1991). Certainly, impairment in set-shifting seems consistent with dysfunction in cortical–basal ganglia circuits, which may be associated with an inability to inhibit non-relevant information (Wise and Rapoport, 1989).

Along similar lines, Enright and Beech (1990, 1993) have argued that OCD is characterized by decreased cognitive inhibition. Certainly, electrophysiological studies in OCD have demonstrated the presence of central hyperarousal (Towey et al., 1990). Furthermore, Enright and colleagues found that OCD differs significantly from other anxiety disorders on tests of negative priming. Typically, such a task results in normal negative priming (longer reaction times to previously ignored stimuli). However, OCD patients demonstrate reduced negative priming (shorter reaction times to previously ignored stimuli). Such reduced cognitive inhibition may be consistent with data demonstrating that both the serotonin system and frontal cortex are involved in impulse control (Soubrie, 1986; Stein and Hollander, 1993).

Unfortunately, to date relatively little empirical research has directly explored the relationship between psychological symptoms, neuropsychological impairment, and neurotransmitter dysfunction in OCD. Nevertheless, it is possible to hypothesize a link between core symptoms of OCD, such as a sense of incompleteness and abnormal risk assessment (Rasmussen and Eisen, 1993), and psychobiological findings. Stein and Hollander (1992), for example, have suggested that OCD involves impairment in the determination of goal–response completion. Thus, in some patients a deficit in match–mismatch mechanisms may result in inadequate determination of goal discrepancy with repetitive behaviours prior to goal completion. In other patients, inadequate assessment of goal discrepancy with overestimation of harm associated with possible mismatch may result in exaggerated uncertainty and doubt.

Preliminary data provide partial support for the validity of these kinds of associations. Thus, Hollander et al. (1991) found that responses on the Matching Familiar Figures Test (MFFT) may be useful in delineating the heterogeneity of OCD. This test of reflection–impulsivity involves comparing a set of detailed figures with a background foil that differs in only one detail. Hollander and colleagues reported that one subgroup of OCD patients responded rapidly with a high error rate, whereas a second subgroup responded slowly and with a low error rate. It might be postulated that the first group had difficulty in determining goal–response completion, while the second group was characterized by harm overestimation.

Furthermore, there is preliminary evidence that neuropsychological responses on the MFFT correlate with specific neurobiological deficits (Hollander et al., 1991). Thus, rapid erroneous response correlated with increased neurological soft signs and with poor response to serotonin reuptake blockers. On the other hand, slow correct response correlated with more reactive responses to serotonergic challenge. Thus, there is some suggestion that one subgroup of OCD patients has match—mismatch impairments associated with neurological deficits. while a second subgroup of OCD patients is characterized by harm overestimation associated with serotonin dysregulation (Stein and Hollander, 1992). Clearly, however, further theoretical and empirical work needs to be undertaken to consolidate this framework.

Integration via a neural network model

A crucial task for both the clinician and the researcher interested in OCD, then, is to develop integrated models that incorporate neurobiological and psychological data. A comprehensive understanding of OCD requires attention not only to brain dysfunction, but also to impairment in emergent psychological structures and processes. Certainly, the evidence suggests that effective intervention in OCD can take place at this psychological level, and that this in turn is accompanied by brain changes (Baxter et al., 1992). In this way, OCD provides an outstanding exemplar of 'complex' neuropsychiatric disorders, in which both brain and mind play crucial roles.

Building a rigorous computational model that incorporates both biological and psychological information may be useful in developing such an integration. Stein and Hollander (1994) have previously presented a theoretical approach to developing connectionist models of OCD. They discussed neural networks concerned with modelling inadequate determination of goal discrepancy, and considered a network for the assessment of goal discrepancy as harmful. For example, a high threshold for pattern switching in a neural network, with implementation of only a single response pattern, may be seen as equivalent to behavioural inhibition and high harm avoidance. In contrast, a low threshold for pattern switching with execution of several response patterns may be seen as equivalent to behavioural activation and low harm avoidance. Changes in serotonin activity may be associated with the modulation of thresholds for pattern switching.

Stein and Hollander (1994) noted that additional work was necessary in order to understand the interaction of the neural networks for the determination of goal discrepancy and for pattern switching, perhaps by incorporating data on the interaction of serotonin and dopamine systems in OCD. Furthermore, they provided no computer implementation of their particular neural network models. Such an implementation is the subject of the rest of this chapter. In particular, a neural network is described for simulating neuropsychological data on decreased cognitive inhibition in OCD in order to model the effects of serotonin and dopamine dysfunction in this disorder.

Complex negative priming task

As noted earlier, impaired set-shifting has been a consistent finding in studies of the neuropsychology of OCD (Stein et al., 1994) and OCD has been characterized as a disorder of impaired cognitive inhibition (Enright and Beech, 1990, 1993). Enright and Beech (1990, 1993) found that OCD differs substantially from other anxiety disorders on tests of negative priming, particularly when the complexity of these tests is increased. This experimental paradigm was therefore chosen to provide simulation data for the neural network developed here.

In negative priming tasks, subjects are presented with a priming stimulus (for example, two simultaneously presented figures, one in red, the other in green), and they attempt to identify the target (the red stimulus) and ignore the distractor (the green stimulus). The previously ignored distractor stimulus is then presented as the next target for selective naming. Such a task results in negative priming, and OCD patients were found to demonstrate reduced negative priming.

Enright and Beech (1993) have also presented a more complex negative priming task (which might be called the Temporal Stroop). In this task, the stimuli were ten words, two drawn from each of five semantic categories. Subjects were instructed to ignore the green word in each pair and to categorize the red word into one of the five semantic categories. Stimuli were presented under one of five conditions (Table 9.1). There were 40 randomized trials in each of the five conditions. The amount of negative priming was calculated by subtracting the mean reaction time of the control (CO) condition from the mean reaction time of the ignored repetition (IR) condition. The amount of semantic negative priming was calculated by subtracting the mean reaction time of the CO condition from the mean reaction time of the ignored semantic (IS) condition.

In the Temporal Stroop, Enright and Beech (1993) found that anxiety disorder patients demonstrated negative priming in both the repetition priming and the semantic negative priming condition. In comparison, OCD patients failed to show any priming effects in the repetition priming condition and demonstrated reduced negative priming in the semantic priming condition. The increased complexity of the semantic negative priming task would seem to be reflected by the enhanced difference between OCD patients and anxiety disorder controls on this task.

Table 9.1. *Stimuli were presented under one of the five conditions in the Temporal Stroop task. The stimuli were ten words, two drawn from each of five semantic categories (animals, furniture, body, tool, and music).*

Condition	Description	Example
Attended repetition (AR)	The attended priming stimulus was identical to the subsequent probe	Red DOG Red DOG
Attended semantic (AS)	The attended priming stimulus was semantically related to the subsequent probe	Red DOG Red CAT
Control (CO)	The attended and ignored priming stimuli were unrelated to the subsequent probe	Red DOG/green CHAIR Red FOOT
Ignored semantic (IS)	The ignored distractor prime was semantically related to the subsequent probe	Red CHAIR/green DOG Red CAT
Ignored repetition (IR)	The ignored distractor prime was identical to the subsequent probe	Red CHAIR/green DOG Red DOG

Recurrent network simulation of the Temporal Stroop

A partially recurrent neural network was developed in order to simulate normal performance on the semantic negative priming task. A partially recurrent neural network model was chosen as these are particularly useful for the storage and recognition of temporal processes and are not as computationally expensive as fully recurrent networks. The model consisted of two coupled Elman partially recurrent neural networks (Elman, 1988, 1990) in order to have a so-called 'left word pathway' (with its own colour input unit, word units, context units and hidden units) and a similar 'right word pathway' (Fig. 9.1). This was necessary because the network was not only required to learn to give the correct current and previous semantic categories, but also to 'switch off' (i.e. ignore) the green word's pathway, whether it was left or right.

The training data consisted of 200 temporal patterns (where each temporal pattern consisted of two pairs of red/green words), with 40 randomized trials in each of the five conditions. The coupled Elman partially recurrent neural network was trained with a back-propagation learning algorithm with a learning rate of 0.1. The network was trained until the root mean square error was less than 0.005 and the percentage of correct responses on the training set was 100 per cent. A response was classified

Neural network modelling in obsessive–compulsive disorder   239

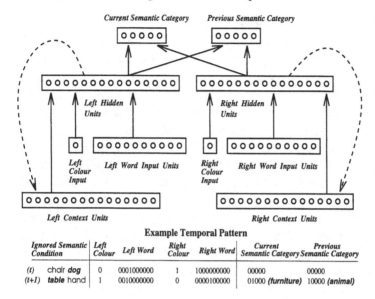

Fig. 9.1 Recurrent neural network model for the Temporal Stroop.

as correct if the current and previous semantic category output units with maximum activation values matched their respective desired targets. This was achieved after 6000 epochs.

A simulation consisted of a run through the entire test set of 200 temporal patterns. The following were the processing steps for a particular temporal pattern in a simulation.

1. After presenting the first pair of red/green words, the hidden and output units were activated in a normal single processing step.
2. For the second pair of red/green words, the context layers contained a copy of the previous hidden unit activation values, and a gradual build-up of activation over time was allowed for the hidden and output units.

Reaction time was implemented in the network as a function of the number of cycles (single processing steps in the gradual build-up of activation) it takes to accumulate the specified amount of activation according to the response threshold. This was to simplify the comparison between the empirical reaction times (obtained by Enright and Beech, 1993) and the model's performance.

Lesioning the recurrent neural network

Three kinds of lesions were made to the recurrent network, each representing changes to a single monoamine neurotransmitter system. First, gain of the colour module was decreased in order to simulate serotonergic dysfunction. There is sound evidence that serotonergic modulatory effects in frontal cortex play a key role in harm assessment. Thus, in both preclinical and clinical paradigms, serotonergic dysfunction typically results in impaired impulse control, leading to increased self-directed and other-directed aggression (Soubrie, 1986). Specifically, decrease in serotonergic transmission leads to an inability to accept situations that necessitate or create strong inhibitory tendencies or to adopt passive or waiting attitudes (Soubrie, 1986). In a general sense, Jacobs and Fornal (1995) argue that serotonin facilitates gross motor output and inhibits sensory information processing. In the recurrent neural network described here, the colour module plays a specific role in representing information about the colour of the current stimulus, effectively ensuring the representation of information about the dangerousness of the current stimulus (green being a colour that must be ignored, and red being a colour that must be focused on).

Second, gain of the context module was decreased in order to simulate dopaminergic dysfunction. As Le Moal (1995) has argued, dopamine neurons are thought to regulate and allow integrative functions in the areas onto which they project. Lesioning of dopamine neurons results in a decreased facilitation of response sequencing in preclinical paradigms, and impaired executive functioning in patients (Lyon and Robbins, 1975). It is also possible that dopamine projections of the striatum are involved in the filtering of signals relating to sensorimotor processing (cortex) and basic biological drives (limbic area), which are then synchronized and translated into behaviour via the pallidal and pontine motor nuclei (Le Moal, 1995). Fuster (1980) and Goldman-Rakich (1989) described dopamine as having a modulatory effect on the responsivity of cells in prefrontal cortex, where it mediates the representation of goals. In the neural network described here, the context module played a particular role in representing information about differences between previous and current goals.

Simulation results reported are the mean of 50 simulations for each combination of parameters. Results were tabulated (Table 9.2) for normal simulation, reduction of context gain, reduction of colour gain, and combined reduction in context and colour gain. Reduction of context

Table 9.2. *Mean results of 50 simulations for normal performance, only context gain reduction, only color gain reduction, and combined context and colour gain reduction compared to OCD experimental results.*

Lesion type	Normal	Colour	Context	Combined	OCD
Colour gain	1.0	0.6	1.0	0.6	
Context gain	1.0	1.0	0.8	0.8	
Reaction times (ms)					
Attended repetition (AR)	424.7 (6.4)	436.4 (8.0)	578.8 (7.9)	561.1 (7.1)	447.4
Attended semantic (AS)	455.6 (7.4)	487.8 (8.7)	579.6 (6.3)	597.6 (4.1)	558.1
Control (CO)	463.6 (9.1)	475.0 (7.9)	605.2 (5.5)	590.3 (8.4)	602.0
Ignored semantic (IS)	469.6 (10.0)	472.0 (8.0)	597.5 (7.4)	569.4 (7.3)	565.9
Ignored repetition (IR)	456.3 (9.9)	480.4 (7.4)	607.4 (4.5)	590.6 (6.3)	602.1
Derived priming data					
RNP = IR − CO	−7.3	5.4	2.2	0.4	0.2
SNP = IS − CO	6.0	−3.1	−7.7	−20.9	−36.1
Correct performance (%)	100.0	99.8	98.9	99.1	97.1

SNP, semantic negative priming; RNP, repetition negative priming; standard deviation indicated in brackets.

gain, colour gain, or both, results in significantly slower reaction times ($F = 48.6$, df = 199, $p < 0.0001$) and more error responses ($F = 54.2$, df = 199, $p < 0.0001$) than in the normal case. Enright and Beech (1993) found that anxiety disorder patients demonstrated negative priming in the semantic negative priming (SNP) condition, whereas OCD patients exhibited positive priming (reduced negative priming) on the same measure. The simulation results indicate that the normal performance exhibits negative priming in the SNP condition, whereas lesioning the colour and/or context gain results in reduced negative priming on this condition.

Interestingly, reduction of both context and colour gain resulted in responses that correspond nicely with those obtained by Enright and Beech, i.e. OCD patients failed to show any priming effects in the repetition priming and demonstrated reduced negative priming in the semantic priming condition (the amount of repetition negative priming is respectively 0.4 and 0.2, whereas the amount of semantic negative priming is, respectively, −20.9 and −36.1). Thus, the hypothesis that serotonin and dopamine are both involved in OCD and that they are known to have significant functional interactions is further emphasized by the result that lesions to both dopamine and serotonin units in the neural network more accurately reflect the experimental data than lesions to only dopamine or only serotonin units.

The third lesion was to increase the maximum time cycle during network training in order to simulate noradrenergic discharge. Several theories have been presented to explain noradrengergic function (Robbins and Everitt, 1995). An early idea was that the locus coeruleus was involved in alarm systems, increasing attention and vigilance (Aston-Jones et al., 1991). Similarly, Cole and Robbins (1992) described the locus coeruleus as resulting in focused rather than automatic functioning. Thus, according to Robbins and Everitt (1995), the noradrenergic system seems to play a role in focusing attention onto salient events in demanding or threatening situations. In the neural network developed here, the maximum time cycle sets a limit on the number of processing steps allowed during the build up of activation over time, with an increase in maximum time cycle effectively allowing increased concentration on the task at hand.

It was found that increasing the maximum cycle number under ordinary conditions resulted in a further increase in semantic negative priming, whereas increasing the maximum cycle number in OCD during context or colour gain reduction resulted in a significant further decrease in semantic negative priming. Although the role of the noradrenergic system in OCD has not been fully elucidated, these results are consistent with evidence for significant interactions between the noradrenergic, serotonergic, and dopaminergic systems.

Conclusion

Empirical psychiatric researchers may offer a general objection to the theoretical nature of the research reported here, expressing dissatisfaction that neural network modelling of psychopathology fails to uncover new knowledge about either the neurobiology or the neuropsychology of psychiatric disorders. Although this is possibly an accurate criticism, it fails to see the advantages and strengths of the neural network approach. Connectionist models do not necessarily aim to uncover new neurobiological or psychobiological mechanisms; rather, they often aim at integrating biological and psychological data in a particularly rigorous way in order to shed new light on these data.

In the authors' view, the model described here supports an interesting theoretical view of OCD and suggests further avenues for empirical research on this disorder. The model is based on data that OCD is characterized by impairment in cognitive inhibition, with involvement of monoamine regulatory neurotransmitters. The success of the simulation thus supports a view that emphasizes the failure of impulse control in OCD (Lopez-Ibor, 1990; Stein and Hollander, 1993). In addition, the simulation leads to the suggestion that heterogeneity of OCD may be explained in terms of variance in neurobiological (serotonergic and dopaminergic) dysfunction and neuropsychological (harm assessment and goal discrepancy) impairment. The evidence for the heterogeneity of OCD is increasing, and a differentiation between the psychobiology of harm assessment and goal discrepancy determination may provide a way of further researching this issue.

Our recurrent neural network model does not necessarily support a definitive division of OCD subtypes. However, one speculative way of subtyping OCD may be to divide patients into those with predominantly serotonergic and those with both serotonergic and dopaminergic involvement. OCD patients with predominantly serotonergic deficits may have increased harm avoidance, more exacerbation of OCD symptoms on m-CPP challenge, decreased neurological soft signs, and a better response to SRIs. In comparison, OCD patients with both serotonergic and dopaminergic abnormalities may have increased executive function impairment, less exacerbation of OCD symptoms on m-CPP challenge, increased neurological soft signs, and a poorer response to SRIs unless these are combined with dopamine blockers. While this division is clearly speculative, there are some supporting data for it (Hollander et al. 1991; Stein and Hollander, 1992; Hollander et al., 1993; McDougle et al., 1994).

Research in this area challenges the creative imagination of clinicians and connectionists to develop increasingly elaborate mechanisms and quantitative parameters to account for disorders. Computer implementation provides a rigour that many approaches towards psychobiological integration lack. In particular, a recurrent neural network model of OCD may allow a novel account of how neurobiological dysfunction (of serotonergic and dopaminergic systems) mediates neuropsychological impairment (of harm assessment and goal determination) characteristic of OCD, so providing a rigorous integrative psychobiological approach to this disorder.

Summary

This chapter presents advances in the neurochemistry, neuroanatomy, and neuropsychology of OCD, and develops a neural network model for integrating neurobiological and neuropsychological data. A connectionist simulation of a semantic negative priming task on which patients with OCD have reduced negative priming, but in which anxiety disorder patients do not, allowed an investigation of the effects of lesioning of each of the monoamine neurotransmitter systems. The temporal nature of this task demanded a complex recurrent neural network, which led to a more comprehensive neural network simulation of neurotransmitter dysfunction in OCD than has previously been offered. Lesions of the recurrent neural network that corresponded to dopaminergic and serotonergic dysfunction resulted in reduced semantic negative priming, while modifications of the network that corresponded to noradrenergic dysfunction resulted in enhancement of effects that had been present beforehand.

Acknowledgement

Dr Ludik is supported by a grant from the Foundation of Research Development and Dr Stein by a grant from the South African Medical Research Council.

References

Aston-Jones, G., Chiang, C. & Alexinsky, T. (1991). Discharge of noradrenergic locus coeruleus neurons in behaving rats and monkeys suggests a role in vigilance. *Progress in Brain Research*, **88**, 501–20.

Baer, L. & Minichiello, W. E. (1990). Behavior therapy for obsessive–compulsive disorder. In *Obsessive–Compulsive Disorders: Theory and Management*, 2nd edn, ed. M. A. Jenike, L. Baer & W. E. Minichiello. Chicago: Year Book Medical Publishers.

Baxter, L. R., Schwartz, J. M., Bergman, K. S. et al. (1992). Caudate glucose metabolic rate changes with both drug and behavior therapy for OCD. *Archives of General Psychiatry*, **49**, 681–9.

Borcherding, B. G., Keysor, C. S., Rapoport, J. L. et al. (1990). Motor/vocal tics and compulsive behaviors on stimulant drugs: is there a common vulnerability? *Psychiatry Research*, **33**, 83–94.

Cole, B. J. & Robbins, T. W. (1992). Forebrain norepinephrine: role in controlled information processing in the rat. *Neuropsychopharmacology*, **7**, 129–41.

Elman, J. L. (1988). *Finding Structure in Time*. CRL Technical Report 8801. San Diego, University of California.

Elman, J. L. (1990). Finding structure in time. *Cognitive Science*, **14**, 179–211.

Enright, S. J. & Beech, A. R. (1990). Obsessional states: anxiety disorders or schizotypes? An information processing and personality assessment. *Psychological Medicine*, **20**, 621–7.

Enright, S. J. & Beech, A. R. (1993). Reduced cognitive inhibition in obsessive–compulsive disorder. *British Journal of Clinical Psychology*, **32**, 67–74.

Frye, P. E. & Arnold, L. E. (1981). Persistent amphetamine-induced compulsive rituals: response to pyridoxine (B6). *Biological Psychiatry*, **16**, 583–7.

Fuster, J. M. (1980). *The Prefrontal Cortex*. New York: Raven Press.

Goldman-Rakic, P. S. (1989). Circuitry of primate prefrontal cortex and regulation of behavior by representational memory. *Handbook of Physiology – The Nervous System*, **5**, 373–417.

Goodman, W. K., McDougle, C. J., Price, L. H., Riddle, M. A., Pauls, D. L. & Leckman, J. F. (1990). Beyond the serotonin hypothesis: a role for dopamine in some forms of obsessive compulsive disorder? *Journal of Clinical Psychiatry*, **51S**, 36–43.

Greist, J. H., Jefferson, J. W., Kobak, K. A., Katzelnick, D. J. & Serlin, D. C. (1995). Efficacy and tolerability of serotonin transport inhibitors in obsessive–compulsive disorder. *Archives of General Psychiatry*, **52**, 53–60.

Head, D., Bolton, D. & Hymas, N. F. S. (1989). Deficit in cognitive shifting ability in patients with obsessive–compulsive disorder. *Biological Psychiatry*, **15**, 929–37.

Hollander, E., DeCaria, C., Nitescu, A. et al. (1992). Serotonergic function in obsessive–compulsive disorder: comparison of behavioral and neuroendocrine responses to oral m-CPP and fenfluramine in patients and healthy volunteers. *Archives of General Psychiatry*, **49**, 21–8.

Hollander, E., Liebowitz, M. R. & Rosen, W. T. (1991). Neuropsychiatric and neuropsychological studies in obsessive compulsive disorder. In *Psychobiology of Obsessive Compulsive Disorder*, ed. J. Zohar, T. R. Insel & S. Rasmussen, pp. 126–45, New York: Springer.

Hollander, E., Stein, D. J., DeCaria, C. M., Saoud, J. B., Klein, D. F. & Liebowitz, M. R. (1993). A pilot study of biological predictors of treatment outcome in obsessive–compulsive disorder. *Biological Psychiatry*, **33**, 747–9.

Insel, T. R. (1992). Toward a neuroanatomy of obsessive–compulsive disorder. *Archives of General Psychiatry*, **49**, 739–44.

Jacobs, B. J. & Fornal, C. A. (1995). Serotonin and behavior: a general hypothesis. In *Psychopharmacology: the Fourth Generation of Progress*, ed. F. E. Bloom & D. J. Kupfer, pp. 461–9. New York: Raven Press.

Jenike, M. A. (1992). Pharmacologic treatment of obsessive compulsive disorders. *Psychiatric Clinics of North America*, **15**, 895–919.

Karno, M., Goldin, J. M., Sorenson, S. B. & Burnam, M. A. (1984). The epidemiology of obsessive compulsive disorder in five US communities. *Archives of General Psychiatry*, **45**, 1094–9.

Le Moal, M. (1995). Mesocorticolimbic dopaminergic neurons: functional and regulatory roles. In *Psychopharmacology: the Fourth Generation of Progress*, ed. F. E. Bloom & D. J. Kupfer, pp. 283–94. New York: Raven Press.

Lopez-Ibor Jr, J. J. (1990). Impulse control in obsessive–compulsive disorder: a biopsychopathological approach. *Progress in Neuro-Psychopharmacology and Biological Psychiatry*, **14**, 709–18.

Luxenberg, J., Swedo, S., Flament, M., Friedland, R., Rapoport, J. & Rapoport, S. I. (1988). Neuroanatomical abnormalities in obsessive–compulsive disorder detected with quantitative X-ray computed tomography. *American Journal of Psychiatry*, **45**, 1089–93.

Lyon, M. & Robbins, T. W. (1975). The action of central nervous system stimulus drugs: a general theory concerning amphetamine effects. In *Current Developments in Psychopharmacology*, Vol. 2, ed. W. Essman & L. Valzelli, pp. 79–163. New York: Spectrum Publications.

Martinot, J. L., Allilaire, J. F., Mazoyer, B. M. et al. (1990). Obsessive–compulsive disorder: a clinical, neuropsychological and positron emission study. *Acta Psychiatrica Scandinavica*, **82**, 233–42.

McDougle, C. J., Goodman, W. K., Leckman, J. F., Lee, N. C., Heninger, G. R. & Price, L. H. (1994). Haloperidol addition in fluvoxamine-refractory obsessive–compulsive disorder: a double-blind placebo-controlled study in patients with and without tics. *Archives of General Psychiatry*, **51**, 302–08.

Pauls, D. L. & Leckman, J. (1986). The inheritance of Gilles de la Tourette's syndrome and associated behaviors: evidence for autosomal dominant transmission. *New England Journal of Medicine*, **315**, 993–7.

Rasmussen, S. & Eisen, J. L. (1993). Assessment of core features, conviction and psychosocial function in OCD. Paper presented at the First International Obsessive–Compulsive Disorder Conference, Capri, Italy.

Robbins, T. W. & Everitt, B. J. (1995). Central norepinephrine neurons and behavior. In *Psychopharmacology: the Fourth Generation of Progress*, ed. F. E. Bloom & D. J. Kupfer, pp. 363–72. New York: Raven Press.

Robinson, D., Wu, H., Munne R. A. et al. (1995). Reduced caudate nucleus volume in obsessive–compulsive disorder. *Archives of General Psychiatry*, **52**, 393–8.

Soubrie, P. (1986). Reconciling the role of central serotonin neurones in human and animal behavior. *Behavioral Brain Science*, **9**, 319–64.

Stein, D. J. & Hollander, E. (1992). Cognitive science and obsessive–compulsive disorder. In *Cognitive Science and Clinical Disorders*, ed. D. J. Stein & J. E. Young, pp. 235–47. San Diego: Academic Press.

Stein, D. J. & Hollander, E. (1993). Impulsive aggression and obsessive–compulsive disorder. *Psychiatric Annals*, **23**, 389–95.

Stein, D. J. & Hollander, E. (1994). A neural network model of obsessive-compulsive disorder. *Journal of Mind Behavior*, **15**, 25–40.

Stein, D. J., Hollander, E. & Cohen, L. (1994). Neuropsychiatry of obsessive–compulsive disorder. In *Current Insights in Obsessive–Compulsive Disorder*, ed. E. Hollander, J. Zohar, D. Marazzati & B. Olivier, pp. 137–52. Chichester: Wiley.

Stein, D. J., Spadaccini, E. & Hollander, E. (1995). Meta-analysis of pharmacoltherapy trials for obsessive compulsive disorder. *International Clinical Psychopharmacology*, **10**, 11–18.

Thoren, P., Asberg, M., Bertilsson, L., Mellstrom, B., Sjoqvist, F. & Traskman, L. (1980). Clomipramine treatment of obsessive–compulsive disorder. II. Biochemical aspects. *Archives of General Psychiatry*, **37**, 1289–94.

Towey, J., Bruder, G., Hollander, E. et al. (1990). Endogenous event-related potentials in obsessive–compulsive disorder. *Biological Psychiatry*, **28**, 92–8.

Weissman, M. M., Bland, R. C., Canino, G. J. et al. (1994). The cross national epidemiology of obsessive compulsive disorder. *Journal of Clinical Psychiatry*, **55S**, 5–10.

Wise, S. P. & Rapoport, J. L. (1989). Obsessive–compulsive disorder: Is it basal ganglia dysfunction? In *Obsessive–Compulsive Disorders in Children and Adolescents*, ed. J. L. Rapoport, pp. 327–44. Washington, DC: American Psychiatric Press.

Zohar, J. & Insel, T. R. (1987). Obsessive–compulsive disorder: psychobiological approaches to diagnosis, treatment, and pathophysiology. *Biological Psychiatry*, **22**, 667–87.

Zohar, J., Mueller, E. A., Insel, T. R. et al. (1987). Serotonergic responsivity in obsessive–compulsive disorder: comparison of patients and healthy controls. *Archives of General Psychiatry*, **44**, 946–51.

10

The fables of Lucy R.: association and dissociation in neural networks

DAN LLOYD

According to Aristotle, 'to be learning something is the greatest of pleasures not only to the philosopher but also to the rest of mankind.' But even as he affirms the unbounded human capacity for integrating new experience with existing knowledge, he alludes to a significant exception: 'The sight of certain things gives us pain, but we enjoy looking at the most exact images of them, whether the forms of animals which we greatly despise or of corpses.' Our capacity for learning is happily engaged in viewing representations of painful objects, but not, it seems, in viewing the objects themselves. When an experience is intensely painful, what then is a rational animal to do? We can neither disable our learning process, nor erase its traces. In the face of intense pain, horror, or terror, learning and remembrance cause no pleasure but rather persistent psychological pain and disruption. The memorious mind reverberates with trauma.

The traumatized mind responds in diverse ways to the recurrent crises of reminiscence, responses which lead at the extreme to the symptoms of various disorders. These reactions fall into two broad categories: the associative and the dissociative. The first is exemplified by some (but not all) of the symptoms of post-traumatic stress disorder, in cases in which even a trivial element associated with the painful event becomes an evocative cue for reliving the experience. In contrast, dissociation is characterized by subjective distancing from the initial pain and its remembrance, often with secondary effects. In dissociative amnesia, for example, subjects fail to recall critical spans of their lives, often seeming to obliterate the traumatic memory. The erasure is only apparent; in diverse ways the trauma continues to oppress even if it cannot be consciously recalled.

There are, of course, many (too many) occasions of trauma. That diversity, and the diversity of responses in its aftermath, imply that the causal mechanisms of traumatized cognition are manifold. Understanding post-traumatic psychopathology is further complicated by the compounded effects of multiple or repeated trauma. With this complexity in mind, this chapter explores connectionism as a unifying framework for understanding the traumatized mind. The first motive for this attempt is already apparent. Trauma is an occasion for a kind of learning, and connectionist models are most adept at simulating learning. In addition, a connectionist model offers extraordinary flexibility in representation. Arrays of neural processing units afford subtlety and precision in simulating the contents of mind. With learning, these representations change. 'Traumatic learning' can thus be modeled, and a network observed in its initial responses, and then subjected to further simulated trauma with further testing. In this way, a narrative of traumatic experience and its diverse psychological manifestations can be condensed, simplified, and examined. Even a simple network allows many variations. For a first foray into the simulation of psychogenic psychopathology, the author followed a well-known case study, using the concrete history and experienced symptoms of a patient (and her therapist) as a guide for a network model. The case study is exemplary of the 90s – the 1890s, that is. In various ways, it is emblematic of a century of clinical thinking that followed.

Sometime in the fall of 1892 a governess working in the outskirts of Vienna visited her doctor with an unusual complex of symptoms. The patient presented a physical symptom, a chronic suppurative rhinitis, combined with a 'psychological' symptom, a persistent olfactory hallucination, the smell of burnt pudding. Her doctor referred the case to Sigmund Freud, who ultimately told the patient's story as the case study of 'Lucy R.,' in Freud and Breuer's *Studies on Hysteria* ([1895] 1955). Freud described the case as 'a model instance of one particular type of hysteria, namely the form of this illness which can be acquired even by a person of sound heredity, as a result of appropriate experiences' ([1895] 1955, p. 122). Looking back on the case from the other end of Freud's career, it seems to be a model instance of more than just a type of hysteria. It anticipates Freud's own evolution toward psychoanalysis, as well as developments in clinical approaches to psychopathology both before and after Freud. In the early 1890s, Freud and Breuer hypothesized that 'hysterics suffer mainly from reminiscences' (p. 7).[1] In *Studies on Hysteria*, the mind of the hysteric is seen to be fending off painful memories and wishes, with unintended symptomatic side-effects. This basic process of thoughts repressed and resurgent would soon be applied in pathologies other than hysteria, and ultimately be read into every detail of twentieth-century life. Even more ubiquitous in our time is the presupposition implied by repression, namely, that there is something to repress, in the form of thoughts exerting causal powers without entering consciousness. The conception of an active-but-unconscious realm of mind reigns in both clinical and cognitive psychology. The study of Lucy R. explicates these ideas in terms that are familiar still. In addition, the psychoanalytic method seems already implicitly at work with Lucy R. Unlike Breuer's treatment of Anna O., for example, with Lucy, Freud abandoned hypnotism as a diagnostic and therapeutic aid, probing instead for remembered associations and achieving a 'talking cure.'

Yet at the same time the case of Lucy R. is not yet laden with the apparatus and theory that Freud would later develop. Ego, id, superego, and the specific complexes from infancy all lay in Freud's future. More important, in *Studies on Hysteria*, Freud still clearly conceived of psychopathology as originating in traumatic experience. Later, he would relocate the origins of pathology in repressed fantasies and wishes, a reorientation that decisively influenced the subsequent development of psychoanalysis. In the earlier, 'experiential,' conception Freud showed his affinity with the great nineteenth-century theorists Charcot (with whom Freud studied) and Janet. Conveniently, this orientation has re-emerged as a central contemporary issue. Although hysteria has fallen out of terminological favor, both its symptoms and traumatic etiology still echo in contemporary clinical taxonomy and theory (Kihlstrom, 1994). For the dissociative disorders in particular, a frequent cause is real, not merely imagined, trauma. Lucy R., as Freud interpreted her experience, provides a straightforward example.

For these reasons the author turned to Lucy R. as a model to approach within the connectionist framework. As in all of his case studies, Freud used his subject as an object lesson from which he drew specific conclusions. As we revisit Freud's fable, we will examine the conclusions he drew and draw some new ones as well.

'Lucynet,' the simulation of Lucy R.

Representing Lucy R.'s phenomenology

Lucy R. also enjoys the curious distinction of having been the target of an earlier attempted computer simulation, which was described but not implemented by Cornelis Wegman (1985). In the epilogue to his heroic effort, Wegman estimated that the actual implementation of the model would require at least five years of programming work. How did the case of Lucy R., one of Freud's briefest, get so complicated? This author suggests that the complexity reflects the limitations of the approach taken, which was drawn entirely from classical artificial intelligence (AI) in its heyday, before the re-emergence of connectionism. A brief look at Wegman's work shows the limits of classical AI as a concrete modeling tool, suggests the unique powers of connectionism, and offers an initial foot-hold on 'Lucynet,' our sequel to Freud's study.

Wegman based his efforts on a sophisticated theory of 'knowledge structures' and their modifications, Roger Shank's theory of scripts (Shank and Abelson, 1977). A script is a framework for knowledge about actions or other sequences of events. To define a script, one draws from a repertoire of actions (of which some are basic), each action having specified effects on the world. The problem unfolds from the words 'define' and 'specify:' every change, and all its relevant or probable consequences, must be programmed by hand. Any genuine interaction in the world demands a huge script for its description. The one event from the Lucy saga that Wegman fully scripts accordingly implicates 17 separate actions fulfilling ten distinct goals and plans for their achievement. Being an outline and not an implemented program, there is no guarantee that even this level of detail will be enough. His initial scripting is certainly not enough, Wegman notes, to incorporate the proposed mechanisms of hysteria, and thence he carefully and explicitly adds each of the following to the expanding model: affect, arousal, facial expression, abreaction, working-over, episodic memory, and several others. Significantly, a separate component called 'consciousness' appears in the flowchart in order to enable the functions of attention and repression. (For a similar exegesis, but much less sympathetic to Freud, see Cummins, 1983.)

The exercise has the enormous value of flushing out unnoticed ambiguities in Freud's hypotheses. But even if the model led to a working implementation, it would leave open the question which, if any, of the many installed modules was real. Like the epicycles of Ptolemaic astronomy, every module in this sort of model is a kludge, hand-built to do just what Freud (as interpreted by the would-be modeler) supposes. A more powerful demonstration, in contrast, would be one that requires less programming intervention, operates according to a few highly general principles, and yet exhibits several of the symptoms and responses in parallel with the case study. A model of this sort has the capacity to exhibit the target phenomena as emergent side-effects of more basic and general functions, rather than as the explicit result of a deliberate program. This in turn suggests new hypotheses and tests in the target domain. Connectionist models, when they work, have these attractive features. Indeed, connectionism makes a virtue of simplicity. The simpler the model, the more basic and general will be the mechanisms explaining its functional behavior, resulting in more powerful explanatory hypotheses in the real world.

To construct Lucynet, then, the author took the minimalist approach of radical simplicity, as afforded by connectionism. Network design was guided by the observations reported by Freud, which were taken at face value (*pace* Crews, 1993; Grünbaum, 1984; and other critics of Freud's self-fulfilling observations). Lucy's primary symptoms, unlike those reported elsewhere in *Studies on Hysteria*, were perceptual hallucinations, a smell of burnt pudding and the smell of cigar smoke. To understand these symptoms, Freud probed Lucy's conscious memories and eventually uncovered episodes that Lucy had apparently repressed. But although Lucy would not easily recall them, these episodes were initially fully conscious. The goal of the model, then, could be initially restricted to capturing the conscious world of Lucy's perceptions, representing both a sequence of perceived events, some of them traumatic, and the recollection of those events later on, including their 'conversion' into symptoms. The case study mentions many details of Lucy's background and current life, but the specific and significant players in Freud's reconstruction of the case turn out to be few. As a prelude to setting the simulated psychodynamics in motion, the author compiled the salient elements from Lucy's reports. The first is the head of the household, a widower, and director of a factory outside Vienna (the 'Director,' for short). No less important in Lucy's narrative are the Director's two children, Lucy's pupils. Although each of the two girls would have been separately and complexly represented in Lucy's consciousness, for the purposes of understanding her neurosis it was sufficient to treat them as a single element ('Children'). The several servants working alongside Lucy can be similarly conflated. One other role repeats in important moments in the study, a guest of the Director, in one case female and in another male. But as the study unfolds, these two also occupy an interchangeable functional role, abbreviated as 'Guest.' In Lucy's experience, these key players are not inert, but among their many deeds just one plays a recurrent and significant role in her story: the attempt by each of the guests to kiss the children. These events ('Kissing,' in short) will be narrated below. Lucy's 'lived world' also features intense feelings. 'Love' and 'Distress' are prominent, along with the subjective sensations of her chronic rhinitis. Last, but not least, is her perception of burnt pudding and cigar smoke, both the real percepts during moments explicitly identified in the case study, and the later recurrent hallucinations.

In sum, these ten explicit elements within Lucy's unfolding experience compose an initial 'alphabet' for Lucynet. Each would have been a complex internal representation but, in pursuit of the minimal model, we can regard each as a distinct whole, with varying degrees of prominence from moment to moment in Lucy's history. Different scenes from the saga, then, can be represented by combining subsets of these, as letters might combine to form words. However, in Lucynet as in Lucy herself, the elements are not isolated. Connectionism borrows from a long psychological tradition a single highly general conception of the interaction of ideas, namely, association. Potential 'elements' in conscious thought can be activated by associated thoughts, or by inputs from the external world. Which elements are most active at any moment depends on the combination of these influences. In keeping with the radical minimalism of the approach, the activation of any unit at any time was proportional to the sum of its immediately preceding inputs only – units retained no activation from the previous cycle. By these broad strokes, we have built an architecture for Lucynet consisting of ten elements – ten processing units – suggested by Lucy R., with the potential for interaction both among the elements themselves and from the outside. This architecture is shown in Figure 10.1. (For a similar approach to modeling memory, see McClelland and Rumelhart, 1986.)

The narrative of learning, and the lessons of trauma

Experience changed Lucy. Whether trivial or traumatic, each episode in the case study left its traces, and so each may be regarded as an occasion of learning. Connectionism captures these experience-driven changes through a process of changing association strength governed by overarching 'learning rules.' In a network with the simple architecture of Lucynet, we can use a simple form of a very general learning rule known as the delta rule (McClelland and Rumelhart, 1986). To a first approximation, the delta rule works as follows. For each cycle of processing, the current level of activity in a unit is compared to the current sum of all inputs to the unit. The connection strengths among the units involved are adjusted so as to reduce this difference (for details, see

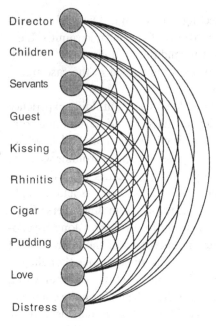

Director

Children

Servants

Guest

Kissing

Rhinitis

Cigar

Pudding

Love

Distress

Fig. 10.1 Architecture of Lucynet. Ten elements prominent in the phenomenal reports of Lucy R. are represented by ten neuron-like processing units. The network is fully interconnected; units also have recurrent self-connections (not shown).

Lloyd, 1994). In general, delta rule learning produces networks that are good at associative learning. When Lucynet receives the paired inputs, 'Director' and 'Children,' the delta rule increases the connection strengths between these two units. Subsequently, if Lucynet is presented with either input alone, it will tend to reproduce their combination, the learned association.

The extent of learning with each cycle of operation is governed by a crucial variable, the learning rate coefficient. In connectionist models, this learning rate is kept very low (usually around 0.05) to prevent the learning of one association interfering with the learning of others. As a consequence, network learning traditionally requires massive repetition of inputs to be learned. With a low learning rate, the same network can learn a number of associations. As a prelude to Lucynet's bumpy ride, the network was trained on a number of background associations that would have characterized Lucy's regular associations in her job. (Some examples: 'Director + Children,' due to the obvious familiar links; 'Rhinitis +

Distress,' reflecting Lucy's chronic complaint; 'Children + Love,' following Lucy's repeated statements of fondness for her charges). The network had no trouble learning these associations and reproducing them when partial inputs were provided. In terms of the model, for any given sensory input, Lucynet 'recognizes' it (= corresponding unit activation) and experiences 'conscious associations' with it (= secondary, weaker activations), both in plausible correspondence to a simple associative psychology conjectured for Lucy herself. During testing, these associations were manifest with the processing cycle immediately following the test input. The network did not need to 'settle' through multiple cycles to display its associative pattern completions.

Both Lucy and Lucynet are severely challenged by several subsequent events. Freud identified these episodes as traumatic, although weakly so. To represent these in the changeable web of Lucynet, a crucial hypothesis was tested, the sole modification of connectionist minimalism: *an essential concomitant of traumatic experience is learning at an abnormally high learning rate*. One main effect of a high learning rate is obvious. Patterns of inputs presented with a high learning rate will be 'branded' into a network, swamping prior learning with new associations. In Lucynet, the 'traumatic learning' effects occurred with learning rates over 0.3. These effects were increasingly complex, as the subsequent stages of the network will show. Furthermore, at a high learning rate, large effects follow *single* exposures of patterns to be learned. In this respect, the learning-rate hypothesis corresponds to a fortunate fact about most traumas – the traumatic event is isolated in its intensity among more ordinary, nontraumatic experiences. The story of Lucy R., then, was reduced in Lucynet to a prelude of unexceptional associative pattern learning, followed by a sequence of single exposure learning trials, where each of Lucy's traumas was modeled by just one exposure, at a 'traumatic' high learning rate, to a pattern corresponding to each trauma from the case study.

First, the author followed Freud in a slight romantic excess. Lucy's troubles began with falling in love with her boss, the factory director and father of the children in Lucy's care. Freud imagined Lucy's passion beginning with a single meaningful conversation, a sudden and dramatic psychological change. The first pattern for 'traumatic learning' was accordingly 'Director + Love.' The results were as expected. After learning, the background associations involving both units were overwhelmed by the new mutual association of love. Table 10.1, row I displays Freud's account of the moment and its effects, together with their recreation in Lucynet.

Lucy's love for her employer infuses her reactions to several other events. The first of these is a scene that 'crushed her hopes' (p. 118) of a real relationship with the director. The blow came following a visit from a female acquaintance. As the guest prepared to leave, she kissed the two children on the lips. Later, the director shouted at Lucy that such a breach of sanitation was intolerable. If Lucy permitted it to happen again, she would be dismissed. Freud describes this moment as traumatic, the 'operative trauma' in the case. The case study is unclear about the immediate effect of the episode (which occurred well before the encounter with Freud). The Lucynet simulation of the event suggests some plausible conjectures. The input for learning is the complex 'Director + Guest + Kissing-children + Distress.' As expected, subsequent tests after learning showed a pronounced pattern completion effect: presentation of any one element of the 'trauma' led to a pronounced 'recall' of the other elements. The sole modulation of this emphatic recall showed a continuing influence of the already established association of units representing the Director and Love. The episode model appears in row II of Table 10.1.

DSM-IV (American Psychiatric Association, 1994) lists the following phenomenological symptoms for post-traumatic stress disorder (PTSD):

B. The traumatic event is persistently re-experienced in one (or more) of the following ways:

1. Recurrent and intrusive distressing recollections of the event, including images, thoughts, or perceptions. . . .
2. Recurrent distressing dreams of the event. . . .
3. Acting or feeling as if the traumatic event were recurring (includes a sense of reliving the experience, illusions, hallucinations, and dissociative flashback episodes). . . .
4. Intense psychological distress at exposure to internal or external cues that symbolize or resemble an aspect of the traumatic event.
5. Physiological reactivity on exposure to internal or external cues that symbolize or resemble an aspect of the traumatic event.

All of these are plausible elaborations of the pattern completion effects observed in Lucynet. Thus, the basic mechanism of PTSD suggested is a mechanism for associative learning and recall operating in a disruptively emphatic way. In Lucynet, the learned complex has no internal structure and every element is equally effective in recreating or 'reliving' the experience. As a result, a range of inputs, including trivial reminders of the event, may be sufficient to kindle the whole traumatic pattern.

Table 10.1. *Turning points in the case history, and their simulation.*

Lucy R.: 'Traumatic' events*	Lucynet representation: patterns for 'traumatic learning'	Lucy R.: Symptoms	Lucynet after learning: test inputs →	→ Resulting activations (by decreasing magnitude)
I. Sudden love 'He looked at her meaningly. . . . Her love for him had begun at that moment.' (p. 118)	Director Love	'She even allowed herself to dwell on the gratifying hopes which she had based on this talk.' (p. 118)	1. Director → 2. Love →	→ Director, Love → Love, Director
II. The operative trauma '. . . A lady who has an acquaintance of her employer's came to visit them, and on her departure kissed the two children on the mouth. . . His fury burst on the head of the unlucky governess. . . This had happened at a time when she still thought he loved her. . . The scene had crushed her hopes.' (p. 118).	Director Guest Kissing children Distress	'For a time, however, that scene had no manifest effect. . . Her hysterical symptoms did not start until later, at moments which may be described as "auxiliary".' (p. 123)	1. Director → 2. Guest → 3. Kissing → 4. Distress → 5. Love →	→ Director, Kissing, Guest, Distress, Love → Guest, Distress, Kissing, Director → Kissing, Distress, Guest → Distress, Kissing, Guest, Director → Love, Director

Table 10.1. *Continued*

Lucy R.: 'Traumatic' events'*	Lucynet representation: patterns for 'traumatic learning'	Lucy R.: Symptoms	Lucynet after learning: test inputs →	→ Resulting activations (by decreasing magnitude)
III. *1st auxiliary trauma* 'There is a guest . . . it's the chief accountant . . . As the children say good-bye, the accountant tries to kiss them. My employer flares up and actually shouts at him. . . I feel a stab at my heart; and as the gentlemen are already smoking, the cigar-smoke sticks in my memory.' (p. 119)	Director Guest Kissing children Cigar smoke Distress	'She was being bothered by [a] smell resembling cigar smoke. . . She did not know where the subjective olfactory sensation came from.' (p. 119)	1. Director → 2. Guest → 3. Kissing → 4. Cigar → 5. Distress →	→ Director, Cigar, Love → Cigar, Guest, Director → Cigar, Kissing → Cigar, Love → Cigar, Distress, Rhinitis
IV. *2nd auxiliary trauma* '"The thought of leaving the dear children made me feel so sad." . . . The conflict between her affects had elevated the moment. . . into a trauma . . . Just at that time she had once more been suffering from such a heavy cold in the nose that she could hardly smell anything. Nevertheless, while she was in her state of agitation she perceived the smell of burnt pudding, which broke through her organically-determined loss of her sense of smell.' (p. 115)	Children Rhinitis Burnt pudding Distress	'Ever since this I have been pursued by the smell. It is there all the time and becomes stronger when I am agitated.' (p. 114)	1. Children → 2. Rhinitis → 3. Pudding → 4. Distress →	→ Children, Pudding, Distress, Rhinitis → Rhinitis, Pudding, Distress, Children → Pudding, Distress, Rhinitis, Children → Distress, Pudding, Rhinitis, Children, Cigar

* Page references from Freud and Breuer ([1895], 1955).

These observations were very much as expected, given the initial understanding of the delta rule and the effects of increased learning rates. Moreover, the apparent analogy between network learning and PTSD symptoms has been independently noted by Li and Spiegel (1992), who proposed (but did not implement in a model) that trauma be modeled as pattern-completion effects following unusually strong constraints that are imposed on the net from the environment (Li and Spiegel, 1992, p. 146). However, Li and Spiegel did not anticipate the side-effects of traumatic learning when traumas compound. For Freud, Lucy, and Lucynet, the more interesting and complex developments lay ahead.

Associations dissociated: effects of multiple traumas

As it happened, the unpleasantness in Lucy's household recurred. Some weeks after the director's outburst, another guest repeated the attempt to kiss the children. This time the director flared up at the guest, the chief accountant at the factory and a regular visitor. To Lucy, however, the scene was 'a stab at my heart' (p. 120). One other feature was prominent in Lucy's eventual memory of the scene, the smell of cigar smoke. As in the case study, the Lucynet representation of this scene (which Freud called an 'auxiliary trauma') closely parallels the previous traumatic scene, with the noted addition of the smell of cigars. The learned pattern, then, was the complex 'Director + Guest + Kissing-children + Cigar-smoke + Distress.'

For Freud, it was this scene, rather than the first, that was the origin of Lucy's hysterical symptoms. One might expect that the large overlap between the operative trauma and its auxiliary echo would only reinforce the emphatic learning and pattern completion effects. Yet in Lucynet, the responses to the next cycle of traumatic learning departed from the PTSD-like symptoms observed earlier. The first surprise is the nearly complete disappearance of the pattern completion effects (row III, Table 10.1). None of the elements of the two traumatic scenes evokes the others. The recall of 'Distress' and of the main event, the attempt to kiss the children, both seem to vanish. *This paradoxical loss of exactly the pattern expected to be retained is the neural network analogue of repression.*

Instead of accurate recall of the learned pattern, the network exhibited an unexpected replacement. To several input probes, Lucynet responds with the activation of the unit representing the smell of cigar smoke. Prior to this point in the simulation, when an input was sent to a single unit of the network, the strongest response was invariably in that same unit; we interpreted that response as the perceptual registration of the input. Now, after compounded trauma, the strongest network activation no longer corresponds to the input, but is found in another unit altogether, the 'Cigar' representation. An input is thus converted into a new percept, an activation formed in the absence of its appropriate input. Lucy experienced a recurrent hallucination of cigar smoke. Lucynet exhibited an 'inappropriate' activation of its 'Cigar' unit, without the corresponding input. *The paradoxical emergence of a maximal activation without the corresponding input is the neural network analogue of hallucination.*

What is going on here? Freud drew his principal morals from the case study at this point, offering a mechanism to explain the twin observations of repression and symptom formation. Repression begins with a deliberate and conscious effort to banish a painful memory from recall. Memories cannot be erased, however. Instead, they are merely isolated (p. 123):

When this process occurs for the first time there comes into being a nucleus and center of crystallization for the formation of a psychical group divorced from the ego – a group around which everything which would imply an acceptance of the incompatible idea subsequently collects. The splitting of consciousness in these cases of acquired hysteria is accordingly a deliberate and intentional one.

This effort to repudiate the hated memory is thwarted when something in the environment strongly reminds one of the original trauma. In the case of Lucy R. (p. 123):

Her hysterical symptoms did not start until later, at moments which may be described as 'auxiliary'. The characteristic feature of such an auxiliary moment is, I believe, that the two divided psychical groups temporarily converge in it.

The 'convergence' is unbearable, however (pp. 122–3):

The hysterical method of defense . . . lies in the conversion of the excitation into a somatic innervation; and the advantage of this is that the incompatible idea is repressed from the ego's consciousness. In exchange, that consciousness now contains the physical reminiscence that has arisen through conversion (in our case, the patient's subjective sensations of smell) and suffers from the affect which is more or less clearly attached to precisely that reminiscence.

In short, Freud imagines a dual process: repression, followed by conversion. His conception of these processes posits a discrete 'nucleus of thoughts,' explicit mental representations ('reminiscences') that are driven from consciousness, but nonetheless reassert themselves in disguise as symptoms. Because these unbearable thoughts continue to exist, Freud cheerfully posited an explicit unconscious 'system' to house them. This conception would be elaborated throughout his career (e.g., Freud [1915] 1957), but is already presupposed here.

Lucynet models the significant symptoms of Lucy R., and develops those symptoms through a consistent analogue of Lucy's experience in the months before her visit to Freud. But, as Figure 10.1 makes clear, Lucynet utterly lacks the mechanism Freud imagined. Connectionism thus offers a different way of thinking about what occurred in Lucy R., and in cases of compounded trauma in general, Lucynet's 'symptoms' are explained by the conjoint effects of the 'traumatic learning' of overlapping patterns and the delta learning rule. With a single trauma, the delta rule leads to a pronounced increase in connection strength among the units involved in the traumatic pattern. A single exposure leads to 'overlearning,' as discussed above. When that same pattern partly repeats, units involved in the pattern receive a flood of input as the external input combines with the massive lateral inputs along the positive, overlearned connections. The delta rule accordingly compensates for this overload by driving *down* the weights on connections. Since subsequent patterns are also traumatic (that is, are learned at a high learning rate), this inhibitory effect is dramatic. When subsequent patterns partly overlap, the maelstrom of delta rule effects rapidly becomes intractable. In this case, the new element, 'Cigar smoke,' is exempt from the inhibition affecting the other units, and the network develops the tendency to respond as if that element were present in response to several unrelated inputs.

Lucy's story did not end with the episode just modeled, however, nor was the hallucinated cigar smoke her initial complaint. One more 'traumatic' scene followed. In part because of her troubles in her household, Lucy considered quitting her post, but at the price of losing her ties to the children. This conflict of emotions was particularly acute one day as she played with the children just after receiving a letter from her mother, back in Scotland. Just at that moment a pot of pudding on the stove began to burn. Freud reasoned that the conflict of feelings at just that moment was intense enough to constitute a trauma (p. 115), and the smell of burnt pudding its conspicuous marker. As a result, Lucy would hallucinate that smell, her principal complaint henceforth.

Although the pudding only burns once, it seems likely that the emotional tumult that accompanied the smell recurred throughout this period in Lucy's life. If a prior moment of conflict had already been traumatic, then the scene with burnt pudding might have been a repeating, 'auxiliary' trauma. In that case, the psychodynamics underlying this symptom would be parallel to the origin of the cigar smoke hallucination, where the first trauma creates massive association, but its repetition massive inhibition and dissociation, save for new elements, which 'pop out' as conspicuous new symptoms. Alternatively, Freud proposes that in general an initial trauma and its auxiliary repetition can 'coincide,' with conversion occurring as an immediate effect (p. 124). In this case, the immediate recall of trauma would itself be traumatic, and even an isolated trauma would become self-compounding.

Each of these interpretations suggests different simulations at this stage in Lucynet. Rather than pursue them, however, the author kept as close as possible to the case study itself. Freud recounts a single traumatic moment on the theme of leaving the children, a moment also marked, as it happens, by Lucy's rhinitis, and so for Lucynet one pattern was input for traumatic learning: 'Children + Rhinitis + Burnt-pudding + Distress.' Row IV of Table 10.1 shows the results of this next stage of Lucynet traumatic learning. The four elements of the traumatic pattern are bound into a tight associative unit, and the responses parallel the PTSD-like responses also shown in row II. Unlike the cigar smoke hallucination, the smell of burnt pudding does not dominate the response to other inputs. Thus, in the Lucynet framework, it is a pronounced association rather than a clear 'hallucination.' However, the association is very strong, and elicited by single inputs which Lucy might have encountered routinely: children, her rhinitis, and her ongoing distress. This simulation also suggests that the memory of the traumatic scene would be readily available, if not intrusive. So it was for Lucy. Freud began his interrogation by asking whether the smell of burnt pudding reminded her of anything, and she was quick to recount just this scene. But that is another story, one of therapy and cure.

Remembrance and catharsis

Having created what may be the world's only neurotic neural network, the author felt compelled to restore his creation to full (simulated) mental health. Again, he turned to Freud and Breuer for guidance (p. 6, repeated on p. 225, emphasis in the original):

Each individual hysterical symptom immediately and permanently disappeared when we had succeeded in bringing clearly to light the memory of the event by which it was provoked and in arousing the accompanying affect, and when the patient had described that event in the greatest possible detail and had put the affect into words.

In *Studies on Hysteria*, this was called the 'cathartic technique,' which Freud would later call 'the immediate precursor of psycho-analysis; and, in spite of every extension of experience and of every modification of theory . . . still contained within it as its nucleus' (Freud [1924] 1955, p. 194).

The network version of catharsis, then, will consist of the re-exposure to the traumatic stimuli. Freud and Breuer stress that the reminiscence of the scene must be accompanied with its original affect. Thus, within the connectionist framework, at least some of the original traumatic intensity must accompany the catharsis. The overall catharsis was modeled by re-exposing the network once to each of the traumatic patterns, using a learning rate coefficient set at half that of the original traumatic learning. As in the case study, the patterns were presented in reverse order, as Lucy herself (with Freud's prompting) recounted them.

Catharsis led to cure for Lucynet as for Lucy. Re-exposure to the second auxiliary trauma led to a reduction of associative intensity of inputs to the 'burnt pudding' unit (in Lucynet), and a gradual reduction in the hallucination (for Lucy). Re-exposure to the earlier traumas led to a more dramatic reversal. In Lucynet, the 'hallucination' of cigar smoke and the accompanying 'repression' of the traumatic pattern both disappeared completely, replaced with a normal set of associative links among parts of the traumatic pattern. (For example, the input 'Guest' yields activation in 'Guest,' 'Kissing-children,' 'Cigar-smoke,' 'Director,' and 'Distress.') For Lucy, too, the hallucinated cigar vanished at once. However, one trauma neither patient nor network could overcome. Both finished their histories with an abiding (if secret) love for their boss. Lucy confessed as much in her last session with Freud; Lucynet showed an implacable two-way association between 'Director' and 'Love.'

To re-experience a trauma one must first remember it. Usually, any number of cues leads to retrieval of a learned pattern. But when a memory is repressed, whether in artificial or human neural networks, many of those associative paths are blocked. How, then, is the repressed pattern recovered? Lucy R. made her way back to the operative trauma by patient association. 'At my insistence,' Freud wrote, 'a picture gradually emerged before her, hesitatingly and piecemeal to begin with' (p. 119). So far, Lucynet only displays its immediate response to any input, its 'first associations.' This made the 'repression' of the operative traumatic pattern a barrier to its recall that could not be overcome by any combination of inputs. To further explore this issue, Lucynet was redesigned to simulate a purely internal sequence of thoughts, a simulated 'stream of consciousness.' To do this, the author took the current activation following an initial input, and re-input this activation as a new input. In essence, each pattern of internal activation in the network thus generates its successor, following only the associative paths established between units in the course of the network history. Each of these activation states was recorded over ten cycles of recurrent network 'reflection.'

Examples of the network's changing internal operations are shown in Figure 10.2. Each panel shows the initial input to the network in the leftmost column, labeled 'I.' The columns labeled 'A' then show ten cycles of response. (The size of the dark squares indicates the magnitude of positive activation. Light squares signify negative activation values, i.e., inhibition). Cycle 1 is the net's 'percept' or immediate response to the input; this is the activation the author has interpreted as an analogue to Lucy's state of consciousness at turning points in the case study. Each subsequent cycle is the network's purely internal response to its previous state of activation. For comparison, Figure 10.2 depicts just the evolving responses to input in the 'Cigar' unit. Until far along in the traumatized training, the net displays a fairly predictable associative 'psychology,' in which the network settles into a stable state of self-sustaining activation. Two of the background associations (prior to any trauma) are initially apparent: 'Director + Guest' (reflecting the director's noted propensity to entertain visitors) and 'Director + Guest + Cigar' (following the favorite pastime, noted explicitly by Lucy, of her boss and his male acquaintances). The cigar input 'reminds' Lucynet of these associations, and the net settles into a stable recreation of those associative patterns, with echoes of other connections (e.g., 'Children + Love').

Following the overlearning of 'Director + Love,' Lucynet's soliloquy changes. The cigar still reminds it initially of guests and the director, but once the latter is 'in mind,' all further thoughts follow the love connection. That stable association is then overthrown by the operative trauma, 'Director + Guest + Kissing-children + Distress.' As soon as the background associations carry the network toward 'Guest' and 'Director,' it is this most recent 'trauma' that dominates, modulated by the prior strong associations between 'Director' and 'Love.'

Up to this point, the network behaves like most connectionist models in that it 'settles' into a stable pattern of activation in the absence of further inputs. Simple assumptions about associative psychology and the intense learning of a traumatic pattern explain its behavior. But all this changes in panel D, showing the network's internal processing following

A. Background Associations

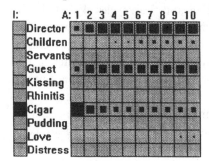

B. Sudden Love

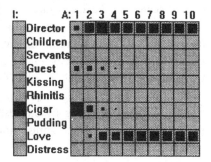

C. Operative Trauma

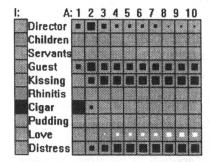

D. 1st Auxiliary Trauma

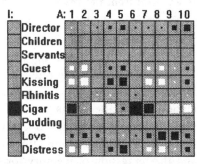

Fig. 10.2 Lucynet 'stream of consciousness.' Each panel shows ten cycles of recurrent activation. After the initial external input, indicated by column I, each column A1 through A10 indicates the activation pattern based solely on the previous state of activation, without further external input. Dark tiles indicate positive activation values; light tiles indicate negative values. Each test panel reflects a different state of network learning: A. following background associative training, prior to episodes of 'traumatic learning;' B. following the emphatic learning of 'Director + Love,' C. following the emphatic learning of 'Director + Guest + Kissing-Children + Distress;' D. following the emphatic learning of 'Director + Guest + Kissing-Children + Cigar + Distress.' Panels A through C exhibit 'settling' toward stable states reflecting the dominant associations at that point in network training. Panel D shows oscillation as a result of interference through compounded traumatic learning. At cycle 1, the traumatic input pattern has been inhibited, but it rebounds around cycle 5, and again at cycle 10. This rebound effect may model recall of repressed or dissociated content.

the auxiliary trauma, which repeated the preceding trauma with the addition of the smell of cigars. First, the 'Cigar' input fails to recreate the traumatic pattern (as discussed above). But rather than settling into a stable response, even without new input the 'neurotic' network oscillates between states of excitation and inhibition, each cycle a flashback to an earlier scene in the case study. Significantly, at cycles 4 and 5, the 'repressed' traumatic pattern briefly reappears, to be promptly canceled in cycle 6. The compounding of traumatic inputs has not simply erased the history of network learning. That history has radically altered network function, and even left a path for its explicit reconstruction. But the path is a tortuous one. Despite its simplicity, Lucynet captured this aspect of the case study by suggesting the possibility of the recall of repressed content. (Other implications of recurrent processing are considered below.)

Discussion: from the 1890s to the 1990s

To summarize, the history of Lucynet follows the case study of Lucy R. by simulating the learning of plausible background associations followed by a series of 'traumatic' inputs, learned via single exposures with an abnormally high learning rate coefficient. A second sequence of learning followed the course of therapy, re-exposing the network to the 'traumatic' input patterns via single exposures at an intermediate learning rate. As a result, the network exhibited robust analogues of three of Freud's most salient observations of Lucy: two olfactory hallucinations and the repression of memory for key episodes of symptom formation. These symptoms emerged and disappeared from the network at moments corresponding to their emergence and disappearance in Freud's chronology of the case. The pattern of symptoms emerged as a side-effect of the simulation of Lucy's experience and the operation of the neural network, rather than as a direct result of programming or explicit training to produce these responses.

These are intriguing results given the radical simplicity of Lucynet – ten units only, governed by a single activation equation and a single learning rule. From ten processing units to the tens of billions in the human brain is a sobering leap. We would not wisely conclude anything about the specific psychology or physiology of Lucy R. or anyone else based on Lucynet. But we can use Lucynet as a heuristic model and foil for theories of hysteria and dissociation. Its simplicity leaves no place for special processes to hide, and thus reveals and questions some widespread assumptions about the mechanisms and etiology of hysteria and its modern descendants.

Perhaps the most useful lesson of Lucynet lies in its deep challenge to what might be called the archival model of memory. By this is meant the conception of memories as fixed records or 'reified contents' that can pass in and out of consciousness, and be variously influential or dormant over time. Even in *Studies on Hysteria*, Freud clearly conceived of ideas of all sorts in this way (p. 300):

It remains, I think, a fact deserving serious consideration that in our analyses we can follow a train of thought from the conscious into the unconscious (i.e. into something that is absolutely not recognized as a memory), that we can trace it from there for some distance through consciousness once more and that we can see it terminate in the unconscious again, without this alternation of 'psychical illumination' making any change in the train of thought itself, in its logical consistency and in the interconnection between its various parts.

Once thoughts are reified as special sorts of fixed objects to be manipulated by the mind, most of the Freudian mechanics follows as a matter of course. If thoughts exert influences on behavior and consciousness without themselves becoming conscious, then they must sometimes exist in the unconscious (a sort of specialized processing module) and, moreover, some sort of mental executive must take on the task of moving thoughts in and out of consciousness, and in and out of conscious or unconscious play. This way of thinking about thoughts certainly meshes smoothly with the computational model of mind that has long dominated cognitive science (Erdelyi, 1985).

These days, the archival model of memory has been explicitly disavowed by all. Extensive work in cognitive psychology has shown recall to be *construction* of a memory rather than its retrieval. Connectionists have certainly encouraged this reconception of memory by showing how explicit patterns of activation can be stored implicitly in the form of matrices of connection weights. Memory to a connectionist is a disposition to reform patterns of activation, rather than extract them from some form of storage.

Yet, in discussions of psychopathology, the archival model and its attendant mechanisms still operate, even if covertly. For example, in his excellent review of dissociative disorders, Kihlstrom (1994) notes that a number of disorders involve failures of recall, but the failures are temporarily or permanently reversible. (This characterizes the DSM-IV disorders of dissociative amnesia, dissociative fugue, and dissociative identity disorder.) 'Reversible memory disorders are disorders of retrieval; they occur because the individual cannot, at the moment, gain access to memories that have been adequately encoded, and remain available in storage' (Kihlstrom, 1994; p. 379). Here, the image of the archive is explicit, although one could alter the terminology to depict storage as a merely dispositional, connectionistic storage. But what Kihlstrom concludes from his observation requires an archival view: 'Retrieval and accessibility are phenomena of consciousness as they entail bringing available memories into phenomenal awareness' (Kihlstrom, 1994). Memories, in short, move in and out of the spotlight of awareness; with the reification of memory comes the reification of a special processor, 'consciousness.' Kihlstrom and Hoyt (1990, p. 201) make this explicit as follows:

The essential distinction between what is conscious and what is not is that conscious mental contents are both activated (by perception or thought) and linked with activated representations of the self, its goals, and the local environment. Preconscious mental contents are latent: not activated (or, more properly, not activated above some threshold) and perforce not linked to the activated mental representation of the self. Dissociated, subconscious mental contents, while fully activated, are not linked with either an active mental representation of the self or the active mental representation of the context, or both.

Thus, a conception of memories as fixed records brings along with it a model of mind in which conscious and unconscious mental processes can unfold in parallel, passing thoughts back and forth. The evidence of disintegrated cognition has suggested to a long line of researchers the existence of parallel executives. The first to argue along these lines is probably Plato, who interpreted conflict of the will as evidence for distinct faculties of mind (*Republic*, Book IV). It persists at the origins of clinical psychology, not only in Freud but also in Janet and James, and in numerous contemporary sources (e.g., Hilgard). Even the psychopathologists Li and Spiegel, in their discussion of the import of connectionism for understanding dissociation, declare a need for the parallel operation of two or more information processors (Li and Spiegel, 1992; p. 145).

Lucynet gets away with much less. One processor accommodates both Lucynet's preserved 'normal' associative processing and its dissociated dislocations. Yet, for all its simplicity, once a certain learning history has transpired, the network ceases to be a passive responder to input stimuli. Figure 10.2D depicts a new stage in Lucynet evolution and an intriguing moment in connectionist modeling. At this point, patterns vie for expression. While some strut and fret their hour upon the stage, others are (temporarily) heard no more. When various trains of network thought exclude each other, we observe the network analogue of dissociation. But, as always in this study, there is no off-stage orchestration. There are just the thoughts on the surface, interacting with each other. The functions of integration or disintegration, making conscious or repressing, are not administered by an agency separated from the thoughts (patterns) themselves.

Instead of a special processing system to monitor and manipulate explicit unconscious representation, through learning Lucynet undergoes widespread changes in the *connection weights* between conscious elements. These weights define the dispositions of elements to activate one another. They are 'unconscious' in the sense that they are part of the implementation of the network rather than its explicitly represented content, analogous to the physiology of synapses in the brain. But this remains a different and less robust conception of the unconscious than that of the archival model.

In addition to its dispositional, connectionist storage of memories, Lucynet exhibits a further break from the archival model: in Lucynet, *encoding of new memories alters the encoding of the old.* Previously learned patterns change as an immediate side-effect of traumatic learning; no special re-enactment of old memories is required. Connectionist modelers usually go to great lengths to *prevent* the interference of old learning by new, with the goal of accurate reconstruction of discrete learned patterns (Hetherington and Seidenberg, 1989; Kortge, 1990; Murre, 1992). But in Lucynet this interference is exactly the source of both the negative and positive 'symptoms' – dissociation from the overlearned past, and the insertion of a 'perceptual hallucination.' In most models, interference effects are meaningless noise, but within the guiding framework of a clinical study, Lucynet's wild ride remains interpretable.

The study of Lucy R. has thus become a twice-told tale. Its second telling, as Lucynet, has elided much of the humanity of the first, but it has preserved the main episodes and the main effects noted in Freud's version. The new tale has added a crucial subtext, the fundamental hypothesis that one form of psychogenic pathology can originate when stimulus patterns are subject to intense single-exposure learning. But a single episode of 'traumatic learning' did not generate the dissociative effects typical of hysteria. For this, our simulated subject needed a history of simulated suffering. Only then did the network become both neurotic and interesting.

Like any story, the new fable of Lucynet is open to many interpretations. Given its simplicity, Lucynet provides no direct evidence about any aspect of human psychology. But it does show something of what is possible on a shoestring. In that spirit, it suggests a few *possible* morals – avenues of inquiry worth noting for future clinical research.

1. *Psychopathology is a narrative.* The scientific emphasis on efficient
   causation, experimental method, and statistical significance leads to
   a search for 'stories' of pathology in which there are just two episodes, a single cause and its particular effect. Lucynet developed its
   most revealing syndrome only after a sequence of unique events,
   each contributing to a complex outcome. In the huge networks
   that are each of us, every experience and every response reflects
   the remembrance of things past. Our past experience may not merely
   provide a general backdrop, but instead contribute in specific ways
   to otherwise inexplicable responses. Freud, of course, would agree,
   as would most clinicians (but not most insurers). This complicates
   the understanding of pathology in general, as well as diagnosis and
   treatment of specific cases. It also threatens the rigor of clinically
   based science, leading to charges (such as those leveled at psychoanalysis) that it is pseudoscience (e.g., Grünbaum, 1984, 1993).
   Connectionism may offer a middle ground, by allowing for models
   sensitive to the cumulative effects of personal history, but still constrained by the basic computational capacities of networks. Such
   models afford further controled exploration of several variables
   that may be clinically important.

2. *To interpret a clinical narrative, one must understand the perceptual,
   cognitive, and affective world of the subject.* Models like Lucynet are
   'loose' in several senses. First, they rest on an initial assignment of
   meanings to network architecture and possible patterns of activation. Second, the traumatic learning is indiscriminate, branding both
   the central and the trivial elements of a horrific scene into the traumatized memory. But a compounded trauma has the further effect
   of inhibiting some links within the repeated trauma while enhancing
   others, leading (in Lucynet, and perhaps in humans) to modifications in subsequent encodings and ultimately to dissociative phenomena. *These complex effects in turn depend on the perceptual
   categories that underlie the recognition of elements as 'same' or 'different' from one exposure to the next.* This category assignment will
   be sensitive to the ramifying effects of compounded trauma, and to a
   host of developmental and idiosyncratic differences. If retroactive
   memory interference occurs in us as well, unravelling a dissociated
   life narrative may be even more difficult. Event memory traces may
   not merely be hidden but altered.

3. *Connectionism is a multilevel modeling tool.* Connectionists often
   celebrate the 'neural inspiration' of their approach, and in recent

years have worked toward ever-increasing biological realism. The connectionist approach naturally lends itself to the simulation of biological and neural networks. But it nonetheless also lends itself to the simulation of other complex phenomena, especially systems subject to multiple simultaneous constraints or internal interactions. Our minds, described at the psychological level as arenas for the interplay of thought, are such systems. It does not matter that Lucynet is biologically unrealistic, or that the delta rule probably does not describe the waxing and waning of synaptic efficacy. What does matter is that the model offers a consistent representation of a domain, so that the model's behavior can be compared with that of entities in the domains. As models become sufficiently general, they become theories of the domain. Lucynet, as a pilot study, cannot pose as a theory of dissociation. But it could indicate a family of psychological models that may ultimately cohere as a theory of some aspect of psychology. That ultimate theory will be no more biological than Lucynet, but none the worse as a theory at its own level.

4. *Without a central executive, anything is possible.* Just as digital computers suggest (falsely) an image of unfailing and unflappable rationality, connectionist networks project the image of steady pattern completion and solid, predictable, rote association. They are built to work. But no law enforces this expectation. In fact, these networks are delicate hot-house flowers, reared in the most rigid and contrived learning environments. In the erratic climates of human experience, such nets would fail. Lucynet became a failure as a pattern associator, but an interesting and suggestive one. After his reading of Charcot, Janet, Breuer, and Freud, William James ([1896] 1982, pp. 71–2) commented:

> The enigmatic character of much of all this cannot be contested, even though there is a deep and laudable desire of the intellect to think of the world as existing in a clean and regular shape. The mass of literature growing more abundant daily, from which I have drawn my examples, consisting as it does almost exclusively of oddities and eccentricities, of grotesqueries and masqueradings, incoherent, fitful, personal, is certainly ill-calculated to bring satisfaction either to the ordinary medical mind or that of a psychological turn. The former has its cut and dried classifications and routine therapeutic appliances of a material order; the latter has its neat notions of the cognitive and active powers, its laws of association and the rest. Everything here is so lawless and individualized that it is chaos come again; and the dramatic and humoring and humbugging relation of operator to patient in the whole business is profoundly distasteful to the

orderly characters who fortunately in every profession most abound. Such persons don't wish a *wild* world, where tomfoolery seems as it were among the elemental and primal forces. . .

Between 'chaos come again' and the 'neat notions of cognitive and active powers,' we find the vast middle ground of connectionism. In its mechanics and its poetics we may oneday find a new understanding of both psychopathology and everyday mental life.

Endnote

1 Undated page references are from *Studies on Hysteria* (Freud and Breuer, [1895] 1955).

References

American Psychiatric Association (1994). *Diagnostic and Statistical Manual of Mental Disorders*, 4th edn. Washington, DC: APA.
Crews, F. (1993). The unknown Freud. *New York Review of Books*, **40**(19), 55–65.
Cummins, R. (1983). *The Nature of Psychological Explanation*. Cambridge, MA: MIT Press.
Erdelyi, M. (1985). *Psychoanalysis: Freud's Cognitive Psychology*. San Francisco: Freeman.
Freud, S. ([1924] 1955). A short account of psycho-analysis. In *The Standard Edition of the Complete Psychological Works of Sigmund Freud*, Vol. 19, ed. J. Strachey, pp. 191–209. London: Hogarth.
Freud, S. ([1915] 1957). The unconscious. In *The Standard Edition of the Complete Psychological Works of Sigmund Freud*, Vol. 14, ed. J. Strachey, pp. 159–217. London: Hogarth.
Freud, S. ([1895] 1966). *Project for a Scientific Psychology*. The Standard Edition of the Complete Psychological Works of Sigmund Freud, Vol. 1, ed. J. Strachey. London: Hogarth.
Freud, S. & Breuer, J. ([1895] 1955). *Studies on Hysteria. The Standard Edition of the Complete Psychological Works of Sigmund Freud*, Vol. 2, ed. J. Strachey. London: Hogarth.
Grünbaum, A. (1984). *The Foundations of Psychoanalysis: A Philosophical Critique*. Berkeley: University of California Press.
Grünbaum, A. (1993). *Validation of the Clinical Theory of Psychoanalysis*. Madison, CT: International Universities Press.
Hetherington, P.A. & Seidenberg, M. (1989). Is there 'catastrophic interference' in connectionist networks? In *Program of the 11th Annual Conference of the Cognitive Science Society*, pp. 26–33. Hillsdale, NJ: Lawrence Erlbaum.
James, W. ([1896] 1982). Hysteria. In *William James on Exceptional Mental States*, ed. E. Taylor, pp. 53–72. New York: Scribner's.
Kihlstrom, J. (1994). One hundred years of hysteria. In *Dissociation: Clinical and Theoretical Perspectives*, ed. S.J. Lynn & J.W. Rhue, pp. 365–94. New York: Guilford Press.

Kihlstrom, J. & Hoyt, I.P. (1990). Repression, dissociation, and hypnosis. In *Repression and Dissociation: Implications for Personality Theory, Psychopathology, and Health*, ed. J.L. Singer, pp. 181–208. Chicago: University of Chicago Press.

Kortge, C.A. (1990). Episodic memory in connectionist networks. In *Program of the 12th Annual Conference of the Cognitive Science Society*, pp. 764–71. Hillsdale, NJ: Lawrence Erlbaum.

Li, D. & Spiegel, D. (1992). A neural network model of dissociative disorders. *Psychiatric Annals*, **22**(3), 144–7.

Lloyd, D. (1994). Connectionist hysteria: Reducing a Freudian case study to a network model. *Philosophy, Psychiatry, and Psychology*, **1**(2), 69–88.

McClelland, J. & Rumelhart, D. (1986). A distributed model of human learning and memory. In *Parallel Distributed Processing: Explorations in the Microstructure of Cognition*. Vol. 2: *Psychological and Biological Models*, ed. J. McClelland, D. Rumelhart, & the PDP Research Group, pp. 170–216. Cambridge, MA: MIT Press.

Murre, J. (1992). Effects of pattern presentation on interference in back-propagation networks. In *Program of the 14th Annual Conference of the Cognitive Science Society*, pp. 54–9. Hillsdale, NJ: Lawrence Erlbaum.

Shank, R.C. & Abelson, R.P. (1977). *Scripts, Plans, Goals, and Understanding*. Hillsdale, NJ: Lawrence Erlbaum.

Wegman, C. (1985). *Psychoanalysis and Cognitive Psychology*. London: Academic Press.

11

Neural network analysis of learning in autism

IRA L. COHEN

Goldilocks . . . dipped a spoon into Father Bear's bowl, but the porridge in it was too hot. . . Then she tried some from Mother Bear's bowl, but that was too cold. The porridge in Baby Bear's bowl was just right. . .
Robert Southey, *Goldilocks and the Three Bears*

Even though autism is a relatively infrequent disorder, occurring in about 1.5 to 2 cases/1000 in the population (Sugiyama and Abe, 1989), it has attracted the attention of many researchers since the time of Kanner's (1943) initial description of the syndrome. This curiosity reflects, in part, the fact that the bizarre and puzzling behaviors shown by individuals with autism present a challenge to theorists. More urgently, the fact that age-appropriate learning and social–communicative behavior is not present in these children has a devastating impact on their families and on the children's later social, emotional and cognitive development. Understanding the biological mechanisms responsible for autism may help to shed light on the best way to treat this syndrome.

Autism has an age of onset that is, typically, between 12 and 30 months of age, although some mothers report noticing abnormalities in their child's behavior from birth. The first behavioral disturbances noted include lack of response to the child's name being called, acting as if deaf, despite other evidence of apparent normal hearing (e.g., dashing to the kitchen from another room when a candy bar is unwrapped); failure to anticipate being picked up; failure to cuddle when held; poor eye contact and lack of interest in social interaction; failure to use normal gestures such as pointing to communicate (instead pulling others to desired objects); lack of speech development or speech regression; failure to develop appropriate play skills; and later development of repetitive/ritualistic behaviors such as unusual hand movements, visual fixations, rocking, resistance to change, etc. (Gillberg and Coleman, 1992).

Unless exposed to highly intensive intervention (e.g., Lovaas, 1987), most show persistent problems in language, cognition and social interaction throughout their lives. If speech is acquired, it is not used for sharing experiences and conversational purposes but, instead, is often literal, repetitive (on words, phrases or topics), echoic, emitted with an odd rhythm (prosody) and/or solely used to make requests for desired objects. Additionally, many individuals display disturbances in sleep or arousal, hypersensitivity to tactile, taste, or auditory stimuli, and incongruous affect (American Psychiatric Association, 1994).

This vast variety of behavioral disturbance in autism and similar syndromes such as Asperger's disorder (Wing, 1981) suggests that multiple systems are affected, hence the use of the term 'pervasive developmental disorder' (American Psychiatric Association, 1994). Most affected persons are male (about three to four males for every one female) and have sub-average intellectual functioning (about 70 percent with IQs less than 70). However, it is often the case that not all aspects of cognition are equally affected. On standardized tests, many persons with autism tend to do poorly on tests of vocabulary and comprehension but do quite well on tests of rote memory and visual pattern recognition (Frith and Baron-Cohen, 1987). Abstract concepts of language and social interaction such as pronouns, prepositions, humor, and empathy typically elude such individuals, irrespective of IQ. A few, however, display islets of normal to exceptional abilities (so-called savant skills) such as calendar calculating skills, hyperlexia, rote memorization of extensive lists of information on idiosyncratic topics, memorization of locations and routes to various places, etc. In addition, unusual learning styles have been consistently demonstrated. Many of these children can be highly distracted by task-irrelevant stimuli yet appear highly focused at other times. Frequently, what they have been taught fails to generalize well to other teachers, situations, or environments (Koegel and Koegel, 1995).

This list of unusual behaviors presents a challenge for the development of theories as to how such patterns could exist or coexist. Why are such inconsistencies present? Why are some complex associations easily memorized and performed while others, such as the desire to share experiences or feedback from others, are not acquired despite the fact that such behaviors are displayed by typically developing infants? Why is it that behaviors acquired in one situation fail to generalize to others?

The purpose of this chapter is to review and elaborate upon the implications of a previously published model of the learning characteristics of people with autism (Cohen, 1994). This model attempts to integrate recent neuropathological observations with some of the attentional and learning characteristics described above. Unlike other models, the linkage between the neuropathological observations and behavior that is drawn here is more direct in the sense that the observed pathology is qualitatively 'simulated' with a neural network in which the effects of abnormal neuroanatomy on learning (relative to a given problem type) can be simulated. The model is, admittedly, speculative, but it does have an advantage in its parsimony in addition to its ability to simulate and tie together a diverse set of data about autism – neuroanatomy, neuropathology, pathogenesis, behavioral characteristics, learning, generalization, and behavior modification – in one single framework as well as making specific, testable predictions.

The neuropathology of autism

Several researchers have identified neuropathological changes in the brains of individuals diagnosed with autism. The specificity of these observations to autism has yet to be elucidated, i.e., it has not been clearly demonstrated that the observations are unique to autism. However, if they are, then the findings are potentially interesting because they help to explain some of the phenomena, as described below. These abnormalities have been revealed primarily by two means: neuropathological observations of the brains of deceased individuals and magnetic resonance imaging (MRI).

Although earlier neuropathological investigations provided inconsistent findings (Williams et al., 1980), Bauman and Kemper (1985; 1986) and Kemper and Bauman (1993) have more recently reported abnormalities in the 'wiring patterns' of several individuals who had been diagnosed with autism. Specifically, increased neuronal density along with smaller neurons was observed in several limbic structures including the hippocampus, entorhinal cortex, amygdalae, mammillary body, medial septal nucleus (pars posteriori), and cingulate cortex. Neuronal loss was reported in the diagonal band of Broca and the biventer, gracile, tonsile, and inferior semilunar lobules of the neocerebellar cortex (Purkinje and granule cells) as well as the fastigial, globose, and emboliform nuclei. Raymond, Bauman and Kemper (1989) have reported, in hippocampal pyramidal cells, reduced dendritic branching in CA1 and CA4 and reduced area of the perikaryon in CA4 neurons. Kemper (1988) has also reported finding polymicrogyria in the orbital frontal cortex and operculum. In a different laboratory, Ritvo et al. (1986) reported finding lower Purkinje cell counts in the cerebellum in four cases. One of these cases also showed microgyria of the left occipital and temporal lobes, asymmetry of the ventral–medial temporal lobes, and asymmetry of the cerebellar tonsils.

MRI studies have revealed problems in the forebrain and hindbrain consistent with some of these neuropathological studies, in particular those related to aberrant cerebellar development (Courchesne et al., 1987, 1988, 1993, 1994; Gaffney et al., 1987a, 1987b, 1988, 1989; Murakami et al., 1989; Hashimoto et al., 1991, 1992, 1993, 1995). Others were unable to replicate some of these observations, or had methodological concerns (Ritvo and Garber, 1988; Nowell et al., 1990; Hsu et al., 1991; Filipek, 1995; Piven and Arndt, 1995).

These MRI and neuropathological observations are suggestive of abnormal wiring patterns in various brain regions and have been hypothesized to be due to deficits in neuronal migration during fetal development (Courchesne et al., 1988; Piven et al., 1990), curtailment of normal neuronal growth (Bauman, 1991) and/or aberrant development (Courchesne et al., 1993). Despite variability in location, the structural deficits, as noted by Bauman (1991), appear to be of two types: 'too few' neurons in one area, e.g., the cerebellum, and apparently 'too many' in other areas, e.g., the amygdala and hippocampus.

Explanations of the meaning of these structural abnormalities for the behavior and learning characteristics of people with autism have been based on the behavioral sequelae of lesion experiments in animals and/or on clinical human neuropsychological studies of patients with lesions in these same areas of the brain (Bauman and Kemper, 1985; Courchesne et al., 1988; Gaffney et al., 1989; Hashimoto et al., 1992). However, it is often not the case that lesioning an intact or developing nervous system is functionally the same as an aberration in neuronal wiring patterns resulting from some prenatal insult or genetic anomaly.

For example, the above autopsy studies implicate the hippocampus in the pathology of some cases with autism. One of the functions the hippocampus serves is to provide the ability to form spatial maps of the environment (Wilson and McNaughton, 1993), and lesioning the hippocampus in primates disrupts the acquisition of spatial maps of the environment and the control of spatially directed movements (Rolls, 1990a, 1990b). However, many people with autism seem to be especially adept at encoding, discriminating and recalling spatial maps, such as complicated routes to various places, and can be very upset if these routes are not followed precisely (Wing and Attwood, 1987).

In 1994, Cohen discussed the ramifications of an abnormal wiring pattern for a theory of autism in which the presenting deficit was one of having too many or too few neurons and/or neuronal connections from a connectionist perspective. The a priori assumption in this model is that the problem of 'too many' and/or 'too few' neurons or neural connections (whether pathological or a 'normal' variant) is a reliable observation, at the cellular level, in autism. A review and an elaboration of these implications are now presented, following a brief discussion of back-propagation models, simulations of which form the basis for the arguments that follow.

Back-propagation analogues of learning in autism

Neural networks come in a variety of architectures, with some having more 'biological realism' than others. One of the most frequently used multilayer associative networks is one that uses a back-propagation training algorithm to adjust the strengths of the weighted connections among the layers (Rumelhart, Hinton and Williams, 1986). Figure 11.1 shows a typical feed-forward network consisting of at least three layers: (1) an 'input layer' in which the number of neurons usually corresponds to the number of distinct features of the input pattern; (2) one or more 'hidden layers,' the first of which receives connections from the input layer; and (3) an 'output layer' which arrives at a prediction or classification based on input from the hidden layer(s). The number of neurons in the output layer usually depends on the number of categories in a classification problem or on the output pattern that is to be represented in prediction problems. The quantitative relation (i.e., the 'transfer function') between output from and input to a neuron is nonlinear in such models (typically sigmoidal), as shown in Figure 11.2. This type of architecture is known as a feed-forward model because information flows in one direction only. Weight changes occur based on the error that is 'back-propagated' first to the hidden layer–output layer connections and then to the input layer–hidden layer connections – hence the name. Each individual neuron can have both excitatory and inhibitory influences on elements to which it is connected. Thus, this anatomy is not very similar to a biological nervous system. Nevertheless, back-propagation networks have been extensively used in nervous system models. Why is this the case? As Churchland and Sejnowski (1992, p. 135) have stated:

FEED-FORWARD NEURAL NETWORK

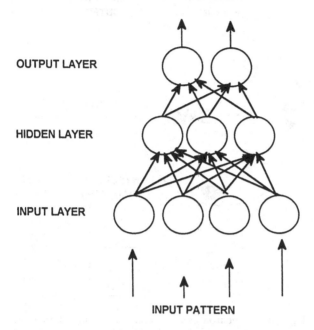

Fig. 11.1 A typical multilayer, feedforward neural network is shown with four input-layer neurons, three hidden-layer neurons and two output-layer neurons. In this network, all of the input-layer neurons are connected to all of the hidden-layer neurons, which are, in turn, connected to all of the output-layer neurons. These multiple connections allow for distribution of information in the network. (Reprinted, with modification, by permission of the publisher from Cohen, I.L. (1994). An artificial neural network analogue of learning in autism. *Biological Psychiatry*, **36**, 5–20. Copyright 1994 by Elsevier Science, Inc.)

(1) It is reasonable to assume that the evolution of nervous systems can be described by a cost function; development and learning in nervous systems are probably also describable by a cost function. In other words, by dint of parameter-adjusting procedures, nervous systems. . . appear to be finding minima in their error surfaces. (2) Model nets that are highly constrained by neurobiological data concerning architecture and dynamics of the neural circuit being simulated may use backprop as a search procedure to find local minima. (3) Identical nets using the same cost function and sliding into error minima will nonetheless vary considerably in the specific values assigned to their para-meters. . . (4) There is no guarantee that the local minima found by the model net will overlap the local minima found by the real neural network, but it is reasonable to assume so. . . (5) That assumption can be tested against the nervous system itself. . . (6) Thus the model nets can be viewed as hypoth-esis generators.

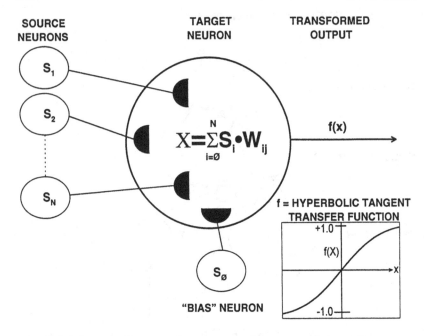

Fig. 11.2 Schematic diagram of a neuron as the target with input from source neurons and a bias neuron that always provides a constant input. Also shown is the equation for combining weights (W_{ij}) with inputs (S_i), yielding a value (X) which is, in turn, the parameter in the transfer function. The transfer function shown here produces an S-shaped, nonlinear, hyperbolic tangent output, which is a function of the input X. (Reprinted, with modification, by permission of the publisher from Cohen, I.L. (1994). An artificial neural network analogue of learning in autism. *Biological Psychiatry*, **36**, 5–20. Copyright 1994 by Elsevier Science, Inc.)

Relevant to points (4) and (5), Lehky and Sejnowski (1988, 1990; cited in Churchland and Sejnowski, 1992) have been able to use a back-propagation network to extract information on curvature of objects from shaded image input to an artificial retina. In learning this task, the hidden-layer neurons developed properties similar to the receptive fields of simple cells in the visual cortex. Therefore, even though such back-propagation models are not that similar to biological nervous systems, they mimic, and may help to explain, some of their properties (Churchland and Sejnowski, 1992).

Thus, there would seem to be enough similarities for one to begin to ask questions about a back-propagation network that could have importance for understanding parts of a biological nervous system.

However, the analogy extends much further. Back-propagation models can successfully mimic some of the learning characteristics of people with autism, once the task and neuropathological observations suggestive of too few or too many neurons are taken into account. How is this possible?

Neural network anatomy and problem type

As one of its functions, the brain maps its environment, as exemplified by the tonotopic organizational map of the auditory cortex. Neural networks also perform such a mapping function, i.e., they compute mathematical functions that relate a set of data in one domain (e.g., presence or absence of symptoms elicited from a diagnostic interview) to another domain (e.g., internal representations of symptom clusters at the hidden layer(s) or predicted diagnoses at the output layer). For example, in a classification problem, a suitably constructed network can identify complex, multidimensional, nonlinear boundaries separating one class from another. As it turns out, the effect of having too many, as opposed to too few, neurons and neural connections on learning in computer-generated neural networks depends on the anatomy of the network and the type of problem the network is asked to solve.

Linear classification problems

Linear classification problems, by definition, have linear boundaries, i.e., groups can be separated by a line, plane or hyperplane. These problems are fairly easy to solve, do not require, and are not helped by, hidden layers with nonlinear transfer functions. For such problems, a two-layer network is sufficient, i.e., one with an input layer and an output layer. Such a 'network' is functionally identical to linear discriminant analysis, multiple linear regression or multiple logistic regression (if a logistic transfer function is used at the output layer). Therefore, for such problems, only the number of inputs devoted to the input layer is critical during the learning process. Too many noninformative inputs that are spuriously correlated with other inputs or with the outputs can affect both learning and generalization.

In working with young children with autism, it is not unusual for teachers to present their pupils with such linear discrimination problems. Consider the problem of teaching such a child to discriminate between cartoon pictures of happy and sad faces, as shown in Figure 11.3. If we

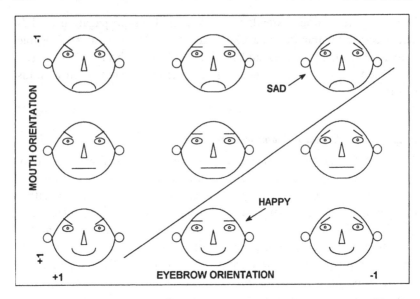

Fig. 11.3 Cartoon happy and sad faces are shown as two of nine possible outcomes in a two-dimensional coordinate system in which mouth or eyebrow orientation is manipulated. Note that these two categories can easily be separated by a single line. Hence, this is an example of a linear classification problem. Also note that these expressions emerge as qualitatively distinct configurations as a result of quantitative variation in their component features. Neural networks are quite good at this type of pattern recognition.

assume that the nonlinear downstream perceptual systems of such children are functioning properly, such that issues of rotation and translation are not of concern, then one output neuron is sufficient to discriminate these faces as long as that neuron receives pertinent preprocessed information such as the orientation of the mouth and/or slant of the eyebrows. Such a problem is linearly separable because, as shown in Figure 11.3, a line can easily separate these faces based on eyebrow and/or mouth orientation. Why, then, do some children with autism seemingly have difficulty with learning such easy problems? The answer may be that for such children: (1) stimuli such as eyebrow or mouth orientation are as salient or less salient than any other stimulus present in the learning situation such as prompts provided by the teacher, extraneous noise, visual distracters etc., i.e., a true 'blank state' is present for facial cues (Weeks and Hobson, 1987); and (2) the decision-making neuron(s) may be receiving too many connections from downstream neurons that process these other, often extraneous, inputs.

Why would facial cues be equally or less salient than extraneous stimuli for people with autism? The autopsy data described above indicate that there are too many neurons in the amygdalae of some of these individuals. The amygdalae are important in acquiring and remembering affective associations and in facial recognition (Rolls, 1992). If having too many neurons has a deleterious effect on such associative learning, then the affective value of facial cues important to effective and meaningful social communication could be impaired. The effect of having too many neurons on the learning and generalization of complex, fuzzy, nonlinear pattern recognition problems, such as the meaning of facial expressions, is described in more detail below. For the simple linear classification problem described here, however, lack of salience of relevant cues means that other cues may have relatively greater salience, even extraneous ones, depending upon their attention-grabbing value. Should such extraneous stimuli become spuriously correlated with the requirements of the learning situation, then they would serve as potential sources of information for problem solution. Since the correlation is spurious, however, any learning that takes such stimuli into account will fail to generalize if such spurious stimuli are not present in the to-be-generalized testing situation.

The author has simulated such a situation with a three-layer feed-forward network that employs a back-propagation training algorithm for weight change (NeuralWare, 1993). The problem involved differentiating between a 'happy' and a 'sad' face by presenting two numbers describing the orientation of the 'mouth' or 'eyebrows.' These numbers varied from -1.0 to $+1.0$ for mouth orientation, with negative numbers corresponding to the corners of the mouth downward, and from 0 to -1.0 for eyebrow orientation, with negative numbers indicating that the part of the eyebrows closest to the ears was lower than the part closest to the nose (see Fig. 11.3). Thus, the mouth input was more 'salient' in that it had greater variation in range than did the less salient, and redundant, eyebrow input. In addition to these salient, but redundant, cues, 1, 3, 5 or 10 extraneous inputs were also added to the input. These consisted of random numbers (from 0 to 1.0) derived from a uniform random numbers distribution. The number of neurons in the middle or hidden layer was varied as follows: 1, 2, 4 and 8. The number of neurons in the output layer was two, corresponding to the presence of a happy or sad face. The transfer function at the hidden and output layers was a hyperbolic tangent (see Fig. 11.2). In keeping with typical classroom-type situations, a small data set was used. Sixteen data points were used in the training set and eight in the test set. Nets were run for 100 trials and stopped every ten trials to record classification accuracy. Four additional replications were run for each permutation by initializing a net to a different set of starting connection weights so that each would converge on the solution from a different starting point in weight space.

Contrary to expectation, even though this was a simple linear problem, hidden-layer size affected performance in the training set. Specifically, the net with only one hidden-layer neuron acquired the discrimination at a slower rate than the other anatomies, which did not differ from each other $(F(30,800) = 3.44, p < 0.001$ for the hidden neurons by trials interaction). However, all nets eventually achieved the same level of accuracy, i.e., percentage correct classification. Thus, although accuracy was not affected by hidden-layer size in this problem, acquisition rate was influenced by this variable.

The number of extraneous inputs also affected learning speed $(F(40,800) = 2.72, p < 0.001$ for the number of extraneous inputs by trials interaction) such that, up to a point, the greater the number of extraneous stimuli, the faster learning took place, as shown in Figure 11.4. Why was this the case? Although the extraneous inputs were random numbers,

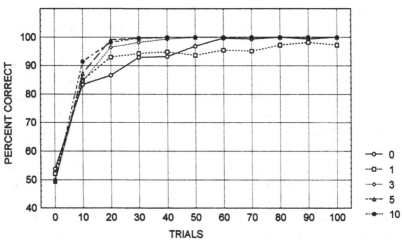

Fig. 11.4 Acquisition rate is shown as a function of number of training trials, with number of extraneous inputs as the manipulated parameter for the happy–sad discrimination problem.

some were spuriously linearly correlated with the output. Thus, extra input numbers 1, 3, 5 and 7 had Pearson correlations of 0.47, 0.39, −0.47, and −0.39, respectively, with one of the outputs (the signs were reversed for the other output). This is somewhat analogous to the teacher who provides, on some trials, cues to the correct answer by pointing to the relevant stimulus. While this speeds up learning, it can cause problems with generalization. Indeed, this was the case.

For the test set, the rate of generalization was also affected by hidden-layer size (F(30,800) = 2.64, p < 0.001). Generalization occurred at the fastest rate for the network with two hidden neurons and was slowest for the network with only one hidden neuron. However, as above, all networks eventually achieved the same accuracy.

The number of extraneous inputs had a marked effect on both the rate and pattern of generalization (F(40,800) = 12.93, p < 0.001). As shown in Figure 11.5, the addition of one extraneous cue had no significant effect on generalization. Three extra inputs led to a lower asymptote. Five or more extraneous inputs had minimal effects on generalization initially, but then had a marked deleterious effect as training proceeded. These data suggested that the networks were

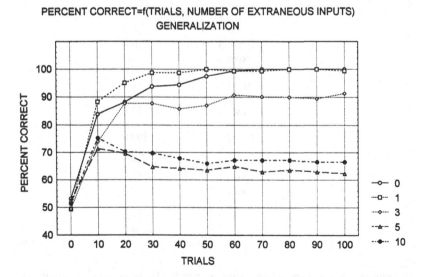

PERCENT CORRECT=f(TRIALS, NUMBER OF EXTRANEOUS INPUTS)
GENERALIZATION

Fig. 11.5 Generalization rate is shown as a function of number of training trials, with number of extraneous inputs as the manipulated parameter for the happy–sad discrimination problem.

'attending to' or utilizing the spurious inputs in the training set as
learning proceeded and that reliance on such data had a deleterious
effect on generalization. Indeed, this was evident when the effect of
systematic deletion of successive neurons in the input layer on generalization was examined. Table 11.1 shows the effect of successive deletion
of input neurons, for each fully trained network that had eight neurons
in the hidden layer, as a function of increasing numbers of extraneous
inputs. This hidden-layer size was arbitrarily chosen since hidden-layer
size, by itself, had no overall effect on generalization.

Table 11.1. *Effects of deletion of successive inputs on generalization in nets with
eight hidden neurons.**

Number of extraneous inputs	Inputs deleted	Generalization impact (%)[†]
1	Brow	0.6
1	Mouth	−41.5
1	Extra 1	−1.4
3	Brow	−28.8
3	Mouth	−117.6
3	Extra 1	−42.0
3	Extra 2	−0.4
3	Extra 3	5.6
5	Brow	−17.3
5	Mouth	−146.5
5	Extra 1	−27.3
5	Extra 2	16.5
5	Extra 3	100.0
5	Extra 4	5.1
5	Extra 5	73.6
10	Brow	14.5
10	Mouth	−263.3
10	Extra 1	17.9
10	Extra 2	−7.1
10	Extra 3	199.9
10	Extra 4	36.6
10	Extra 5	259.1
10	Extra 6	−15.5
10	Extra 7	42.5
10	Extra 8	−1.6
10	Extra 9	15.2
10	Extra 10	−29.2

*See text.
[†]Percentage difference in generalization accuracy relative to baseline conditions
with no inputs deleted. Negative numbers signify deterioration in generalization
when that input is deleted; positive numbers signify improvement in generalization
when that input is deleted.

As shown in Table 11.1, all of the networks relied on the more salient input of mouth orientation for categorization, in that elimination of this input had marked deleterious effects on generalization. In most instances, elimination of successive extraneous input neurons caused marked improvements in generalization accuracy, with numbers 3 and 5 (corresponding to random inputs 3 and 5, respectively) having the most influence – two of the four extraneous inputs that showed a moderate linear correlation with the training set outputs.

By analogy, if all inputs have equal initial salience, biological nervous systems may also attend to all available information that is correlated, even spuriously, with the problem that is to be solved. If those spurious stimuli are not present in novel test sets, generalization will be hampered. Up to a point, the greater the number of connections from such downstream inputs, the greater the problem. This same phenomenon is pervasive amongst children with autism.

It has been repeatedly demonstrated that such children are notoriously poor at generalization, and the need to train generalization is built into behavior-modification programs (Koegel, Rincover and Egel, 1982). Lovaas et al. (1971) have attributed this generalization decrement to a problem with 'stimulus overselectivity.' In this study, children with autism were found to attend to only one of three components of a redundant compound cue (as in the above simulation), whereas nonhandicapped children responded to all three, and those with mental retardation responded to two. Subsequent studies have replicated this phenomenon but have also shown that when such children are taught stimulus discriminations involving multiple stimulus attributes, they will learn the discrimination by focusing on a characteristic of the stimulus that may be relevant to the discrimination at hand but irrelevant for generalization to a related but dissimilar stimulus (Schreibman and Lovaas, 1973).

This stimulus overselectivity effect is remarkably similar to the effects of extraneous, irrelevant information on learning and generalization just described. Indeed, when cues are presented to aid discrimination learning (so-called extrastimulus prompts), children with autism have marked difficulty in maintaining their task performance when such cues are eliminated (Schreibman, Charlop and Koegel, 1982). Solutions to this problem have included increasing the salience of the stimuli by exaggerating their features – so-called within-stimulus prompts (Schreibman, 1988) – as in the present simulation. In the model described above, this can also be mimicked by increasing the size of the weights for the two relevant cues, relative to the extraneous stimuli, prior to training. When this (prebiasing) was done with one of the networks described above, generalization was facilitated in a manner proportional to the size of the preset weights.

The network with five extraneous input neurons and four hidden neurons was arbitrarily selected for modification. The pretrained weights connecting the two salient inputs with the four hidden neurons were set to either 0.5, 1.0, 2.0 or 4.0. At each weight level, the network was trained for 100 trials, with training and generalization results checked every ten trials. This process was replicated four additional times at each weight level, with all weights except the prebiased ones randomly initialized to values between $+/-0.1$.

As shown in Figure 11.6, the higher the preset weight, the higher the asymptote ($F(30, 160) = 2.55$, $p < 0.001$) in the test set. Thus, by pre-enhancing 'attention' to relevant stimuli in a neural network, generalization is enhanced, much as it is with children with autism. Presumably, typically developing children are already biologically 'prebiased' or 'prepared' to attend to relevant facial cues such as mouth or eyebrow orientation, and would not therefore need this additional help. Similar arguments could be made for so-called 'higher-functioning'

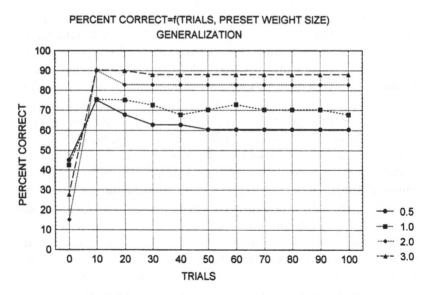

Fig. 11.6 Generalization rate is shown as a function of number of training trials, with preset weight size as the manipulated parameter for the happy–sad discrimination problem, with pre-biasing of the eyebrow and mouth orientation stimuli.

children with autism who appear to be less susceptible to these overselectivity problems (Koegel and Koegel, 1995).

Well-defined nonlinear classification problems

There exist other classification problems that children with autism are asked to learn that are not linearly separable. Consider teaching such a child the concept of the prepositions 'inside' *vs* 'outside'. Here, a teacher might give the child a block and tell him to put it inside or outside of a circle placed on a table top. In this case, there is no linear mapping contour that divides these two categories. However, the circular border separating these categories, in this problem, is well defined. To solve such nonlinear pattern classification problems requires a more complex neural network. In this case, a simple three-layer network will do, with nonlinear sigmoidal functions at the hidden and output layers governing the relation between output and input to a cell. Such a network can readily solve this problem, also known as the 'circle in the square' problem (NeuralWare, 1993) – as long as irrelevant distracters are not present. Since it has been shown that a single hidden layer with enough neurons can fit almost any mathematical function (Hornik, Stinchcombe and White, 1989), complex but well-defined borders can be described quite well with three-layer, feed-forward models. Indeed, the more complex the function that describes the border regions, the more neurons are required in the hidden layer. By extrapolation, aberrant neural development that results in an excessive number of neurons in a given region should result in enhanced ability to define and map out complex patterns. However, presenting a child with new inside/outside problems with differently shaped or localized borders requires learning to map new contours. If too many neurons and neural connections are present, the possibility of 'cross-talk' problems developing, with degradation of previously acquired memories as more and more new, but similar, problems are introduced, becomes of concern.

Some studies have indicated that the brain size of people with autism is above average (Piven et al., 1995). These observations, coupled with the subcortical autopsy results, suggest that some affected individuals have more neurons and/or neural connections than average in selected brain areas. It is hypothesized, therefore, that this is the basis for the above-average to savant-like skills shown by some individuals when it comes to learning and memorizing well-defined, nonlinear patterns such as routes to various places or musical selections. As Kanner (1943) described, some people with autism have an extraordinary ability to encode and recall complex patterns, be they visual, auditory, spatial, or temporal. For example, in the visual modality, the child known as Nadia (Selfe, 1977) had an exceptional ability to draw pictures from memory with exquisite detail. Other children have a facility with reproducing detailed geographic maps from memory or show unusual fascination with diverse visual patterns such as lines and edges, their hands or their face in the mirror. Auditorially, many such children precisely echo what they hear, including the intonation pattern, and they can be better than matched controls when asked to recall random word strings (Hermelin and O'Connor, 1967). Spatially, as noted above, many other children with autism call recall complicated routes and locations of significant objects in space. Temporally, some readily learn routines and can become quite upset if those routines are altered. Therefore, it would follow from the above that, for so-called savants, the number of neurons and neural connections is increased in those networks responsible for learning visual, auditory, spatial and/or temporal patterns, depending on the particular skills of the savant. In other words, those with savant visual memory skills should have enlarged development of visual, but not haptic, memory circuits. However, if this is the case, then the danger of spatial or temporal cross-talk is problematic and could be the basis for the reported 'resistance to change' shown by people with autism when they are asked to modify their rituals or tolerate change in their environment.

In neural network construction, various solutions to this cross-talk problem have been proposed. One of these is to have 'sparse' connectivity where fewer neurons are used to represent information (Churchland and Sejnowski, 1992). This notion of an optimal connectivity size for a given problem is discussed in more detail below.

Fuzzy nonlinear classification problems

Most categorization problems that we face in everyday life are not so easily classified. The border regions are not only nonlinear, but they are subtle or 'fuzzy' (Kosko, 1993) and depend on context. What, for example, defines a chair? A four-legged structure that people can sit on equally describes a table, as well as a chair, and excludes sofas, ottomans, tree stumps, etc. Laughter can indicate delight as well as hysterical fear, sarcasm, etc., depending on the context or the actors' point of view. Differentiating between shapes requires attending to their invariant properties, irrespective of their physical location or rotation in space. Solving such nonlinear, ill-defined problems requires complex neural network structures. In some less complex instances, multilayer back-propagation models will suffice, as when such models are used for hand-writing recognition (Sejnowski and Rosenberg, 1987), diagnosis (Cohen et al., 1993), etc. Fuzzy boundary problems are precisely the types of problems that people with autism have difficulty resolving, irrespective of degree of intellectual functioning. For example, semantic comprehension is often problematic, with many having quite literal interpretations of words and sentences (Kanner, 1943) and a concomitant inability to comprehend their world. Some normally intelligent people with autism have difficulty with higher abstractions such as perceiving situations from another's point of view (Frith and Baron-Cohen, 1987). Why? Analysis of the anatomy of back-propagation models may provide a clue.

As noted above, back-propagation networks employ a hidden layer (or layers) that can form higher order representations of the input pattern. In forming these representations or boundary regions, the hidden layer performs a type of curve fitting, i.e., trying to find the best curve that will fit all of the data points (or separate out groups in a classification problem) in the set on which it is trained (Churchland and Sejnowski, 1992). As in any other curve-fitting procedure, one desires the simplest function that will best describe the data. Why? Because, as noted by Cohen (1994) and many others, a complex curvilinear function may fit a training set too well, i.e., it describes the training set so perfectly that it is relatively poorer than a simpler function at describing a different, albeit conceptually similar, sample, the 'test set.' (This problem is known as 'overfitting.') In a back-propagation network, this curve-fitting problem translates into determining the number of neurons needed in the hidden layer, as well as the number of hidden layers to use, in order to (a) best fit the data set, and (b) best describe the test set. As the number of neurons and connections increases, the fit to the test set may deteriorate (NeuralWare, 1993). Thus, while too few neurons may not be able to solve a problem to begin with, having too many may impair generalization. This problem in overfitting the data set is also a function of the number of training trials (NeuralWare, 1993) because, as the network learns, it will modify connection weights so as to minimize error on the training set. To the extent that the test set does not precisely resemble the training set and to the extent that the boundaries between groups are fuzzy, generalization will worsen as training progresses. Similar effects were also present in the linear classification problem described above as the number of noisy inputs increased.

An illustration of how this would apply to autism is exemplified by the problems autistic individuals have with speech and language comprehension. It has been argued (Lovaas, Koegel and Schreibman, 1979) that a stimulus overselectivity problem can, in part, explain this deficit. That is, if a child attends to irrelevant parts of a verbal cue, such as the pitch contours to which infants attend (Mehler et al., 1978), instead of those features that are important in discriminating one type of word from another, then comprehension will be impaired. In a related manner, the same or different people may pronounce the same words in different ways, depending on their age, gender, states of health, regional accent etc., i.e., word recognition is a complex, nonlinear, fuzzy classification problem. Consider a more basic problem than word recognition – vowel recognition, a phenomenon that is very likely evident in early infancy (see Rosser (1994) for a review). Figure 11.7 shows a plot of the first two formants of different speakers (males, females, and children) saying ten different vowels in an hVd format (Nowlan, 1990): (1) 'ee' as in 'heed'; (2) 'ih' as in 'hid'; (3) 'eh' as in 'head'; (4) 'aah' as in 'had'; (5) 'uh' as in 'hud';

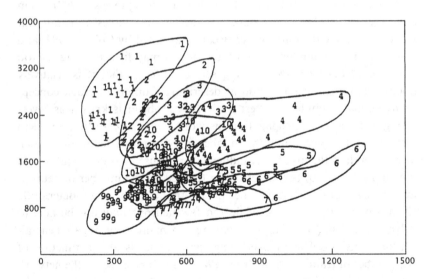

Fig. 11.7 Samples of the first and second formant values of all vowels spoken by different speakers. The abscissa is the first formant value and the ordinate is the second formant value. Axes are labeled in cycles per second. The solid-line boundaries of each vowel class were estimated from the training data. (Reprinted, with modification, by permission of the author from Nowlan, S.J. (1990). Competing experts: An experimental investigation of associative mixture models. Technical Report CRG-TR-90-5, University of Toronto, Copyright 1990.)

(6) 'ah' as in 'hod'; (7) 'aw' as in 'hawed'; (8) 'uuh' as in 'hood'; (9) 'oo' as in 'who'd'; and (10) 'er' as in 'heard.' Note that there is wide variation in the way different speakers pronounce the same vowel, and a great deal of overlap amongst the different vowel clusters. Even if a child with autism were to attend to relevant features such as the first two to four formants of vowel production and did not find some frequencies more salient than others, a problem with too many or too few neural connections could still impair generalization, albeit for different reasons.

Too few connections would limit the complexity of the boundaries that must be computed in order to differentiate one vowel from another. Here, a generalization problem is secondary to limited classification ability. The problem with too many connections is more complex. To the extent that the child's experience with attending to a variety of different speakers is limited (the 'training set'), generalization to other speakers (the 'test set') could be impaired, especially if the spectral characteristics of the vowels that they produce differ from the child's experience and/or if those vocal characteristics overlap with other vowels spoken by familiar speakers. Why? Because too many connections would compute boundaries that fit the training set 'too well' and this would therefore limit generalization under the conditions specified. This would result in a child who could accurately recognize (and, perhaps, reproduce) sounds or words spoken by his or her teacher but not some of the same sounds or words when spoken by an unfamiliar person.

This effect was modeled with a three-layer, feed-forward network. The data for the network were approximated from a replotting of some of the recognizable data points in Figure 11.7. The first two formants served as the inputs, and five of the ten vowel sounds (numbers 1, 2, 3, 4, and 10) served as the predicted outputs. In order to model a 'limited experience' situation, one-half of the data was set aside for the training set and the rest served as the test set. Two experiments were run. In the first, the number of neurons in the hidden layer was systematically manipulated as follows: 3, 6, 9, 12, and 15. Nets were run for 50 000 trials. Four additional replications were run for each hidden-layer size by initializing a net to a different set of starting connection weights so that each would converge on the solution from a different starting point in weight space. In the second experiment, nets with hidden-layer sizes of 2, 3, and 12 were run on the same problem (each with five replications) with the nets stopped at 2000, 4000, 8000, 16 000, 32 000, and 64 000 trials in order to track the effects of experience on both learning and generalization.

In the first experiment, as hidden-layer size increased during training, classification accuracy increased from 81 percent with three hidden-layer neurons to over 88 percent with 9 to 15 hidden-layer neurons ($F_{(16,80)} = 27.66$, $p < 0.0004$). Further, some vowels were easier to recognize than others ($F_{(16,60} = 90.23$, $p < 0.0001$), as shown (on the left) in Figure 11.8. Recognition of vowels 3 and 10, for example, required increasingly larger hidden-layer sizes, with the former achieving levels of 90 percent accuracy at hidden-layer sizes of nine or more, and the latter requiring a hidden-layer size of 15 to reach 77 percent accuracy. The latter is not surprising since, as shown in Figure 11.7, vowel 10 ('er') showed significant overlap in cluster areas with some of the other vowels, particularly 3 ('eh') and 4 ('aah').

Results for generalization testing were the opposite of those seen during acquisition. Overall, the larger the hidden-layer size, the worse the generalization ($F_{(4,20)} = 16.49$, $p < 0.007$). However, this effect depended on vowel type ($F_{(4,80)} = 8.75$, $p < 0.0001$). As shown on the right in Figure 11.8, generalization was quite good (over 90 percent) for vowels 1 and 4, irrespective of hidden-layer size; increased from 69 percent to 78 percent for vowel 2; and decreased from 82 percent to about 50 percent for vowel 3 as hidden-layer size increased. Thus, as the hidden-layer size

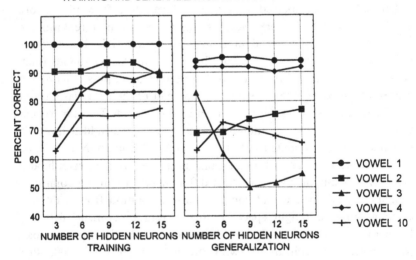

Fig. 11.8 Acquisition (left) and generalization (right) rates are shown as a function of number of hidden neurons for each vowel type.

increased, the border isolating the training set data for vowel 3 became more complex. This increasingly complex border led to a progressive generalization decrement for the test set with increases in hidden-layer size. The results for vowel 10 were more complex. Generalization improved as hidden-layer size increased from three to six, but declined with further increases in hidden-layer size. Thus, as the border for this vowel became more complex in order to describe its training set data, generalization to the test set deteriorated markedly, once network size had exceeded some 'optimal' range. These observations, and the results for vowel 3, are examples of how exposure to a limited data set can impair generalization in those whose nervous systems may be 'too complex.' If this concept is extended beyond vowels to words, phrases and sentences, it could, perhaps, account for the idiosyncratic reactions of some children with autism to the statements of others.

Results for the developmental progression of this phenomenon were examined in Experiment 2. As shown in Figure 11.9, learning accuracy was low (65 per cent overall) and did not improve with trials for the net with two hidden-layer neurons. Learning accuracy monotonically increased with trials for the other two hidden-layer sizes, eventually reaching almost 90 percent correct for the largest network $(F(10,60) = 2.69, p < 0.0076)$.

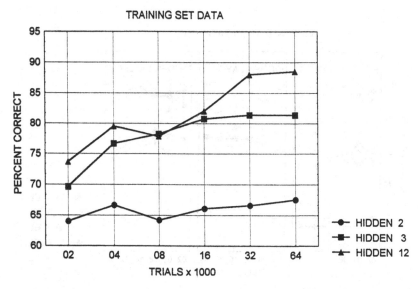

Fig. 11.9 Acquisition rate is shown as a function of trials, with hidden-layer size as a parameter.

The generalization data were complex, with the results affected by hidden-layer size, vowel type and trials ($F(40,240) = 1.79$, $p < 0.005$), as shown in Figure 11.10. A hidden-layer size of two clearly could not generalize because, as evident from Figure 11.9, it was unable to learn to classify all five patterns. That is, a system with too few neurons has limited capacity to learn and therefore generalize, as noted above. Further, there were small, but consistent declines in generalization performance as training proceeded. By contrast, hidden-layer sizes of three or 12 generalized quite well, depending on when generalization was assessed during training. A hidden-layer size of three actually resulted in increased generalization accuracy, for four of the five vowels, with extended training. Thus, this network size, which appeared to be almost optimal for generalization in the previous study, did not show a generalization decrement with extended training. Put in other terms, an optimal brain size improves with experience.

The networks with a hidden-layer size of 12 showed excellent generalization early on in training (about 4000 to 8000 trials), equaling that of the more optimal network size. However, with continued exposure to the same vowels, one of the vowels, vowel 3, showed a marked decrement from 85 percent to 45 percent accuracy with extended training. Therefore, the effects on generalization of having too many neurons and neural

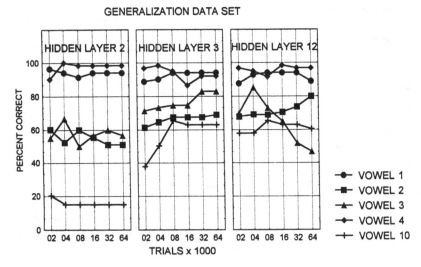

Fig. 11.10 Generalization rate is shown as a function of trials and hidden-layer size for each vowel type.

connections depends on when, in the course of learning or development, generalization is assessed. Had training been stopped for this network size between 4000 and 8000 trials, and inappropriate or irrelevant connections deleted or pruned (as in Table 11.1), excellent learning and generalization could have been maintained with continued exposure to the training set.

It should also be noted that the variability in generalization outcome was a function of hidden-layer size for four of the five vowels, in Experiment 1, and all five vowels at the end of training, in Experiment 2, based on tests for homogeneity of variance across hidden-layer size. As shown in Table 11.2, variance was lowest at both the near-optimal and largest hidden-layer sizes, relative to the other hidden-layer sizes. Thus, with too few neurons, overall learning and generalization are weak and responses are inconsistent. With an optimal number of neurons, both learning and generalization are good and correct responding is consistent and predictable. With too many neurons, learning is good but generalization is poor and shows relatively little variation, i.e., incorrect answers tend to be reproduced in such systems.

Accordingly, unpredictability in outcome is inevitable with such dynamical systems but the degree of variation in generalization ability is a function of network complexity for a given type of problem. This observation is consistent with the typically stereotyped and inflexible responses of children with autism to verbal requests from others. As several parents have said to the author, 'He doesn't understand it when you ask him that way, you have to say. . .'. Such children must be truly puzzled and frustrated (or depressed) by their efforts at trying to fathom the rules behind fuzzy problems. This could encourage some (depending on arousal state, 'temperament,' and prior history) to try harder by memorizing ever-more irrelevant details (see Carpenter and Grossberg's (1991) discussion of arousal effects in their ART-1 model). This is an instance of not being able to 'see the forest for the trees.'

Of course, vowel comprehension is much more complicated than the simple vowel discrimination model described here. Rule-governed 'top-down' expectancies play a large role in phoneme or word recognition, as in the phonemic restoration effect (Warren, 1984). However, such top-down rules must be based on a history of having received reasonably consistent 'bottom-up' information. Should the latter be error laden, appropriate top-down rules should be particularly difficult to abstract. Similarly, too many or too few neurons in certain top-down networks could lead to a system that fails to develop appropriate rules, develops

Table 11.2. *Percentage correct means (M) and standard deviations (SD) of vowel generalization as a function of hidden-layer size in Experiments 1 and 2.**

Vowel		Hidden-layer size				
		3	6	9	12	15
Experiment 1 (50 000 trials)						
1	M	94.0	95.2	95.2	94.0	94.0
	SD	0.0	2.7	2.7	0.0	0.0
2	M	69.0	69.2	73.8	75.4	77.0
	SD	0.0	5.3	7.2	3.6	0.0
3	M	83.0	61.8	50.0	51.6	54.8
	SD	0.0	7.7	13.3	6.7	4.4
4	M	92.0	92.0	91.8	90.2	91.8
	SD	0.0	0.0	6.0	4.0	6.0
10	M	63.0	72.6	70.2	67.8	65.4
	SD	0.0	5.4	6.6	6.6	5.4

Experiment 2 (64 000 trials)				
Vowel		Hidden-layer size		
		2	3	12
1	M	94.0	94.0	89.0
	SD	0.0	0.0	11.2
2	M	51.0	69.0	80.0
	SD	28.7	0.0	6.7
3	M	56.6	83.0	46.8
	SD	13.9	0.0	4.4
4	M	98.4	92.0	96.8
	SD	3.6	0.0	4.4
10	M	15.0	63.0	60.4
	SD	33.5	0.0	5.8

*See text.

extremely limited rules, or develops rules that are incorrect or bizarre because they include spuriously correlated information in the input pattern. Such a developmental history could be responsible for the higher-order 'theory of mind' deficits noted in children with autism (e.g., Leslie and Thaiss, 1992).

Implications and predictions

The above data for vowel classification illustrate several well-known properties of neural networks when they are presented with complex problems that have ill-defined borders. In general, the more hidden neurons, the better the network is at classifying data in the training set. Generalization to a novel test set is a bitonic function of hidden-layer size in which an optimal size (the 'Goldilocks size') exists for maximizing both training and test set predictions. Also, because neural networks are dynamical systems, substantial variability in performance exists that depends upon the initial state and size of the network. Finally, since the system attempts to minimize error on the training set, test set predictions may deteriorate with extended training.

Thus, it can be seen that quantitative variation in one basic parameter, number of neurons and neural connections, can result in complex effects on learning and generalization. These complex outcomes mimic several well-validated characteristics of the learning style of children with autism: (1) greater attention to idiosyncratic than to socially relevant stimuli; (2) stimulus overselectivity; (3) problems in acquiring fuzzy concepts; (4) development of savant skills; (5) problems with generalization of previously acquired skills; (6) rigidity and resistance to change; (7) stereotyped responses to others; and (8) difficulty in learning complex higher-order concepts. By extension and analogy, these basic learning and generalization effects have implications for a variety of other issues in autism, and these are outlined below.

Lack of awareness of the affective meaning of facial expressions

Discriminating context-specific differences in facial expressions is an example of the type of fuzzy classification problem that people must learn to respond to every day. Having too few or too many neurons for such problems should, by extension, interfere with learning and generalization of these affective cues. This is illustrated in Figures 11.11 and 11.12.

Imagine a two-dimensional weight space exists for discriminating between angry and sad facial expressions. Further, imagine that the border between these states is noisy or fuzzy, as pictured by the closed triangles. A typically developing child with an optimal number of amygdalar neurons and neural connections establishes a nonlinear boundary that 'satisfies' (to use Churchland and Sejnowski's (1992) term) the distinction between these two emotional states, as illustrated by the quadratic function. A child with too few neurons (Fig. 11.11) in this structure does not possess enough computational power adequately to differentiate these states and so his or her boundary is linear, with substantial overlap amongst the two true states. The child with too many neurons (Fig.

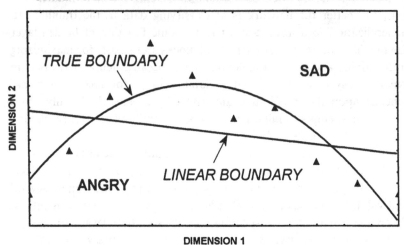

CONCEPTUAL FEATURE SPACE OF CHILD WITH "TOO FEW" CONNECTIONS

DIMENSION 1

Fig. 11.11 A hypothetical two-dimensional weight space for the problem of differentiating between angry and sad faces with a noisy or fuzzy boundary (closed
triangles). The quadratic function 'satifices' the discrimination between these two
states (true boundary). The child with too few neurons in a relevant brain structure lacks the computational power to identify this curvilinear boundary (represented by the linear boundary) and so has difficulty discriminating these states.
(See text.)

11.12) has the opposite problem. He or she attends to all of the noisy
aspects of the border between these two states, as illustrated by the spline
curve. As a result, this child learns to attend to too many irrelevant
details and, so, generalization of these affective associations is hampered.
In either situation, knowledge concerning affective associations is idiosyncratic and fails to generalize well. Therefore, other normally developed neural structures that rely on this information may show poor
performance because they lack relevant information concerning the affective salience of evolutionarily significant stimuli in the child's environment (see Churchland and Sejnowski's (1992, pp. 317–29) discussion on
Damasio hierarchies, and Eichenbaum, 1993). Without such salience
information, overselective attention to irrelevant cues can result, as illustrated above.

   Accordingly, the following pathogenic scenario suggests itself. For a
variety of possible reasons, the development of the brain of a child with
autism is altered in such a manner that regions that are important for
processing of affective and other associations have either too few or too

CONCEPTUAL FEATURE SPACE OF CHILD WITH "TOO MANY" CONNECTIONS

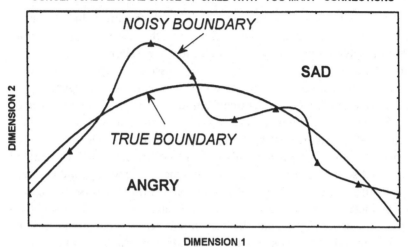

Fig. 11.12 A hypothetical two-dimensional weight space for the problem of differentiating between angry and sad faces with a noisy or fuzzy boundary (closed triangles). The quadratic function 'satifices' the discrimination between these two states (true boundary). The child with too many neurons attends to all of the noise in this curvilinear boundary (represented by the spline function noisy boundary) and so has difficulty in generalizing these states. (See text.)

many neurons and/or neural connections. Too few neurons and neuronal connections will set an upper limit on the number and quality of affective associations that can be acquired. If too many neurons and neuronal connections exist, then the number and quality of affective associations that can be learned and stored may be limited, associations could be highly idiosyncratic, and there may also be deterioration in the quality of these associations with time (the stability–plasticity dilemma discussed in Carpenter and Grossberg, 1991), depending on the memory storage capacity of the network. This deficiency in processing of affective responses from others could readily account for the unusual social learning and performance deficits shown by these children, such as lack of awareness about when to establish eye contact, how close to stand next to others, stereotyped questioning of strangers, etc. In a causal chain, failure to comprehend the function of fuzzy social cues, and to associate *affective meaning* with them, would be expected to lead to failure of the child to have a desire to share experiences with others – so-called joint attention deficits (Mundy, Sigman and Kasari, 1990).

Self-stimulatory behaviors

It has been known for quite some time that the reward value of a given environmental stimulus is judged relative to the reward value of stimuli that compete for the individual's attention (e.g., Herrnstein, 1970). It is also the case that organisms tend to be biased or 'prepared' to acquire associations at a faster rate to some stimuli than to others, suggesting the presence of an 'attending hierarchy' (Baron, 1965). For example, Warren (1953) reported that monkeys learn visual discriminations best when cues are based on color; next best when cues are based on form; and least when they are based on size. Advertisers have learned that people attend to visual stimuli that are bright, flashy, repetitive, moving, and colorful. Such stimuli are easily detectable, controllable (in some instances), and/ or predictable and they also tend to be interesting to children with autism, as evidenced by the fact that they often focus too intently on flashing lights, brightly colored signs, television cartoons, spinning wheels, their own moving fingers, etc. Precisely which stimulus a child with too many connections chooses to focus on is likely to be highly idiosyncratic and dependent, in part, on 'superstitious' associations that may have been established with that stimulus in the past. The relative reward value of attending to such 'concrete' stimuli should be especially high if competing fuzzy stimuli lack affective meaning. It would be predicted, therefore, that the frequency of repetitive behaviors should be an inverse function of social–communicative functioning. Based on data collected from caregivers of almost 300 people with autism seen in the clinic of the New York Institute for Basic Research in Developmental Disabilities, caregiver reports of the severity of repetitive behaviors shown by these individuals were weakly, but significantly, negatively correlated with increases in adaptive functioning (partial $r(274) = -0.27$, $p < 0.0001$), but not with increases in age (partial $r(274) = 0.004$), as predicted. Data on repetitive behaviors were gathered with a parent interview developed by Cohen et al. (1993) and adaptive functioning was assessed with the Vineland Adaptive Behavior Scales (Sparrow, Balla and Cicchetti, 1984).

Alternative pathogenetic mechanisms

Aside from the mechanisms discussed at the beginning of this chapter, what else could account for having too many or too few neurons and/or neural connections in selected regions of the brain? The typically developing brain produces more neurons than it needs (Rakic, 1991), and excess neurons are removed through a 'pruning' process. LaMantia and Rakic (1990) have reported that newborn monkeys lose over 70 percent of their axons in the hippocampal commissure. Overproduction of synaptic connections has also been noted in the neocortex by Rakic et al. (1986). While such cell or connection death may be genetically programmed, the death of certain connections may be a Darwinian competitive process in which, as a function of experience, connections that have been strengthened through learning or exposure survive while those that are weak die (Rakic, 1991). The results from the simulations described above suggest that this pruning is necessary for proper learning and generalization. Indeed, pruning of connections in large, overdetermined, artificial neural networks leads to improved generalization of the network (Sietsma and Dow, 1988). Therefore, if not already affected by pathological aberrations such as migration errors, the brains of children with autism could have too many or too few neurons and/or neural connections because they are impaired in their ability to develop or strengthen new connections and/or to prune out weak or interfering connections in critical brain regions (Rapin, 1993). Indeed, had the larger neural networks in the vowel discrimination problem been monitored while they acquired the discrimination, hidden neurons that impaired generalization could have been pruned away, leading to no loss of ability, and, perhaps, improved performance with additional training. Pruning of too many neurons and/or neural connections could lead to deterioration in pre-existing concepts according to Lashley's mass action principle, depending on when in the course of development such pruning occurs, and could account for some cases of autism that are associated with early loss of previously acquired skills and/or the often reported positive or negative changes in functioning at adolescence when cortical pruning of connections accelerates (Hoffman and McGlashan, 1993).

For the child who has problems with too many neurons in some brain structures as a result of insufficient pruning, continued exposure to fuzzy categorical problems should lead to a nonlinear developmental progression (see Fig. 11.10). Initially, learning should proceed well and, eventually, the child will correctly generalize. However, continued exposure to the same experiences will lead to overlearning, attention to idiosyncratic details, deterioration in concept formation, and poor generalization. Perhaps this can explain, in part, the apparent regression in functioning from 'normalcy' shown by some children with autism between 18 and 30 months of age. Those children with too few neurons because of diminished development or excessive pruning may also show a regression, but attainment of age-appropriate social–communicative functioning would not be expected.

Hoffman (Hoffman and Dobscha, 1989; Hoffman and McGlashan, 1993) has explored this same concept of excessive neural pruning to simulate some of the symptoms of schizophrenia using a reciprocally connected, parallel distributed processing model. In Hoffman's model, excessive pruning at adolescence was felt to be localized primarily to cortical regions, with secondary effects on the hippocampus. With excessive amounts of pruning, three consequences were noted in the simulations (Hoffman and McGlashan, 1993). First, outputs 'became bizarre' in that stimuli were found to elicit memories unrelated to the input. Second, subpopulations of neurons were found to become functionally autonomous. Finally, spontaneous outputs that were unrelated to any stored memory in the system were excessively reproduced. The latter was termed a 'parasitic focus.' These unusual consequences were felt to simulate positive symptoms such as thought insertion, loose associations, delusions of control, auditory hallucinations, ideas of reference etc., as well as some negative symptoms such as thought withdrawal.

The present model of autism differs in several ways from Hoffman's model. First, the present model emphasizes the fact that problems in behavioral development can occur in response to too much, as well as too little, neuronal complexity. Second, the cortical brain structures thought to be involved in schizophrenia by Hoffman are unlikely to be involved in autism to the same degree because the two disorders differ markedly in several ways, including age of onset and types of behaviors displayed. As alluded to above, the present model assumes that the most likely neural structures to be involved in autism are those that relate to social–emotional development, with, perhaps, some involvement of those regions that are responsible for certain 'cognitive' behaviors such as language. There are several reasons for this assumption:

1. The earliest appearing symptoms relate to lack of appropriate reactions to social cues (poor eye contact, lack of response to being held, etc.) and these behaviors are the ones that are least likely to be influenced by overall intelligence in these children.
2. Cortical changes are not consistently reported in either autopsy or imaging investigations, as noted above.
3. Differences that have been more consistently observed (at least in one laboratory) involve those brain areas related to social–emotional development, as cited in the section on neuropathology.

These same structures have been speculated to be involved in more general issues of temperament differences in children and adults (Nelson, 1994; Steinmetz, 1994).

4. Some of the deeper structures appear to reach maturity within the first one to two years of postnatal life (Nelson, 1994), close to the time of onset of most cases of autism.

5. It has been found that neonatal amygdalar–hippocampal lesions produce a syndrome in primates that resembles autism in several ways (Bachevelier, 1991). Indeed, the author has evaluated several children with autism who also displayed behaviors reported to occur in Kluver–Bucy syndrome (Kluver and Bucy, 1939), a disorder resulting from damage to the temporal lobes. Thus, in addition to autism, these children also displayed indiscriminate mouthing and ingestion of inedible objects as well as lack of response to stimuli that would be painful to others.

Treatment

Recently, data have become available that would suggest that the aberrant neural development hypothesized to be responsible for autism can, in some instances, be overcome by early, intensive, structured learning experiences (Lovaas, 1987; McEachlin, Smith and Lovaas, 1993). This could be accounted for in the present model if such experiences force activity-dependent or experience-dependent strengthening of appropriate connections and pruning of aberrant ones, as has been demonstrated for development of some parts of the visual system. Hypothetically, this intervention should work best in those cases where the problem is, in pertinent brain structures, one of too many rather than too few neurons or neural connections. This is because neural activity appears to play more of a role in maintenance and elimination of synapses than in their initial formation (Jacobson, 1991). This assumes, of course, that any other normally developed structures that may be present cannot be remapped to 'take over' the function of the malfunctioning structure.

Such intensive behavioral therapy is hypothesized to work by focusing the child's attention on a larger and more varied data set than he or she is used to, thereby forcing the child to attend to all relevant aspects of the problem space. Then, given suitable problems to solve (e.g., those dealing with affective recognition of emotional states or learning to recognize words pronounced by different people), constant repetition of these many different patterns together with immediate feedback should lead

to higher-order recognition by weakening or pruning previously established, irrelevant connections that do not 'pay-off' and maintaining or
strengthening those that do. That is, it is assumed that such intensive
work may stimulate a sluggish neurodevelopmental process. In artificially
distributed neural networks, increasing the size of the data set for a fixed
network size leads to enhanced performance, especially when the data set
is noisy (NeuralWare, 1993). A critical period may exist for such intervention because synaptic patterns that are already established are, theoretically, difficult to change (Munro, 1986).

The present model implies that genes that control (or exogenous
agents that influence) neural growth, migration, differentiation, cell
death or pruning will have treatment as well as etiological significance
for autism. Drugs that facilitate or inhibit nerve growth or pruning in
relevant brain regions or that selectively stimulate or inhibit nerve functioning in these same regions may be of benefit in the treatment of this
syndrome, when given in combination with intensive structured interventions so that experience-dependent plasticity effects can be realized.
Unfortunately, the psychopharmacology literature in autism is limited
in this respect. For example, in the only study of this kind in young
children with autism, Campbell et al. (1978) investigated the therapeutic
efficacy of a combination of behavioral language instruction with haloperidol, a drug that is primarily a dopamine antagonist. They found
that the drug potentiates the effects of language intervention.
Unfortunately, the possible long-term side-effects associated with this
drug limit its usefulness with this population. The mechanism that could
account for the language intervention effect is unclear, but this study
and other research suggest that haloperidol helps such children to suppress impulsive and stereotyped behaviors (e.g., Cohen et al., 1980;
Campbell et al., 1982) that can interfere with learning, perhaps through
its action on those dopamine systems involved in initiation and control
of body movements. As a possible mechanism for the latter, it is relevant to note that dopamine has effects on striatal synaptic plasticity and
has been hypothesized to be involved in determining when such
synapses should be strengthened or weakened (Alexander, 1995). In
fact, neurotransmitters such as dopamine, norepinephrine, serotonin,
and the endogenous opioids have been implicated in synaptogenesis,
neural plasticity, dendritic and dendritic spine development (Jacobson,
1991), axonal pruning and cell death (Soto-Moyano et al., 1991), and
they have also been suggested as possible etiologies for autism
(Panksepp, 1979; Gillberg and Coleman, 1992). Support for the opioid

model, for example, has been developing. Mild beneficial effects of naltrexone, an opiate antagonist, have been observed on a variety of symptoms of autism (e.g., Campbell et al., 1990; Kolmen et al., 1995). The short-acting version of naltrexone, naloxone, has been found in animal studies to enhance memory of an avoidance task through its effects on amygdalar norepinephrine receptors (McGaugh, 1991), and there is evidence that opiates are strongly involved in the development of social attachment (Panksepp, 1979).

Long-term studies examining the possible therapeutic effects of 'safe' pharmacological agents that modify neural development in relevant sites, such as the amygdala, should be initiated. Such studies should be combined with intensive, early intervention in young children with autism so that relevant neural activity can be stimulated by environmental means and, it is to be hoped, enhanced pharmacologically.

Some additional speculations: genetics; neural development and the 'broader phenotype'

It has been hypothesized that the large variations in brain structure seen both within and across species could be caused by genetic mutations that have had no selective survival advantages or disadvantages. Therefore, these mutations would accumulate across generations, because of this neutrality, and result in increased polymorphism of the nervous system. This polymorphism could then lead to survival advantages or disadvantages, depending on the environment (Jacobson, 1991). Rakic (1991) has arrived at similar conclusions regarding numbers of neural connections. Taken together, these hypotheses have significance for the, as yet unknown, numbers of children with autism who, despite the best technology, will never be found to demonstrate pathological aberrations in their neural development. They also relate to observations suggestive of a 'broader phenotype' characterized by learning and social communication deficits in the relatives of children with autism (Folstein and Rutter, 1988). Why?

In the generalization data for the vowel discrimination problem, generalization variance was greatest for the nets with too few or with above-optimal (but not too much above optimal) numbers of hidden neurons (see also Cohen, 1994). Some of the nets that found a good solution at a given network size clearly took a different path in weight space during learning from those whose generalization results were not as good. From a pathogenetic point of view, these observations suggest that the deleterious effects of having many neuronal connections are dependent upon a chaotic process, i.e., resulting from a very complex dynamical system showing strong sensitivity to initial conditions (Abraham, Abraham and Shaw, 1990). In fact, brain maturation has been hypothesized to be such a dynamical system (Mpitsos, 1993). If neurons and neuronal connections increase across successive generations because of the mutations described above and positive assortative mating, behavioral outcomes would be expected to be increasingly varied both within and across generations of family members with good outcomes (e.g., gifted and/or unusually socially adept children), less advantageous ones (e.g., autism and/or mental retardation), or a combination of autism or autistic-like behavior and giftedness (e.g., many typical Asperger's cases). This, of course, assumes that the mutations responsible for variable numbers of neural connections cause such events to happen in brain sites relevant to social–emotional awareness, brain sites involved in higher-order cognitive functioning, or both. The number of neurons in such children would be statistically, but not pathologically, unusual.

This effect is illustrated in Figure 11.13. In this scenario, the numbers of neurons and neural connections are hypothesized to increase across successive generations in brain regions important to both cognitive and social–emotional development. For ease of presentation, the expected increases in variance in the middle ranges are not shown. The two curves differ primarily in their terminal portions. It is assumed that the older subcortical structures important for social–emotional development are affected to a greater extent by excesses in neural complexity than the cortical structures involved in cognitive development. In sections A and B, both types of functioning covary in the same direction, with the differences in these two areas separating average to highly intelligent individuals from their progeny who are in the highly gifted range. As neural complexity in these structures increases across generations, the two curves begin to diverge, with cognitive development stabilizing and social–emotional development declining (section C). This region represents 'eccentric' or relatively socially impaired geniuses. As social development continues to decline with further increases in neural complexity across generations (section D), social pathology develops, perhaps conforming to Asperger's disorder. Beyond these two sections, both cognitive and social development decline together and produce high (section E) and low (section F) functioning people with autism, respectively.

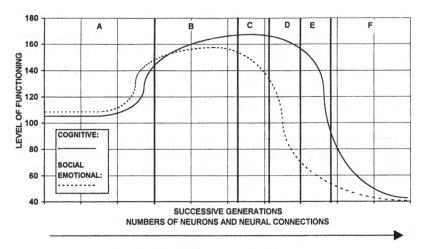

Figure 11.13 A hypothetical graph depicting level of cognitive (solid line) and social–emotional (dotted line) functioning as a function of increasing neural complexity with successive generations of family members. Section A depicts normal to above-normal cognitive and social–emotional functioning; B shows individuals gifted in both social–emotional and cognitive development; C begins to depict gradual declines in social–emotional functioning along with gifted levels of cognitive ability; D shows more severe social impairment with gifted levels of cognitive ability; and E and F depict declines in both functions. (See text.)

The scenario depicted in Figure 11.13 follows directly from the above neural network simulations, assumptions of positive assortative mating, and hypotheses concerning the genetic bases of neural complexity. It predicts increases in the probability of: (1) both social–emotional and cognitive problems in the parents and siblings of low-functioning children with autism; (2) more social–emotional (e.g., Asperger's disorder) than cognitive deficits in the parents and siblings of high-functioning children with autism; and (3) social oddity and high intelligence ('eccentricity' and/or Asperger's disorder) in the parents and siblings of children with Asperger's disorder. In all of these groups, substantial variability in outcome within generations is expected. This scenario 'explains' the broader phenotype of social and cognitive impairment sometimes observed in relatives of the child with autism (Folstein and Rutter, 1988).

There is some empirical support for these predictions. Baird and August (1985) found that the frequency of autism and intellectual impairment was significantly increased amongst siblings of low-functioning children with autism. No such impairment was present in a small sample of siblings of higher-functioning children with autism (IQs > 70). Also, DeLong and Dwyer (1988) found a higher rate of Asperger's disorder and bipolar disorder in family members of high-functioning children with autism than in family members of children with mental retardation and autism.

More well-controlled, large-sample family studies would be needed to support the predictions generated from Figure 11.13. Future genetic, neuropathological, computational and behavioral studies will help to determine the extent to which the predictions generated from the overall model are accurate.

Acknowledgments

This work was supported by funds from the New York State Office of Mental Retardation and Developmental Disabilities. The author wishes to thank Daniel Stein for his helpful comments on an earlier version of this chapter.

References

Abraham, F., Abraham, R.H. & Shaw, C.D. (1990). *A Visual Introduction to Dynamical Systems Theory for Psychology*. Santa Cruz, CA: Aerial Press.

Alexander, G.E. (1995). Basal ganglia. In *The Handbook of Brain Theory and Neural Networks*, ed. M.A. Arbib, pp. 139–44. Cambridge, MA: MIT Press.

American Psychiatric Association (1994). *Diagnostic and Statistical Manual of Mental Disorders*, 4th edn. Washington, DC: APA.

Bachevelier, J. (1991). An animal model for childhood autism. In *Advances in Neuropsychiatry and Psychopharmacology*. Vol. 1. *Schizophrenia Research*, ed. C.A. Tamminga & S.C. Schulz, pp. 129–40. New York: Raven Press.

Baird, J.D. & August, G.F. (1985). Familial heterogeneity in infantile autism. *Journal of Autism and Developmental Disorders*, **15**, 315–21.

Baron, M.B. (1965). The stimulus, stimulus control, and stimulus generalization. In *Stimulus Generalization*, ed. D.I. Mostovsky, pp. 62–71. Stanford: Stanford University Press.

Bauman, M. (1991). Microscopic neuroanatomic abnormalities in autism. *Pediatrics*, **87**, 791–6.

Bauman, M. & Kemper, T.L. (1985). Histoanatomic observations of the brain in early infantile autism. *Neurology*, **35**, 866–74.

Bauman, M. & Kemper, T.L. (1986). Developmental cerebellar abnormalities: A consistent finding in early infantile autism. Abstract. *Neurology*, **36**, 190.

Campbell, M., Anderson, L.T., Cohen, I.L. et al. (1982). Haloperidol in autistic children: Effects on learning, behavior and abnormal involuntary movements. *Psychopharmacology Bulletin*, **18**, 110–12.

Campbell, M., Anderson, L.T., Meier, M. et al. (1978). A comparison of haloperidol and behavior therapy and their interaction in autistic children. *Journal of the American Academy of Child Psychiatry*, **7**, 640–55.

Campbell, M., Anderson, L.T., Small, A.M., Locascio, J.J., Lynch, N.S. & Choroco, M.C. (1990). Naltrexone in autistic children: a double-blind and placebo controlled study. *Psychopharmacology Bulletin*, **26**, 130–5.

Carpenter, G.A. & Grossberg, S. (1991). *Pattern Recognition by Self-Organizing Neural Networks*. Cambridge, MA: MIT Press.

Churchland, P.S. & Sejnowski, T.J. (1992). *The Computational Brain*. Cambridge, MA: MIT Press.

Cohen, I.L. (1994). An artificial neural network analogue of learning in autism. *Biological Psychiatry*, **36**, 5–20.

Cohen, I.L., Campbell, M., Posner, D., Small, A., Triebel, D. & Anderson, L. (1980). Behavioral effects of haloperidol in young autistic children: an objective analysis using a within-subjects reversal design. *Journal of the American Academy of Child Psychiatry*, **19**, 665–77.

Cohen, I.L., Sudhalter, V., Landon-Jimenez, D. & Keogh, M. (1993). A neural network approach to the classification of autism. *Journal of Autism and Developmental Disorders*, **23**, 443–66.

Courchesne, E., Hesselink, J.R., Jernigan, T.L. & Yeung-Courchesne, R. (1987). Abnormal neuroanatomy in a nonretarded person with autism. *Archives of Neurology*, **44**, 335–41.

Courchesne, E., Press, G.A. & Yeung-Courchesne, R. (1993). Parietal lobe abnormalities detected with MR in patients with infantile autism. *American Journal of Roentgenology*, **160**, 387–93.

Courchesne, E., Townsend, J. & Saitoh, O. (1994). The brain in infantile autism: Posterior fossa structures are abnormal. *Neurology*, **44**, 214–23.

Courchesne, E., Yeung-Courchesne, R., Press, G.A., Hesselink, J.R. & Jernigan, T.L. (1988). Hypoplasia of cerebellar vermal lobules VI and VII in autism. *New England Journal of Medicine*, **318**, 1349–54.

DeLong, J.R. & Dwyer, J.T. (1988). Correlation of family history with specific autistic sub-groups: Asperger's syndrome and bipolar affective illness. *Journal of Autism and Developmental Disorders*, **18**, 593–600.

Eichenbaum, H. (1993). Thinking about brain cell assemblies. *Science*, **261**, 993–4.

Filipek, P.A. (1995). Quantitative magnetic resonance imaging in autism: the cerebellar vermis. *Current Opinion in Neurology*, **8**, 134–8.

Frith, U. & Baron-Cohen, S. 91987). Perception in autistic children. In *Handbook of Autism and Pervasive Developmental Disorders*, ed. D.J. Cohen & A.M. Donnellan, pp. 85–102. New York: Wiley.

Folstein, S.E. & Rutter, M. (1988). Autism: familial aggregation and genetic implication. *Journal of Autism and Developmental Disorders*, **18**, 3–30.

Gaffney, G.R., Kuperman, S., Tsai, L.Y. & Minchin, S. (1988). Morphological evidence for brainstem involvement in infantile autism. *Biological Psychiatry*, **24**, 578–86.

Gaffney, G.R., Kuperman, S., Tsai, L.Y. & Minchin, S. (1989). Forebrain structure in infantile autism. *Journal of the American Academy of Child Psychiatry*, **28**(4), 534–7.

Gaffney, G.R., Kuperman, S., Tsai, L.Y., Minchin, S. & Hassanein, K.M. (1987a). Midsagittal magnetic resonance imaging of autism. *British Journal of Psychiatry*, **151**, 831–3.

Gaffney, G.R., Tsai, L.Y., Kuperman, S. & Minchin, S. (1987b). Cerebellar structure in autism. *American Journal of Diseases of Children*, **141**, 1330–2.

Gillberg, C. & Coleman, M. (1992). *The Biology of the Autistic Syndromes*, 2nd edn. New York: Cambridge University Press.

Hashimoto, T., Tayama, M., Miyazaki, M., Murakawa, K. & Kuroda, Y. (1993). Brainstem and cerebellar vermis involvement in autistic children. *Journal of Child Neurology*, **8**, 149–53.

Hashimoto, T., Tayama, M., Miyazaki, M. et al. (1991). Reduced midbrain and pons size in children with autism. *Tokushima Journal of Experimental Medicine*, **38**, 15–18.

Hashimoto, T., Tayama, M., Miyazaki, M. et al. (1992). Reduced brainstem size in children with autism. *Brain Development*, **14**, 94–7.

Hashimoto, T., Tayama, M., Murakawa, K. et al. (1995). Development of the brainstem and cerebellum in autistic patients. *Journal of Autism and Developmental Disorders*, **25**, 1–22.

Hermelin, B. & O'Connor, N. (1967). Remembering of words by psychotic and subnormal children. *British Journal of Psychology*, **58**, 213–18.

Herrnstein, R.J. (1970). On the law of effect. *Journal of the Experimental Analysis of Behavior*, **13**, 243–66.

Hoffman, R.E. & Dobscha, S.K. (1989). Cortical pruning and the development of schizophrenia: a computer model. *Schizophrenia Bulletin*, **15**, 477–90.

Hoffman, R.E. & McGlashan, T.H. (1993). Parallel distributed processing and the emergence of schizophrenic symptoms. *Schizophrenia Bulletin*, **19**, 119–39.

Hornik, K., Stinchcombe, M. & White, H. (1989). Multilayer feedforward networks are universal approximators. *Neural Networks*, **2**, 359–68.

Hsu, M., Yeung-Courchesne, R., Courchesne, E. & Press, G.A. (1991). Absence of magnetic resonance imaging evidence of pontine abnormality in infantile autism. *Archives of Neurology*, **48**, 1160–3.

Jacobson, M. (1991). *Developmental Neurobiology*, 3rd edn. New York: Plenum Press.

Kanner, L. (1943). Autistic disturbances of affective contact. *Nervous Child*, **2**, 217–50.

Kemper, T.L. (1988). Neuroanatomic studies of dyslexia and autism. In *Disorders of the Developing Nervous System: Changing Views on Their Origins*, ed. J.W. Swann & A. Messer, pp. 125–54. New York: Alan R. Liss.

Kemper, T.L. & Bauman, M.L. (1993). The contribution of neuropathologic studies to the understanding of autism. *Behavioral Neurology*, **11**, 175–87.

Kluver, H. & Bucy, P.C. (1939). Preliminary analysis of functions of the temporal lobe in monkeys. *Archives of Neurology and Psychiatry*, **42**, 979–1000.

Koegel, R.L. & Koegel, L.K. (1995). *Teaching Children with Autism*. Baltimore: Brooks Publishing Co.

Koegel, R.L., Rincover, A. & Egel, A.L. (1982). *Educating and Understanding Autistic Children*. San Diego: College-Hill Press.

Kolmen, B.K., Feldman, H.M., Handen, B.L. & Janosky, J.E. (1995). Naltrexone in young autistic children: a double-blind, placebo-controlled crossover study. *Journal of the American Academy of Childhood and Adolescent Psychiatry*, **34**, 223–31.

Kosko, B. (1993). *Fuzzy Thinking: The New Science of Fuzzy Logic*. New York: Hyperion.

LaMantia, A.S. and Rakic, P. (1990). Axon overproduction and elimination in the corpus callosum of the developing rhesus monkey. *Journal of Neuroscience*, **10**, 2156–75.

Lehky, S.R. & Sejnowski, T.J. (1988). Network model of shape from shading: Neural function arises from both receptive and projective fields. *Nature*, **333**, 452–4.

Lehky, S.R. & Sejnowski, T.J. (1990). Neural network model of visual cortex for determining surface curvature from images of shaded surfaces. *Proceedings of the Royal Society of London*, B, **240**, 251–78.

Leslie, A.M. & Thaiss, L. (1992). Domain specificity in conceptual development: neuropsychological evidence from autism. *Cognition*, **43**, 225–51.

Lovaas, O.I. (1987). Behavior treatment and normal educational and intellectual functioning in young autistic children. *Journal of Consulting and Clinical Psychology*, **55**, 3–9.

Lovaas, O.I., Koegel, R.L. & Schreibman, L. (1979). Stimulus overselectivity in autism: A review of research. *Psychological Bulletin*, **86**, 1236–54.

Lovaas, O.I., Schreibman, L., Koegel, R.L. & Rehm, R. (1971). Selective responding by autistic children to multiple sensory input. *Journal of Abnormal Psychology*, **77**, 211–22.

McEachlin, J.J., Smith, T. & Lovaas, O.I. (1993). Long-term outcome for children with autism who received early intensive behavioral treatment. *American Journal of Mental Retardation*, **97**, 359–72.

McGaugh, J.L. (1991). Neuromodulation and the storage of information: involvement of the amygdaloid complex. In *Perspectives on Cognitive Neuroscience*, ed. R.G. Lister & H.J. Weingartner, pp. 279–99. New York: Oxford University Press.

Mehler, J., Bertoncini, J., Barciere, M. & Jassik-Gerschenfeld, D. (1978). Infant recognition of mother's voice. *Perception*, **7**, 491–7.

Mpitsos, G. (1993). Dynamics of brain function and the learning behavior of invertebrates. Paper presented at the Fifth Annual Convention of the American Psychological Society, Chicago, June 25.

Mundy, P., Sigman, M. & Kasari, C. (1990). A longitudinal study of joint attention and language development in autistic children. *Journal of Autism and Developmental Disorders*, **20**, 115–28.

Munro, P.W. (1986). State-dependent factors influencing neural plasticity: A partial account of the critical period. In *Parallel Distributed Processing: Explorations in the Microstructure of Cognition*, Vol. 2, ed. J.L. McClelland & D.E. Rumelhart, pp. 471–502. Cambridge, MA: MIT Press.

Murakami, J.W., Courchesne, E., Press, G.A., Yeung-Courchesne, R. & Hesselink, J.R. (1989). Reduced cerebellar hemisphere size and its relationship to vermal hypoplasia in autism. *Archives of Neurology*, **46**, 689–94.

Nelson, C.A. (1994). Neural bases of infant temperament. In *Temperament: Individual Differences at the Interface of Biology and Behavior*, ed. J.E. Bates & T.D. Wachs, pp. 47–82. Washington, DC: American Psychological Association.

NeuralWare. (1993). *Neural Computing*. Pittsburgh: NeuralWare.

Nowell, M.A., Hackney, D.B., Muraki, A.S. & Coleman, M. (1990). Varied
    MR appearance of autism: Fifty-three pediatric patients having the full
    autistic syndrome. *Magnetic Resonance Imaging*, **8**, 811–16.
Nowlan, S.J. (1990). Competing experts: An experimental investigation of
    associative mixture models. Technical Report CRG-TR-90-5, University of
    Toronto.
Panksepp, J. (1979). A neurochemical theory of autism. *Trends in Neuroscience*,
    2, 174–7.
Piven, J. & Arndt, S. (1995). The cerebellum and autism. (Letter.) *Neurology*,
    45, 398–9.
Piven, J., Arndt, S., Bailey, J., Haverecamp, S., Andreasen, N.C. & Palmer, P.
    (1995). An MRI study of brain size and autism. *American Journal of
    Psychiatry*, **52**, 1145–9.
Piven, J., Berthier, M.L., Starkstein, S.E., Nehme, E., Pearlson, G. & Folstein,
    S. (1990). Magnetic resonance imaging evidence for a defect of cerebral
    cortical development in autism. *American Journal of Psychiatry*, **147**, 734–
    9.
Rakic, P. (1991). Plasticity of cortical development. In *Plasticity of
    Development*, ed. S.E. Brauth, W.S. Hall & R.J. Dooling, pp. 127–61.
    Cambridge, MA: MIT Press.
Rakic, P., Bourgeois, J-P., Eckenhoff, M.E., Zecevic, N. & Goldman-Rakic,
    P.S. (1986). Concurrent overproduction of synapses in diverse regions of
    the primate cerebral cortex. *Science*, **232**, 232–5.
Rapin, I. (1993). Autism: a complex developmental disorder of brain function.
    Paper presented at the 25th Anniversary Celebration of The New York
    State Institute for Basic Research, Staten Island, NY, May 19.
Raymond, G., Bauman, M. & Kemper, T. (1989). The hippocampus in autism:
    Golgi analysis. Programs and abstracts. *Child Neurology Society*, **26**, 483–
    4.
Ritvo, E.R., Freeman, B.J., Scheibel, A.B., Duong, P.T., Robinson, H. &
    Guthrie, D. (1986). Lower Purkinje cell counts in the cerebella of four
    autistic patients: Initial findings of the UCLA–NSAC Autopsy Research
    Report. *American Journal of Psychiatry*, **143**, 862–6.
Ritvo E.R. & Garber, H.J. (1988). Cerebellar hypoplasia and autism. (Letter.)
    New England Journal of Medicine, **319**, 1152.
Rolls, E.T. (1990a). Functions of the primate hippocampus in spatial
    processing and memory. In *Neurobiology of Comparative Cognition*, ed.
    R.P. Kesner, & D.S. Olton, pp. 339–62. Hillsdale, NJ: Lawrence Erlbaum.
Rolls, E.T. (1990b). Functions of neuronal networks in the hippocampus and
    of backprojections in the cerebral cortex in memory. In *Brain Organization
    and Memory: Cells, Systems, and Circuits*, ed. J.L. McGaugh, N.M.
    Weinberger & G. Lynch, pp. 184–210. New York: Oxford University
    Press.
Rolls, E.T. (1992). Neurophysiology and functions of the primate amygdala. In
    *The Amygdala: Neurobiological Aspects of Emotion, Memory and Mental
    Dysfunction*, ed. J.P. Aggleton, pp. 143–65. New York: Wiley-Liss.
Rosser, R. (1994). *Cognitive Development: Psychological and Biological
    Perspectives*. Boston: Allyn and Bacon.
Rumelhart, D.E., Hinton, G.E. & Williams, R.J. (1986). Learning internal
    representations by error propagation. In *Parallel Distributed Processing:
    Explorations in the Microstructure of Cognition*, Vol. 1, *Foundations*, ed.

D.E. Rumelhart & J.L. McClelland, pp. 318–62. Cambridge, MA: MIT Press.
Schreibman, L. (1988). *Autism.* Newbury Park, CA: Sage Publications.
Schreibman, L., Charlop, M.H. & Koegel, R.L. (1982). Teaching autistic children to use extra-stimulus prompts. *Journal of Experimental Child Psychology,* **33**, 475–91.
Schreibman, L. & Lovaas, O.I. (1973). Overselective responding to social stimuli by autistic children. *Journal of Abnormal Child Psychology,* **1**, 152–68.
Sejnowski, T.J. & Rosenberg, C.R. (1987). Parallel networks that learn to pronounce English text. *Complex Systems,* **1**, 145–68.
Selfe, L. (1977). *Nadia: A Case of Extraordinary Drawing Ability in an Autistic Child.* London: Academic Press.
Sietsma, J. & Dow, R.J.F. (1988). Neural net pruning – why and how. *Proceedings, IEEE International Conference on Neural Networks,* **1**, 375–83.
Soto-Moyana, R., Hernandez, A., Perez, H., Ruiz, S., Galleguillos, X. & Belman, J. (1991). Yohimbine early in life alters functional properties of interhemispheric connections of rat visual cortex. *Brain Research Bulletin,* **26**, 259–63.
Sparrow, S.S., Balla, D.A. & Cicchetti, D.V. (1984). *Vineland Adaptive Behavior Scales. Interview Edition. Survey Form Manual.* Circle Pines, MN: American Guidance.
Steinmetz, J.E. (1994). Brain substrates of emotion and temperament. In *Temperament: Individual Differences at the Interface of Biology and Behavior,* ed. J.E. Bates & T.D. Wachs, pp. 17–46. Washington, DC: American Psychological Association.
Sugiyama, T. & Abe, T. (1989). The prevalence of autism in Nagoya, Japan: a total population study. *Journal of Autism and Developmental Disorders,* **19**, 87–96.
Warren, J.M. (1953). Additivity of cues in visual pattern discriminations by monkeys. *Journal of Comparative and Physiological Psychology,* **46**, 484–6.
Warren, R.M. (1984). Perceptual restoration of obliterated sounds. *Psychological Bulletin,* **96**, 371–83.
Weeks, S.J. & Hobson, R.P. (1987). The salience of facial expression for autistic children. *Journal of Child Psychology and Psychiatry,* **28**, 137–52.
Williams, R.S., Hauser, S.L., Purpura, D.P., DeLong, G.R. & Swisher, C.N. (1980). Autism and mental retardation: Neuropathologic studies performed in four retarded persons with autistic behavior. *Archives of Neurology,* **37**, 749–53.
Wilson, M.A. & McNaughton, B.L. (1993). Dynamics of the hippocampal ensemble code for space. *Science,* **261**, 1055–8.
Wing, L. (1981). Asperger's syndrome: a clinical account. *Psychological Medicine,* **11**, 115–29.
Wing, L. & Attwood, A. (1987). Syndromes of autism and atypical development. In *Handbook of Autism and Pervasive Developmental Disorders,* ed. D.J. Cohen & A.M. Donnellan, pp. 3–19. Silver Spring, MD: Winston.

12

Are there common neural mechanisms for learning, epilepsy, and Alzheimer's disease?

GENE V. WALLENSTEIN and
MICHAEL E. HASSELMO

Introduction

Understanding the neurophysiological mechanisms that support learning and memory remains one of the greatest challenges to science today. A major landmark in this area of study occurred some 20 years ago when Bliss and Lomo (1973) discovered a long-term potentiation (LTP) of synaptic excitability in the dentate area of the hippocampal formation due to a brief, high-frequency stimulation of the perforant path. Since then, LTP has become the leading model for the molecular basis of memory. While there is now a growing taxonomy for LTP classification, this chapter is concerned primarily with N-methyl-D-aspartate (NMDA)-dependent potentiation. Recent research has begun to elucidate the manner in which NMDA-dependent LTP induction leads to functional and morphological changes in synaptic structure and ion channel properties that may serve to maintain the increased potentiation (e.g., Desmond and Levy, 1988; Chen and Huang, 1992). Moreover, malfunction in the development of NMDA-dependent LTP may provide insights into our understanding of certain neurological disorders such as epilepsy and, particularly, Alzheimer's disease, both of which seem to be affected by changes in NMDA receptor activation.

In the popular consciousness, Alzheimer's disease is identified as a disorder of memory function. While research on Alzheimer's disease has produced a range of etiological theories, ranging from the improper splicing of the amyloid precursor protein (Selkoe, 1993) to epidemiological factors such as aluminum exposure (Crapper McLachlan and Van Berkum, 1986) or prions (Goudsmit and Van der Waals, 1986), these etiological theories have not explicitly accounted for why this disorder should show its earlier symptoms as a disorder of memory function (Jolles, 1986; Morris and Kopelman, 1986; Albert et al., 1991), and should so severely affect those structures associated with memory function (Hyman et al., 1984; Hyman, Van Hoesen and Damasio, 1990; Arnold et al., 1991; Arriagada, Marzloff and Hyman, 1992). As it stands, the early effect on memory function is attributed to the unexplained specificity of Alzheimer's disease for hippocampal region CA1, the subiculum, and layers II and IV of entorhinal cortex (Hyman et al., 1984, 1990; Arnold et al., 1991; Braak and Braak, 1991). Here, it is proposed that the causality is in fact reversed. The selective cortical neuropathology associated with the progression of this disorder may be rooted in the breakdown of the essential mechanism of cortical memory function.

A major component of this chapter is a computational theory of the initiation of Alzheimer's disease that attempts to account for evidence on the progression of the disease not in terms of a specific etiological factor, but in terms of the processing characteristics of cortical structures, and the stability of the learning mechanisms within these structures. This theory was inspired by the phenomenon of runaway synaptic modification, as demonstrated in models of cortical associative memory function (Hasselmo, Anderson and Bower, 1992; Hasselmo, 1993, 1994; Hasselmo and Bower, 1993; Barkai et al., 1993; Hasselmo and Barkai, 1995). In these models, interference during learning can lead to the exponential growth of a large number of synaptic connections within the network. Runaway synaptic modification of this sort may underlie the neuropathological characteristics of Alzheimer's disease. The theory provides a framework showing why this neuropathology should appear initially in particular cortical regions associated with memory function (Braak and Braak, 1991; Arriagada et al., 1992), and why it should appear to progress into adjacent regions of association cortex along the observed anatomical connections (Pearson et al., 1985; Arnold et al., 1991; Arriagada et al., 1992). Finally, the theory suggests that the apparent degeneration of cortical cholinergic innervation in this disease (Davies and Maloney, 1976; Perry et al., 1977; Whitehouse et al., 1982; Coyle, Price and DeLong, 1983; Saper, German and White, 1985) may result from feedback mechanism placing too great a demand on the cholinergic modulation of learning processes.

Experimental observations

Molecular mechanisms of NMDA-dependent LTP

LTP is characterized by an enhancement of synaptic efficacy following presynaptic activation of a postsynaptic cell above a certain threshold for induction. This potentiation occurs only if presynaptic activation takes place prior to postsynaptic depolarization within a time span of approximately 50 ms (Levy and Steward, 1983), and is locally specific to the active synapse. That is, other inputs to the same postsynaptic cell are not potentiated if they were not active during stimulation (Lynch, Dunwiddie and Gribkoff, 1977). This form of potentiation is consistent with a theory by Hebb (1949) that postulated an increase in synaptic efficacy with repeated co-activation of the cells sharing a single synapse. Approximation of this process in neural models, therefore, has often been referred to as Hebbian learning (Hasselmo, 1995a; 1995c).

Since the primary source of excitatory postsynaptic potentials (EPSPs) in the hippocampus is mediated through glutamate receptors, much attention has focused on their involvement in LTP induction (see Gustafsson and Wigstrom, 1988). There are three classes of glutamate receptors in the central nervous system: (1) those that are NMDA sensitive; (2) those that are activated by alpha-amino-3-hydroxy 5-methyl 4--isoxazole proprionic acid (AMPA); and (3) metabotropic receptors. Each of the conductances associated with channel activation of these classes has different time-dependent properties, which may have a marked influence on membrane dynamics. For instance, in hippocampal pyramidal cells, AMPA-mediated EPSPs have a rapid onset (approximately 2 ms) and short duration (5–8 ms), whereas NMDA receptor-mediated EPSPs have rise times on the order of 5–10 ms and may last 70–100 ms (Jahr and Stevens, 1990). There is now evidence suggesting that NMDA and AMPA receptors are located proximally to each other on dendritic spines and that they may be actively coupled (Wigstrom and Gustafsson, 1986). This anatomical structure may have important functional consequences for the way malfunctions in normal LTP induction may lead to aberrant behavior.

Besides having different conductance properties, a key difference between these receptor types is that the NMDA receptor channel is also voltage sensitive. At resting potentials, NMDA channels are normally blocked by Mg^{2+} (Mayer, Westbrook and Guthrie, 1984). Local depolarization of the membrane in close proximity to the NMDA receptor complex will relieve the Mg^{2+} block and allow the channel to be activated by glutamate or a suitable agonist. During normal low-frequency synaptic transmission, presynaptic spiking leads to glutamate release and subsequent binding at both NMDA and AMPA receptors on the postsynaptic cell. Because low-frequency stimulation does not typically produce a depolarization in the postsynaptic cell of sufficient magnitude to relieve the Mg^{2+} block, only the AMPA receptor channels open initially, which pass both Na^+ and K^+ ions. If presynaptic activity provides sufficient depolarization (through AMPA receptor activation) to relieve the Mg^{2+} block of NMDA receptors, possibly due to bursting in the presynaptic cell or high-frequency single spike firing, NMDA receptor activation will also pass Na^+ and K^+ ions, as well as Ca^{2+} ions which, as is shown below, has been found to be an important step in LTP induction. The fact that NMDA receptor activation depends both on presynaptically released glutamate binding to the channel and postsynaptic depolarization of sufficient magnitude to alleviate the Mg^{2+} block, results in a synapse that operates somewhat akin to a coincidence detector.

Several studies have now shown that the increase in Ca^{2+} in the postsynaptic cell due to NMDA channel activation is a critical step in LTP induction (Dunwiddie and Lynch, 1979; Lynch et al., 1983). Indeed, LTP induction is blocked by intracellular injection of the Ca^{2+} chelator ethylene glycol-bis N, N, N', N'-tetra-acetic acid (EGTA) (Lynch et al., 1983), while transient increases in extracellular Ca^{2+} may induce LTP (Turner, Baimbridge and Miller, 1982). Several Ca^{2+}-activated enzymes (e.g., calpain and calcineurin) and protein kinases have been shown to be important for structural changes to the synapse that maintain LTP. For instance, protein kinase C (PKC) levels have been shown to rise postsynaptically with increased Ca^{2+} (Akers et al., 1986), which, when inhibited, results in a blocking of LTP induction (Malenka et al., 1989). PKC in conjunction with calpain, has been observed to produce changes in cytoskeletal postsynaptic structure (Lynch and Baudry, 1984), which may be responsible for maintaining the sustained potentiation at AMPA receptors. Such structural changes may be related to the reported increase in surface area of postsynaptic spine heads and density following LTP induction (Desmond and Levy, 1988). Moreover, PKC has also been reported to increase NMDA channel conductance and produce alterations in the extent of the Mg^{2+} block, which could have consequences for the proper maintenance of intracellular free Ca^{2+} concentrations (Kelso, Nelson and Leonard, 1992; Chen and Huang, 1992).

NMDA receptor activation and epilepsy

Croucher, Collins and Meldrum (1982) were among the first to point out that NMDA antagonists, while inhibitors of LTP induction, are also potent anticonvulsants. It is also known that hippocampal slices bathed in low Mg^{2+} are prone to seizure behavior (Swartzwelder et al., 1987), presumably through an increase in NMDA receptor activation. Considering these observations, it is perhaps reasonable to postulate a relationship between the processes which support normal LTP induction and those which may lead to epileptiform activity. Such behavior is characterized by a large population of neurons firing in a synchronous and repetitive manner. Indeed, such a firing pattern can be initiated by a process known as kindling, in which seizure activity is induced with repeated applications of brief, high-frequency stimulation similar to what is required for LTP induction. Moreover, even short-lived seizure events have been shown to produce long-lasting changes in synaptic potentiation and morphological changes to cytoskeletal structure such as sprouting, similar to those observed after LTP induction (Ben-Ari and Represa, 1990).

Seizure events have also been reported to produce long-lasting changes to NMDA receptors such as increasing their mean open time (Kohr, DeKoninck and Momdy, 1993), reducing their affinity for Mg^{2+}, and increasing receptor density similar to that observed following LTP induction (Lahtinen et al., 1993). Thus, it seems plausible that a transient alteration of normal NMDA receptor-mediated conductances may play a role in epileptiform development. A classic recipe for epileptic activity in hippocampal slices involves the application of a γ-aminobutyric acid A ($GABA_A$) receptor antagonist such as bicuculine (Traub and Miles, 1991). Removal of local inhibitory effects of this fashion enables tonically active pyramidal cells (mediated by neuromodulatory influences such as acetylcholine from the basal forebrain) to become more depolarized and hence reduce the degree of Mg^{2+} block of NMDA channels. A similar cascade of events has been found to be necessary for LTP induction in the hippocampal slice (Mott and Lewis, 1991). In the case of epilepsy, however, this increase in NMDA channel conductance is left completely unchecked by a block of GABAergic inhibition, resulting in a positive feedback loop where depolarization may spread to other locations, recruiting additional NMDA channels and still further depolarization of the cell. NMDA antagonists such as 2-amino-5-phosphonopentanoic acid (AP5) prevent the development of epileptic activity by reducing this positive feedback and have also been shown to block the induction of LTP (Slater, Stelzer and Galvan, 1985).

NMDA receptor activation and Alzheimer's disease

Given the putative role for NMDA receptors in LTP, a molecular model for memory acquisition, and clinical symptoms of Alzheimer's patients, including an inability to form new memories, several investigators have speculated on a relationship between NMDA receptor malfunction and various forms of neurodegenerative disease (see Krogsgaard-Larsen, 1992, for a review). Some have proposed that hyperactivity of glutamate channel conductances may produce an excitotoxic effect in postsynaptic cells (Maragos et al., 1987; Represa et al., 1988). Indeed, overactivation of NMDA channel conductances would allow a persistent increase in Ca^{2+} inside the postsynaptic cell, which may, through some of the second messengers mentioned earlier, lead to cell death or aberrant changes in cytoskeletal structure (Represa et al., 1988).

Alzheimer's disease is diagnosed post mortem on the basis of the density of the neuropathological characteristics, including neuritic plaques and neurofibrillary tangles (for a review, see Katzman, 1986; Hyman et al., 1990; Selkoe, 1993). Neuritic plaques tend to be broadly distributed, appearing throughout the cortex, with a greater density in regions of frontal, parietal and temporal association cortex distant from the primary sensory and motor cortices (Pearson et al., 1985; Arnold et al., 1991). In addition, neuritic plaques appear in subcortical regions receiving projections from the cortex (Pearson et al., 1985). The distribution and component features of neuritic plaques have led to the suggestion that they reflect the degeneration of axonal processes from the same set of neurons that develop neurofibrillary tangles (Hyman et al., 1984). Here, it is proposed that neuritic plaques result from a breakdown in the normal mechanisms for modification of synaptic strength. In fact, the development of neuritic plaques results from an accumulation of an altered beta-amyloid precursor protein, which has been suggested normally to regulate internal levels of free Ca^{2+} (Mattson et al., 1993). Thus, if internal Ca^{2+} reaches critically high levels, one may expect increases in excitotoxicity. Grenamyre et al. (1987) have, in fact, shown a decrease of 75–87 percent in NMDA-receptor binding in human hippocampal and adjacent parahippocampal cortical slices of Alzheimer's disease patients.

This pattern of degeneration would then be expected to prevail in brain regions associated with high concentrations of NMDA receptors.

Neurofibrillary tangles show a more localized initial distribution than plaques and spread in a characteristic sequence (Hyman et al., 1990; Arnold et al., 1991; Braak and Braak, 1991). Tangles appear initially and attain their highest concentration in layer II of entorhinal cortex, region CA1 of the hippocampus, and the portions of the subiculum adjacent to region CA1 (Ball, 1972; Hyman et al., 1984, 1990; Braak and Braak, 1991; Arriagada et al., 1992). As the severity of the disease progresses, tangles appear in regions receiving projections from these areas, initially in portions of the temporal lobe adjacent to the entorhinal cortex, and later in regions of parietal lobe and frontal cortex that are closely linked to entorhinal cortex (Brun and Gustafson, 1976; Pearson et al., 1985; Arnold et al., 1991; Braak and Braak, 1991; Arriagada et al., 1992). Tangles appear to be distributed in almost columnar fashion, with tangles in layers 2 and 3 appearing in register with tangles in layers 5 and 6 (Pearson et al., 1985). The primary sensory and motor cortices typically show the lowest density of neurofibrillary tangles, suggesting they are the least sensitive to the mechanisms underlying this disorder (Brun and Gustafsson, 1976; Pearson et al., 1985; Esiri, Pearson and Powell, 1986). These patterns of distribution suggest that the disease progresses from the hippocampus along back-projections into cortical regions. In addition, it suggests that susceptibility to degeneration is somehow correlated with the level of involvement in higher-order cognitive processes and associations between modalities – processes that involve ongoing remodeling of cortical representations.

Theories of the progression of Alzheimer's disease

Research into potential causes of Alzheimer's disease at the molecular level does not attempt systematically to describe the spread of pathology between different regions. Many forms of familial Alzheimer's disease have been linked to specific inherited differences in protein structure (Schellenberg et al., 1992), although the fact that monozygotic twins can show different susceptibility for the disease suggests that it is not entirely genetic (Breitner et al., 1993). This class of theories depends upon the assumption that one of the protein components of the Alzheimer neuropathology, such as amyloid or tau, is a causative agent in the disease (see, for example, Hardy and Higgins, 1992). The characteristic distribution of neuropathology places extra demands on this theory, suggesting a particular susceptibility of the hippocampus and association cortex but not of the primary motor and sensory cortices.

Theories based on environmental factors must also account for this selective sensitivity.

The theory presented here focuses on relating initiation and progression of the disease to functional characteristics of cortical regions. In this framework, the initial imbalance of cortical parameters that results in pathology could be due to defects of the genetic code, the spread of toxic factors, an infection by a prion, or a combination of different factors. But this theory proposes that the final effect of this imbalance is the initiation of runaway synaptic modification (an NMDA-dependent process) within cortical regions with a strong capacity for synaptic modification, such as the hippocampal formation. In this context, the progression of the disease depends upon the functional interaction of cortical regions. Rather than depending on the transmission of some substance from the axon terminal of an affected cell to an as yet unaffected postsynaptic neuron, this theory depends only on the normal mechanisms of synaptic transmission and synaptic modification at these connections. The basis of this theory is that the pattern of activity propagated from affected to unaffected regions may be pathological in itself. That is, runaway synaptic modification may cause a breakdown of function in one region, and the patterns of activity elicited can induce runaway synaptic modification in connected regions.

The focus of this model differs from that of other models of Alzheimer's disease (Horn et al., 1993; Herrmann, Ruppin and Usher, 1993), which do not attempt to address the dynamics of spread of cortical neuropathology. These previous models start with the assumption of loss of neurons or synaptic connections within models of cortex, and then analyze how the effects of this loss on memory function may be affected by synaptic compensation mechanisms.

Models of epilepsy and Alzheimer's disease in the hippocampus
Transitions between states of learning and epilepsy

This section presents a biophysical model of hippocampal region CA3, used to investigate the effects of cholinergic modulation from the basal forebrain on population dynamics. Considering that the NMDA-dependent effects mentioned above may be important for regulating LPT induction and the development of epilepsy, how is a stable balance achieved in the hippocampus between conditions that foster accurate associative memory and those that may lead to epileptiform events?

Traub and colleagues (Traub and Jefferys, 1994a, 1994b; Traub, Jefferys and Whittington, 1994; Traub, Colling and Jefferys, 1995) have performed numerous computational investigations of the cellular bases of hippocampal epilepsy. However, to date no one has used a biophysically realistic model to study the manner in which this area is capable of producing accurate associations where limited subsets of neurons exhibit synchronized firing under one condition, but may transition into epileptiform-like activity with globally synchronous behavior under relatively small parameter change. In fact, we show transitions between these two markedly different functional states can occur with changes in a single parameter intrinsic to pyramidal cells. Our network simulations indicate that cholinergic modulation from the medial septum sets the proper 'tonus' of excitability in CA3 pyramidal neurons to promote accurate learning by: (1) blocking a voltage-independent K^+ leak current, $I_{K(leak)}$; (2) suppression of an intrinsic adaptation current, $I_{K(AHP)}$; and (3) reducing synaptic transmission at recurrent excitatory synapses between these cells. Each of these mechanisms has been observed in vitro (Bernardo and Prince, 1982; Cole and Nicoll, 1984; Madison, Lancaster and Nicoll, 1987; Hasselmo, Schnell and Barkai, 1995a). In order to understand how each of these components shapes population activity in area CA3, a biophysical model based on extensive neuroanatomical and electrophysiological findings from this region was developed.

The model consisted of 500 pyramidal cells and 100 inhibitory interneurons. Each pyramidal cell was a reduced Traub model (Traub, Miles and Wong, 1989; Traub et al., 1991), which consisted of a fast sodium current ($I_{Na(fast)}$), a delayed rectifier ($I_{K(DR)}$), a high-threshold calcium current (I_{Ca}), two calcium-dependent potassium currents – ($I_{K(AHP)}$), which is carbachol sensitive, and $I_{K(Ca)}$, which does not appear to be (Madison et al., 1987) – the transient potassium current ($I_{K(A)}$), and a potassium leak current ($I_{K(leak)}$). Each of these currents was located at the soma and proximal dendrites, while the distal dendrites contained I_{Ca}, $I_{K(AHP)}$, $I_{K(Ca)}$, and $I_{K(leak)}$. Calcium buffering was performed in each compartment using a first-order diffusion process (Traub et al., 1991). Each interneuron consisted of $I_{Na(fast)}$ and $I_{K(DR)}$ located at the soma, with the four remaining compartments (two basal and two apical) being passive.

The isolated pyramidal cell reproduced several electrophysiological properties known to exist in real CA3 neurons, including bursting (Fig. 12.1) and the transition to single-spike firing patterns with increasing

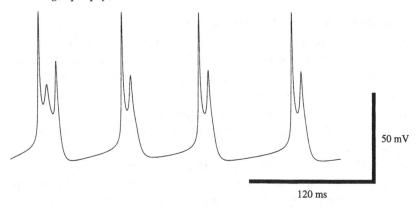

Fig. 12.1 An example of pyramidal cell bursting with a somatic current injection of 0.15 nA.

levels of somatic current injection. Interneurons contained two intrinsic and four synaptic currents. When isolated, these cells displayed high-frequency, single-spike firing with little adaptation as shown in CA3 in-vitro slice preparations (Miles, 1990).

Each cell in the model also included four synaptic currents that were the chloride-dependent GABA$_A$ and potassium-dependent GABA$_B$ inhibitory conductances along with the AMPA and NMDA excitatory conductances. Recurrent excitatory synapses located at the apical dendrites of pyramidal cells included Hebbian modification of NMDA conductances in conjunction with a voltage-dependent Mg^{2+} block based on previous modeling (Zador, Koch and Brown, 1990). The network also included recurrent inhibitory synapses (GABA$_A$ and GABA$_B$) at the soma and proximal dendrites of interneurons. Feedforward inhibition of pyramidal cells occurred via GABA$_A$ receptors situated at the soma and proximal dendrites while slower GABA$_B$ receptor-mediated inhibition was located at distal dendrites (Doi, Carpenter and Hori, 1990). Feedforward excitation occurred through NMDA and AMPA receptors located at the soma of interneurons. Both cholinergic (Frotscher and Leranth, 1985) and GABAergic (Freund and Antal, 1988) projections from the medial septum were included in the model and all synaptic delays, conduction velocities, and connection probabilities were approximated to parameter estimations made previously from in-vivo data (see Traub and Miles, 1991, for a review of these data). Connection probabilities were increased slightly in the model in compensation for the reduced scale compared to slice preparations.

Associative memory and Hebbian learning

Models of cortical associative memory function (Grossberg, 1970; Anderson, 1972; Hopfield, 1982; McClelland and Rumelhart, 1988; Amit, Evans and Abeles, 1990) focus on the anatomical evidence for widely distributed excitatory intrinsic and associational connections linking pyramidal cells within cortical structures, including neocortex and hippocampus. While they differ in detail, the function of all these models depends upon the synaptic modification of excitatory connections using some modification of the Hebb rule (Hebb, 1949; Wigstrom et al., 1986). As mentioned earlier, the basic feature of the Hebb rule is a change in synaptic strength proportional to presynaptic and postsynaptic activity during learning. These modified excitatory synapses can then form the basis for recalling associations between different patterns of activity. A simple example of this associative memory function is shown in Figure 12.2.

Neurophysiological data suggest that Hebbian synaptic modification depends upon combining postsynaptic depolarization with synaptic transmission to activate NMDA receptors at the synapse being modified (Wigstrom et al., 1986). However, if a modifiable synapse can influence postsynaptic activity during learning, strengthening this synapse will increase postsynaptic activity, and thereby increase subsequent strengthening of the synapse. This positive feedback effect can very rapidly lead

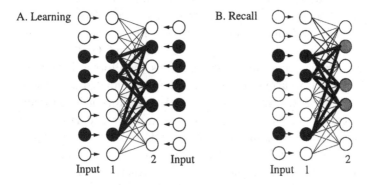

Fig. 12.2 Associative memory function. A. Learning: separate input patterns are presented to regions 1 and 2. The synapses between active neurons are strengthened using a Hebbian learning rule (dependent on presynaptic and postsynaptic activity). Strengthened synapses are represented by thicker lines between neurons. B. Recall: input is presented to region 1 only. The spread of activity along previously strengthened connections (thick lines) induces activity in region 2 resembling the pattern previously associated with pattern 1.

to exponential growth of undesired synapses within the network, i.e., runaway synaptic modification. The mechanism for runaway synaptic modification is illustrated in Figure 12.3. This figure shows that if synaptic transmission at modifiable synapses is allowed during learning, the spread of activity across previously modified connections causes the new synaptic modification to contain elements of proactive interference from previously learned memories (Hasselmo et al., 1992, 1995a; Hasselmo and Bower, 1993; Hasselmo, 1993, 1994). This results in a rather substantial increase in synaptic connections that have been potentiated (Fig. 12.4). Without the proper balance of parameters of cortical function, this interference during learning can have disastrous effects in models of cortical memory function. Though the effect of interference during learning in any particular stage of learning may be small, this phenomenon can severely affect the function of the network over time, because the effects are compounded by subsequent learning. The progressive build up of

A. 1st association   B. 2nd association   C. 3rd association

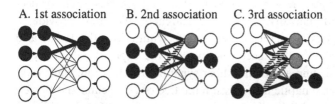

Fig. 12.3 Runaway synaptic modification. As more overlapping memories are stored within the network, greater interference during learning occurs. A. Learning of the first association shows no interference. B. Interference due to recall of the first association during learning of the second association causes strengthening of one additional undesired connection (dashed line). C. Recall of the first and second associations during learning of the third association causes strengthening of two additional undesired connections.

A   B

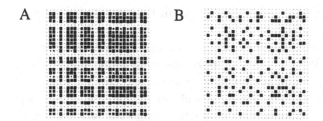

Fig. 12.4 Matrix of synaptic connectivity within an associative memory model. The size of the black squares represents the strength of synapses. A. After runaway synaptic modification. B. After normal learning.

interference from previous retrieval leads to a malignant nostalgia resulting in runaway synaptic modification throughout the whole network. In
this case, severe proactive and retroactive interference results in a complete breakdown of normal memory function. This runaway interference
during learning has been described previously in detail using mathematical analysis (Hasselmo, 1994) and computational models (Hasselmo et
al., 1992; Hasselmo, 1993; Barkai et al., 1993).

Because of the problems caused by synaptic transmission during learning, most associative memory models ignore the effects of synaptic transmission at modifiable synapses during learning (Anderson, 1972;
Hopfield, 1982; McClelland and Rumelhart, 1988; Amit et al., 1990),
allowing synaptic transmission only during recall. In computational models, this suppression of synaptic transmission at intrinsic and association
fiber synapses during learning can prevent runaway synaptic modification
(Hasselmo et al., 1992; Hasselmo, 1993, 1994; Hasselmo and Bower,
1993; Barkai et al., 1993; Hasselmo and Barkai, 1995). Though this suppression of synaptic transmission during learning has been used for decades in neural network models, researchers did not provide a
neurophysiological mechanism for this effect until recently. It has also
recently been shown that acetylcholine has the capacity selectively to
suppress intrinsic and association fiber synaptic transmission, while leaving afferent fiber synaptic transmission unaffected (Hasselmo and Bower,
1992; Hasselmo and Schnell, 1994; Hasselmo et al., 1995a). In addition,
acetylcholine enhances the excitability of cortical neurons to the afferent
synaptic input (Cole and Nicoll, 1984; Barkai and Hasselmo, 1993). In
computational models of cortical associative memory function, application of this selective suppression of intrinsic fiber synaptic transmission
during learning prevents interference from previously learned memories
(Hasselmo et al., 1992; Hasselmo, 1993, 1994; Hasselmo and Bower,
1993; Hasselmo and Barkai, 1995). Prevention of runaway synaptic modification by cholinergic suppression of synaptic transmission is illustrated
in simplified form in Figure 12.5.

In this new framework for learning, synaptic modification must be
maximal during the cholinergic suppression of synaptic transmission.
But how does this allow activation of postsynaptic NMDA receptors?
The activation of NMDA receptors and the mechanisms of synaptic
modification are still possible because the cholinergic suppression of
synaptic transmission is not complete. In neurophysiological experiments, the cholinergic suppression of synaptic transmission is usually
less than 70 percent (Hasselmo and Bower, 1992). Analysis of associative

1st association   2nd association   3rd association

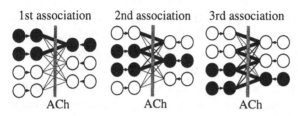

ACh   ACh   ACh

Fig. 12.5 Cholinergic suppression of synaptic transmission during learning can prevent runaway synaptic modification. The thick gray line represents diffuse cholinergic suppression of transmission at modifiable synapses, preventing the spread of excitation across previously modified synapses from bringing post-synaptic neurons above threshold. This allows Hebbian synaptic modification to occur only between neurons receiving direct afferent input (only these neurons have sufficient postsynaptic activity). Strengthening of additional undesired connections does not occur (compare with Fig. 12.3). ACh, acetycholine.

memory models incorporating feedback inhibition, a threshold for synaptic modification and gated decay of synaptic strength shows that this level of suppression is sufficient to prevent interference during learning, while allowing sufficient synaptic transmission for the modification of synapses (Hasselmo, 1993, 1994). In models of cortical associative memory function, interference during learning can be prevented by the proper balance of cortical physiological parameters including: (1) presynaptic cholinergic modulation of synaptic transmission; (2) regulated decay of synaptic connectivity strength; (3) postsynaptic cholinergic modulation of cellular excitability; (4) the level of inhibition within the network; (5) the threshold for synaptic modification; and (6) the nature of the patterns being stored within the network. In addition, cholinergic agonists have been shown to enhance synaptic modification in cortical structures (Hasselmo and Barkai, 1995).

Population oscillations in CA3

Whereas the examples shown here are highly simplified, the prevention of runaway synaptic modification has also been explored in detailed biophysical simulations of cortical associative memory function (Barkai et al., 1993; Hasselmo and Barkai, 1995). To test the manner in which acetylcholine affects associative memory in region CA3, a simple input pattern was presented to the model followed by a degraded version to test recall performance (Wallenstein and Hasselmo, 1997). The input pattern was delivered to the model as a fast AMPA receptor-mediated excitatory input to the apical dendrites of pyramidal cells at 25 Hz for a period of 60 ms every 200 ms. Cholinergic modulation was performed during the 'learning' period and removed during the test of recall performance. At these parameter values, the model partially completed the input pattern during initial recall, with 'waves' of pyramidal cell bursting occurring across the simulated slice. A gradual recruitment of more pyramidal cells into this bursting activity, independent of the particular input pattern, resulted in poor recall performance.

Reasoning that increased excitability in pyramidal cells unique to the input pattern should foster better learning, the maximum conductance underlying $I_{K(AHP)}$ was reduced from a normal value of 0.65 ms/cm^2 to 0.1625 ms/cm^2 to simulate the suppression of this adaptation current by the cholinergic agonist carbachol (Madison et al., 1987). However, during learning the model exhibited a rapid recruitment of pyramidal cells into globally synchronous bursting at approximately 1.5–2 Hz. This effect was most sensitive to shortening the after-hyperpolarizing potential (AHP) that normally follows a calcium-mediated burst. Reduction of the AHP indirectly decreased the bursting refractory period of pyramidal cells, thus creating a condition in which an exaggerated number was available for EPSP-induced firing. Population activity of this sort resembles epileptiform-like behavior observed in hippocampal slice preparations (Swartzwelder et al., 1987), and made learning new patterns impossible because all Hebbian NMDA synapses were systematically increased independent of the given input. Increasing the maximum conductance underlying $I_{K(AHP)}$ to 70 percent of normal resulted in small regions of synchronous bursting, which while not completely blocking recall of learned patterns, still lead to the inclusion of spurious activity. Thus, these results demonstrated that an additional biophysical mechanism was needed to constrain the intercellular spread of excitatory pyramidal cell bursting.

A natural choice for such a mechanism, as alluded to above, was the known cholinergic suppression of recurrent excitatory synapses in stratum radiatum of region CA3 (Hasselmo et al., 1995b). This effect was included in the model during learning by decreasing the maximum conductance underlying the pyramidal cell synaptic current I_{AMPA} to 42 percent of its normal value (1.5 ns), simulating a 38 percent decrement in unitary EPSP height under 20 μm carbachol (Hasselmo et al., 1995b). During learning, this resulted in the attenuation of both globally and partially synchronous pyramidal cell bursting in neurons not related to the input pattern, thus promoting accurate recall performance. At these values, successful recall of a pattern was possible with a learning period as short as a single burst. With further reduction of this conductance to 25 percent of its normal value, a mixture of single bursts and subthreshold oscillations arose, with limited spread of activity beyond cells related to the input pattern. Simulations using multiple, overlapping input patterns were also performed at these parameter values. In one case, three different input patterns were consecutively learned. Each pattern was presented to the model for a period of 60 ms (25 Hz). Successful recall performance was sensitive to the degree of overlap in the patterns. Patterns overlapping by more than 30 percent showed a marked decrement in completion tasks where a degraded version of the pattern was presented.

These results demonstrate the regulatory property of cholinergic modulation in CA3 as illustrated in the $g_{K(AHP)} - g_{AMPA}$ parameter space representation in Figure 12.6. By adjusting the maximum conductances underlying these two currents – one ($I_{K(AHP)}$) an ionic conductance intrinsic to pyramidal neurons, the other a synaptic conductance coupling these cells together – a diverse variety of population behaviors emerges, with substantially different functional implications associated with each. While the parameter space shows a broad region where partial and full recall is possible, state transitions to globally synchronized behavior can occur with changes in a single parameter, depending on the initial location and direction of travel in this space. These results also point to the importance of relating cellular behavior to population activity when investigating the functional aspects of a neuronal system.

From these results, it is clear that at portions of the parameter space where globally synchronous bursting occurs, NMDA-dependent LTP increases markedly since all cells are simultaneously active. As more pyramidal cells are recruited into the rhythm, potentiation is extended to these additional cells, and if the activity becomes epileptic, LTP should also occur more frequently in time as well. This sustained positive feedback could conceivably lead to pyramidal cell excitotoxicity due to an exaggerated level of glutamate in postsynaptic cells. Increased levels of intracellular Ca^{2+} may also trigger aberrant sprouting or other cytoskeletal changes to synapse morphology, which may result in cell death.

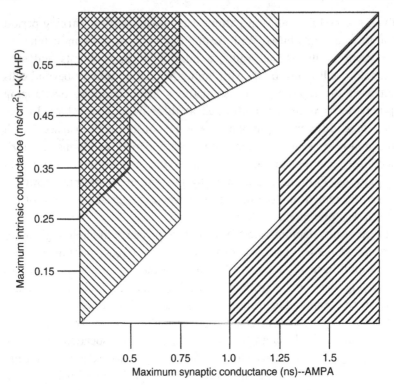

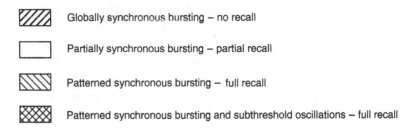

Fig. 12.6 Qualitatively different modes of population behavior were obtained depending on the values for the maximum conductances underlying $I_{K(AHP)}$ and I_{AMPA}. State transitions from accurate recall performance to epileptiform activity were possible with manipulation of a single parameter.

Runaway synaptic modification and the progression of Alzheimer's disease

Selective distribution of neuropathology

From the simulations described above, it is fair to suggest that under conditions of globally synchronous behavior, the resulting exponential increase in NMDA-dependent LTP may induce substantial increases and fluctuations in intracellular free Ca^{2+} levels. In addition to having an impact on the functional electrophysiological characteristics of the cell, this sudden change in intracellular Ca^{2+} dynamics may also trigger excessive sprouting or permanent changes in the protein structure of glutamate receptors in the postsynaptic cell. Thus, the biophysical mechanisms that normally maintain LTP under less active conditions may result in a form of runaway synaptic modification in which intracellular Ca^{2+} levels do not have sufficient time to diffuse.

If the neuropathology associated with Alzheimer's disease results from runaway synaptic modification, this suggests that the apparent early and severe involvement of layers II and IV of the lateral entorhinal cortex, region CA1 of the hippocampus, and the adjacent regions of the subiculum (Hyman et al., 1984, 1990; Arnold et al., 1991; Braak and Braak, 1991; Arriagada et al., 1992) results from a particular sensitivity of these regions to runaway synaptic modification. For example, it is possible that sensitivity to runaway synaptic modification might be associated with two features: (1) a strong capacity for Hebbian synaptic modification, and (2) absence of the cholinergic suppression of synaptic transmission during learning. Indeed, it has been shown that different areas of the hippocampal formation exhibit varying degrees of long-term potentiation with comparable stimulation (Racine, Milgram and Hafner, 1983). Considerable research has focused on how subregions of the hippocampus resemble the structures of associative memory models (Marr, 1971; McNaughton and Morris, 1987). As noted above, this region shows robust Hebbian synaptic modification (Wigstrom et al., 1986) and has been implicated in memory function in extensive research (Scoville and Milner, 1957; Squire and Zola-Morgan, 1991). The greater propensity for synaptic modification could underlie the early sensitivity of the hippocampal formation. The early sensitivity of lateral entorhinal cortex could be linked to the absence of cholinergic suppression at synapses arising from this region and terminating in the outer molecular layer of the dentate gyrus (Kahle and Cotman, 1989), while the relative sparing of region CA3 could result from the robust cholinergic suppression of synaptic transmission at synapses arising from CA3 pyramidal cells (Hasselmo and Schnell, 1994; Hasselmo et al., 1995a).

Spread of degeneration between cortical regions

The neuropathology of Alzheimer's disease appears to spread from the hippocampus into the neocortex along well-established anatomical connections, the back-projections from the subiculum and entorhinal cortex to association cortex (Pearson et al., 1985; Hyman et al., 1990; Arnold et al., 1991). In later stages of the disease, neurofibrillary tangles appear in regions of the temporal, parietal, and frontal neocortex (Hirano and Zimmerman, 1962; Pearson et al., 1985; Arnold et al., 1991). Neurofibrillary tangles primarily spread into cortical regions, though the plaques associated with terminal degeneration appear in subcortical regions as well (Pearson et al., 1985). This spread of degeneration is proposed here to result from the spread of runaway synaptic modification between cortical regions. This would use the same mechanisms that are important for transferring information stored in the hippocampus back into the neocortex – the process of consolidation (Wilson and McNaughton, 1994). A network simulation of the hippocampus (Hasselmo, 1995b) has been used to model the process of consolidation, as shown in Figure 12.7.

Runaway synaptic modification could spread from hippocampus back into neocortical structures using the same mechanisms as consolidation. It has been shown in simulations that if runaway synaptic modification occurs during the initial formation of representations of new memories in the hippocampus, then subsequent retrieval of these representations will result in a spread of runaway synaptic modification. For example, as shown in Figure 12.8, a decrease in the mechanisms of synaptic decay of the input from entorhinal cortex layer II to dentate gyrus results in the initiation of runaway synaptic modification in this pathway. Even if the parameters of other connections have not been altered, the initiation of runaway synaptic modification at these perforant path synapses results in the spread of runaway synaptic modification into back-projections from region CA1 to neocortex. In simulations with multiple interacting layers, the initiation of runaway synaptic modification in one layer results in the progressive spread to other layers, even if those layers would not undergo runaway synaptic modification independently.

Modeling suggests that runaway synaptic modification will spread according to functional boundaries. That is, after occurring in neurons

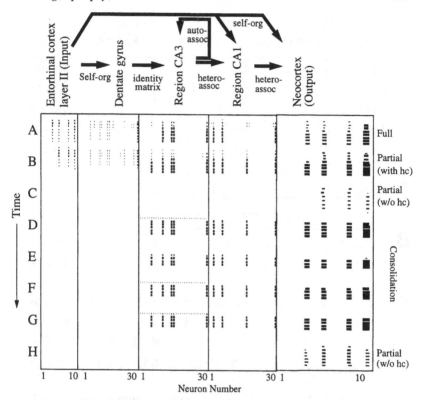

Fig. 12.7 Consolidation of a single pattern in a network model of the hippocampal formation. The size of the black squares represents the activity of individual neurons. A. Presentation of input to entorhinal cortex layer II. Synaptic modification in dentate gyrus forms a sparse self-organized representation, and modification in region CA3 forms an attractor state. B. Testing recall with degraded (partial) input with hippocampus present (with hc). Representations are activated in dentate gyrus and region CA3. Attractor dynamics in region CA3 drive recall activity in CA1 and neocortex. C. With a simulated hippocampal lesion (w/o hc), no recall can occur. Input to neocortex alone does not result in recall before consolidation. This corresponds to temporally limited retrograde amnesia. D–G. Consolidation. Homogeneous depolarization of region CA3 results in activation of the previously stored attractor state. This activates the full pattern in neocortex, allowing gradual strengthening of synapses in neocortex. H. The preceding period of consolidation allows neocortex to respond to the partial input cue with the full learned pattern. Thus, after consolidation, memory recall is not impaired by lesions of the hippocampus.

encoding a particular category of information, it will more rapidly influence similar or strongly associated information before influencing unrelated information. This might explain the apparent heterogeneous distribution of tangles in Alzheimer's disease and the apparent specificity

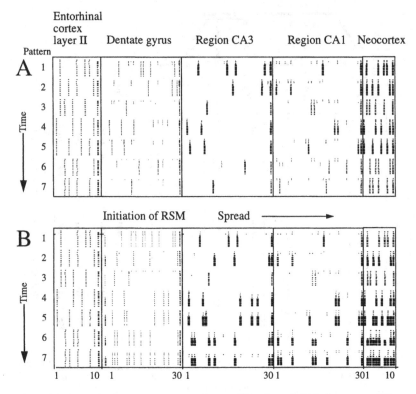

Fig. 12.8 Spread of runaway synaptic modification (RSM) between different regions. A. Normal function of the network. B. Initiation of runaway synaptic modification through regions CA3 and CA1. Excessive strengthening of back-projections from CA1 to neocortex results in broadly distributed activity in response to presentation of later patterns (e.g., pattern 7).

for specific modalities in some cases. In particular, the distribution of neurofibrillary tangles may be of the order of magnitude of cortical columns, with tangles in layers 2 and 3 in register with tangles in layers 5 and 6 (Pearson et al., 1985).

The rate of spread of runaway synaptic modification depends upon the ongoing capacity for Hebbian synaptic modification and the amount of excitatory associative connectivity. Primary sensory and motor cortices have more restricted and specific connectivity of excitatory intrinsic and associational connections (Lund, 1988), and are further removed from the highly plastic structures of the hippocampal formation. This may explain why the neuropathology in Alzheimer's disease is far less pronounced in the primary sensory cortices (Hirano and Zimmerman, 1962; Brun and Gustafson, 1976; Pearson et al., 1985; Esiri et al., 1986).

Conclusions

As has been shown above, in addition to being important for LTP induction, NMDA receptor-dependent events may play a role in the development of certain neurological disorders such as epilepsy and Alzheimer's disease. From a perspective of the symptoms involved, the disorders may seem very distinct, yet may share commonalities when examined at the cellular level. Clearly, a greater understanding of NMDA receptor-mediated changes to synaptic morphology is needed in order to elucidate the mechanisms that may support aberrant glutamatergic activity (AMPA and NMDA) in vivo. The most common symptoms in both disorders involve deficits in the acquisition of new memories. The computational modeling presented here suggests that runaway synaptic modification could cause increased interference between stored representations, causing impairments in short-term memory tasks requiring free recall (Corkin, 1982; Morris, 1986) and increasing the number of intrusions reported in other tasks (Fuld et al., 1982; Troster et al., 1989; Jacobs et al., 1990; Delis et al., 1991). Continued interference effects during learning could eventually lead to the spread of runaway synaptic modification into neocortex via the mechanisms of consolidation. This would lead to impairments of remote memory (Wilson, Kaszniak and Fox, 1981; Corkin et al., 1984) and semantic memory (Huff, Corkin and Growdon, 1986). Although models of the type presented here are far from complete descriptions of the cellular events that may promote such pathological behavior, their use is vital to bridging the gap between the physiological and behavioral study of these disorders.

Summary

Numerous clinical and experimental observations have suggested that the hippocampus is critical to the neural processes believed to underlie learning and memory. At the same time, however, this area has also been shown to be involved in the genesis of certain neurologic disorders such as epilepsy and Alzheimer's disease. By using models of this region at different levels of biophysical detail, this chapter shows that changes in NMDA receptor-mediated excitatory postsynaptic potentials in hippocampal pyramidal cells coupled with alterations in an intrinsic calcium-dependent potassium current can set the stage for transitions between states of learning and neuropathology. Modeling of the CA3 region demonstrates how changes in these parameters can shift the network from a state of associative learning to one in which epileptiform activity dominates. Additional modeling of the entire hippocampal formation also shows how these parameters may contribute to neurodegenerative pathology such as that observed in Alzheimer's disease. Initial sensitivity of the hippocampus and entorhinal cortex to the development of neurofibrillary tangles is proposed to result from an imbalance of parameters regulating the influence of synaptic transmission that may lead to the phenomenon of runaway synaptic modification. It is shown in this chapter that once the disease is initiated, degeneration may spread from the hippocampus into neocortical structures due to the mechanisms of consolidation. Memory deficits are described as due to increased interference effects in recall and the inability of the system to display locally synchronous states of activity.

References

Akers, R., Lovinger, D., Colley, P., Linden, D. & Routtenberg, A. (1986). Translocation of protein kinase C activity may mediate hippocampal long-term potentiation. *Science*, **231**, 587–9.

Albert, M., Smith, L.A., Scherr, P.A., Taylor, J.O., Evans, D.A. & Funkenstein, H.H. (1991). Use of brief cognitive tests to identify individuals in the community with clinically diagnosed Alzheimer's disease. *International Journal of Neuroscience*, **57**, 167–78.

Amit, D.J., Evans, M.R. & Abeles, M. (1990). Attractor neural networks with biological probe records. *Network*, **1**, 381–405.

Anderson, J.A. (1972). A simple neural network generating an interactive memory. *Mathematical Biosciences*, **14**, 197–220.

Arnold, S.E., Hyman, B.T., Flory, J., Damasio, A.R. & Van Hoesen, G.W. (1991). The topographical and neuroanatomical distribution of neurofibrillary tangles and neuritic plaques in the cerebral cortex of patients with Alzheimer's disease. *Cerebral Cortex*, **1**, 103–16.

Arriagada, P.V., Marzloff, B.A. & Hyman, B.T. (1992). The distribution of Alzheimer type pathological changes in non-demented elderly individuals matches the pattern in Alzheimer's disease. *Neurology*, **42**, 1681–8.

Ball, M.J. (1972). Neurofibrillary tangles and the pathogenesis of dementia: A quantitative study. *Neuropathology and Applied Neurobiology*, **2**, 395–410.

Barkai, E. & Hasselmo, M.E. (1993). Modulation of the input/output function of rat piriform cortex pyramidal cells. *Journal of Neurophysiology*, **72**, 644–58.

Barkai, E., Horwitz, G., Bergman, R.E. & Hasselmo, M.E. (1993). Modulation of associative memory function in a biophysical simulation of rat piriform cortex. *Journal of Neurophysiology*, **72**, 659–77.

Ben-Ari, Y. & Represa, A. (1990). Brief seizure episodes induce long-term potentiation and mossy fiber sprouting in the hippocampus. *Trends in Neuroscience*, **13**, 312–18.

Bernardo, L.S. & Prince, D.A. (1982). Cholinergic pharmacology of mammalian hippocampal pyramidal cells. *Neuroscience*, **7**, 1703–12.

Bliss, T.V.P. & Lomo, T. (1973). Long-lasting potentiation of synaptic transmission in the dentate area of the anaesthetized rabbit following stimulation of the perforant path. *Journal of Physiology*, **232**, 331–56.

Braak, J. & Braak, E. (1991). Neuropathological staging of Alzheimer-related changes. *Acta Neuropathologica*, **82**, 239–59.

Breitner, J.C.S., Gatz, M., Bergem, A.L.M. et al. (1993). Use of twin cohorts for research in Alzheimer's disease. *Neurology*, **43**, 261–7.

Brun, A. & Gustafson, L. (1976). Distribution of cerebral degeneration in Alzheimer's disease: A clinicopathological study. *Archiv fur Psychiatrie und Nervenkrankheiten*, **223**, 15–33.

Chen, L. & Huang, L.Y.M. (1992). Protein kinase C reduces Mg^{2+} block of NMDA-receptor channels as a mechanism of modulation. *Nature*, **356**, 521–3.

Cole, A.E. & Nicoll, R.A. (1984). Characterization of a slow cholinergic postsynaptic potential recorded in vitro from rat hippocampal pyramidal cells. *Journal of Physiology*, **352**, 173–88.

Corkin, S. (1982). Some relationships between global amnesias and the memory impairments in Alzheimer's disease. In *Alzheimer's Disease: A Report of Research in Progress*, ed. S. Corkin, K.L. Davis, J.H. Growdown, E. Usdin & R.J. Wutman, pp. 89–101. New York: Raven Press.

Corkin, S., Growdown, J.H., Nissen, M.J., Huff, F.J., Freed, D.M. & Sagar, H.J. (1984). Recent advances in the neuropsychological study of Alzheimer's disease. In *Alzheimer's Disease: Advances in Basic Research and Therapies*, ed. R.J. Wurtman, S. Corkin & J.H. Growdown, pp. 157–73. Cambridge, MA: Center for Brain Sciences.

Coyle, J.T., Price, D.L. & DeLong, M.R. (1983). Alzheimer's disease: A disorder of cortical cholinergic innervation. *Science*, **219**, 1184–90.

Crapper McLachlan, D.R. & Van Berkum, M.F.A. (1986). Aluminum: a role in degenerative brain disease associated with neurofibrillary degeneration. *Progress in Brain Research*, **70**, 399–409.

Croucher, M.J., Collins J.F. & Meldrum, B.S. (1982). Anticonvulsant action of excitatory amino acid antagonists. *Science*, **216**, 889–901.

Davies, P. & Maloney, A.J.F. (1976). Selective loss of central cholinergic neurons in Alzheimer's disease. *Lancet*, **2**, 1403.

Delis, D.C., Massman, P.J., Butters, N., Salmon, D.P., Cermak, L.S. & Kramer, J.H. (1991). Profiles of demented and amnesic patients on the California Verbal Learning Test: Implications for the assessment of memory disorders. *Psychological Assessment*, **3**, 19–26.

Desmond, N.L. & Levy, W.B. (1988). In *Long-term Potentiation: From Biophysics to Behavior*, ed. P.W. Landfield & S.A. Deadwyler, pp. 265–305. New York: Diss.

Doi, N., Carpenter, D.O. & Hori, N. (1990). Differential effects of baclofen and gamma-aminobutyric acid (GABA) on rat piriform cortex pyramidal neurons *in vitro*. *Cellular and Molecular Neurology*, **10**, 559–64.

Dunwiddie, T.V. & Lynch, G. (1979). The relationship between extracellular calcium concentrations and the induction of hippocampal long-term potentiation. *Brain Research*, **169**, 103–10.

Esiri, M.M., Pearson, R.C.A. & Powell, T.P.S. (1986). Cortex of the primary auditory area in Alzheimer's disease. *Brain Research*, **366**, 385–7.

Freund, T.F. & Antal, M. (1988). GABA-containing neurons in the septum control inhibitory interneurons in the hippocampus. *Nature*, **336**, 170–3.

Frotscher, M. & Leranth, C. (1985). Cholinergic innervation of the rat hippocampus as revealed by choline acetyltransferase immunocytochemistry; a combined light and electron microscopic study. *Journal of Comparative Neurology*, **239**, 237–46.

Fuld, P.A., Katzman, R., Davies, P. & Terry, R.D. (1982). Intrusions as a sign of Alzheimer dementia: Chemical and pathological verification. *Annals of Neurology*, **11**, 155–9.

Goudsmit, J. & Van der Waals, F.W. (1986). Scrapie and its association with 'amyloid-like' fibrils and glycoproteins encoded by cellular genes: an animal model for human dementia. *Progress in Brain Research*, **70**, 399–409.

Grenamyre, J.T., Penney, J.B., D'Amato, C.J. & Young, A.B. (1987). Dementia of the Alzheimer's type: changes in hippocampal L-[^{3}H] glutamate binding. *Journal of Neurochemistry*, **48**, 543–51.

Grossberg, S. (1970). Some networks that can learn, remember and reproduce any number of complicated space–time patterns II. *Studies in Applied Mathematics*, **49**, 135–66.

Gustafsson, B. & Wigstrom, H. (1988). Physiological mechanisms underlying long-term potentiation. *Trends in Neurosciences*, **11**, 156–62.

Hardy, J.A. & Higgins, G.A. (1992). Alzheimer's disease: The amyloid cascade hypothesis. *Science*, **256**, 184–5.

Hasselmo, M.E. (1993). Acetylcholine and learning in a cortical associative memory. *Neural Computation*, **5**(1), 32–44.

Hasselmo, M.E. (1994). Runaway synaptic modification in models of cortex: Implications for Alzheimer's disease. *Neural Networks*, **7**(1), 13–40.

Hasselmo, M.E. (1995a). Neuromodulation and cortical function: Modeling the physiological basis of behavior. *Behavioral Brain Research*, **67**, 1–27.

Hasselmo, M.E. (1995b). Modeling the piriform cortex. In *Cortical Models. Cerebral Cortex*, ed. E.G. Jones & P.S. Ulinski, pp. 112–21. New York: Plenum Press.

Hasselmo, M.E. (1995c). Physiological constraints on models of behavior. In *Current Trends in Connectionism*, ed. L. Niklasson & M.B. Boden, pp. 15–32. Hillsdale, NJ: Lawrence Erlbaum.

Hasselmo, M.E., Anderson, B.P. & Bower, J.M. (1992). Cholinergic modulation of cortical associative memory function. *Journal of Neurophysiology*, **67**, 1230–46.

Hasselmo, M.E. & Barkai, E. (1995). Cholinergic modulation of activity-dependent synaptic plasticity in rat piriform cortex. *Journal of Neuroscience*, **15**(10), 6592–604.

Hasselmo, M.E. & Bower, J.M. (1992). Cholinergic suppression specific to intrinsic not afferent fiber synapses in rat piriform (olfactory) cortex. *Journal of Neurophysiology*, **67**, 1222–9.

Hasselmo, M.E. & Bower, J.M. (1993). Acetylcholine and memory. *Trends in Neurosciences*, **16**, 218–22.

Hasselmo, M.E., Rolls, E.T. & Baylis, G.C. (1989a). The role of expression and identity in the face-selective responses of neurons in the temporal visual cortex of the monkey. *Behavioral Brain Research*, **32**, 203–18.

Hasselmo, M.E., Rolls, E.T., Baylis, G.C. & Nalwa, V. (1989b). Object-centered encoding by face-selective neurons in the cortex in the superior temporal sulcus of the monkey. *Experimental Brain Research*, **75**, 417–29.

Hasselmo, M.E. & Schnell, E. (1994). Laminar selectivity of the cholinergic suppression of synaptic transmission in rat hippocampal region CA1: computational modeling and brain slice physiology. *Journal of Neuroscience*, **14**(6), 3898–914.

Hasselmo, M.E., Schnell, E. & Barkai, E. (1995a). Dynamics of learning and recall at excitatory recurrent synapses and cholinergic modulation in hippocampal region CA3. *Journal of Neuroscience*, **15**(7), 5249–62.

Hasselmo, M.E., Schnell, E., Berke, J. & Barkai, E. (1995b). A model of hippocampus combining self-organization and associative memory function. In *Advances in Neural Information Processing Systems*, ed. G. Tesauro, D. Touretzky & T. Leen, Vol. 7, p. 77–84. Cambridge, MA: MIT Press.

Hebb, D.O. (1949). *The Organization of Behavior*, New York: Wiley.

Herrmann, M., Ruppin, E. & Usher, M. (1993). A neural model of the dynamic activation of memory. *Biological Cybernetics*, **68**, 455–63.

Hirano, A. & Zimmerman, H.M. (1962). Alzheimer's neurofibrillary changes: A topographic study. *Archives of Neurology*, **7**, 73–88.

Hopfield, J.J. (1982). Neural networks and physical systems with emergent selective computational abilities. *Proceedings of the National Academy of Sciences of the USA*, **79**, 2554–9.

Horn, D., Ruppin, E., Usher, M. & Herrmann, M. (1993). Neural network modeling of memory deterioration in Alzheimer's disease. *Neural Computation*, **5**, 736–49.

Huff, F.J., Corkin, S. & Growdon, J.H. (1986). Semantic impairment and anomia in Alzheimer's disease. *Brain and Language*, **34**, 269–78.

Hyman, B.T., Damasio, A.R., Van Hoesen, G.W. & Barne (1984). Cell specific pathology isolates the hippocampal formation in Alzheimer's disease. *Science*, **225**, 1168–70.

Hyman, B.T., Van Hoesen, G.W. & Damasio, A.R. (1990). Memory-related neural systems in Alzheimer's disease: An anatomic study. *Neurology*, **40**, 1721–30.

Jacobs, D., Salmon, D.P., Troster, A.I. & Butters, N. (1990). Intrusion errors in the figural memory of patients with Alzheimer's and Huntington's disease. *Archives of Clinical Neuropsychology*, **5**, 49–57.

Jahr, C.E. & Stevens, C.F. (1990). A qualitative description of NMDA receptor channel kinetic behavior. *Journal of Neuroscience*, **10**, 1830–7.

Jolles, J. (1986). Cognitive, emotional and behavioral dysfunction in aging and dementia. *Progress in Brain Research*, **70**, 399–409.

Kahle, J.S. & Cotman, C.W. (1989). Carbachol depresses the synaptic responses in the medial but not the lateral perforant path. *Brain Research*, **482**, 159–63.

Katzman, R. (1986). Alzheimer's disease. *New England Journal of Medicine*, **314**, 964–73.

Kelso, S.R., Nelson, T.E. & Leonard, J.P. (1992). Protein kinase C-mediated enhancement of NMDA currents by metabotropic glutamate receptor in *Xenopus* oocytes. *Journal of Physiology*, **449**, 705–18.

Kohr, G., DeKoninck, Y. & Momdy, I. (1993). Properties of NMDA receptor channels in neurons acutely isolated from epileptic (kindled) rats. *Journal of Neuroscience*, **13**, 3612–27.

Krogsgaard-Larsen, P. (1992). GABA and glutamate receptors as therapeutic targets in neurodegenerative disorders. *Pharmacology and Toxicology*, **70**, 95–104.

Lahtinen, H., Castren, E., Miettinen, R., Ylinen, A., Paltarvi, L. & Riekkinen, P.J. (1993). NMDA-sensitive [^{3}H] glutamate binding in the epileptic rat hippocampus: An autoradiographic study. *Neuroreport*, **4**, 45–8.

Levy, W.B. & Steward, O. (1983). Temporal contiguity requirements for long-term associative potentiation/depression in the hippocampus. *Neuroscience*, **8**, 791–7.

Lund, J.S. (1988). Anatomical organization of macaque monkey striate visual cortex. *Annual Review of Neuroscience*, **11**, 253–88.

Lynch, G. & Baudry, M. (1984). The biochemistry of memory: a new and specific hypothesis. *Science*, **224**, 1057–63.

Lynch, G., Dunwiddie, T. & Gribkoff, V. (1977). Heterosynaptic depression: a postsynaptic correlate of long-term potentiation. *Nature*, **266**, 737–9.

Lynch, G., Larsen, J., Kelso, S., Barrionuevo, G. & Schottler, F. (1983). Intracellular injections of EGTA block induction of hippocampal long-term potentiation. *Nature*, **305**, 719–21.

Madison, D.V., Lancaster, B. & Nicoll, R.A. (1987). Voltage clamp analysis of cholinergic action in the hippocampus. *Journal of Neuroscience*, **7**, 733–41.

Malenka, R.C., Kauer, J.A., Perkel, D.J. et al. (1989). An essential role for calmodulin and protein kinase activity in long-term potentiation. *Nature*, **340**, 554–7.

Maragos, W.F., Greenamyre, J.T., Penney, J.B. & Young, A.B. (1987). Glutamate dysfunction in Alzheimer's disease: an hypothesis. *Trends in Neuroscience*, **10**, 65–8.

Marr, D. (1971). Simple memory: A theory for archicortex. *Philosophical Transactions of the Royal Society*, B **262**, 23–81.

Mattson, M.P., Rydel, R.E., Leiberburg, I. & Smith-Swintosky, V.L. (1993). Altered calcium signaling and neuronal injury: Stroke and Alzheimer's disease as examples. *Annals of the New York Academy of Science*, **679**, 1–21.

Mayer, M. L., Westbrook, G.L. & Guthrie, P.B. (1984). Voltage-dependent block by Mg^{2+} of NMDA responses in spinal cord neurons. *Nature*, **309**, 261–3.

McClelland, J.L. & Rumelhart, D.E. (1988). *Explorations in Parallel Distributed Processing*. Cambridge, MA: MIT Press.

McNaughton, B.L. & Morris, R.G.M. (1987). Hippocampal synaptic enhancement and information storage within a distributed system. *Trends in Neurosciences*, **10**, 408–15.

Miles, R. (1990). Plasticity of recurrent excitatory synapses between CA3 hippocampal pyramidal cells. *Journal of Physiology*, **428**, 61–77.

Morris, R.G. (1986). Short-term forgetting in senile dementia of the Alzheimer's type. *Cognitive Neuropsychology*, **3**, 77–97.

Morris, R.G. & Kopelman, M.D. (1986). The memory deficits in Alzheimer-type dementia: A review. *Quarterly Journal of Experimental Psychology*, **38A**, 575–602.

Mott, D.A. & Lewis, D.V. (1991). Facilitation of the induction of long-term potentiation by GABA-B receptors. *Science*, **252**, 1718–20.

Pearson, R.C.A., Esiri, M.M., Hiorns, R.W., Wilcock, G.K. & Powell, T.P.S. (1985). Anatomical correlates of the distribution of the pathological changes in the neocortex in Alzheimer's disease. *Proceedings of the National Academy of Sciences of the USA*, **82**, 4531–4.

Perry, E.K., Gibson, P.H., Blessed, G., Perry, R.H. & Tomlinson, B.E. (1977). Neurotransmitter enzyme abnormalities in senile dementia. *Journal of Neurological Science*, **34**, 247–65.

Racine, R.J., Milgram, N.W. & Hafner, S. (1983). Long-term potentiation phenomena in the rat limbic forebrain. *Brain Research*, **260**, 217–31.

Represa, A., Duyckaerts, C., Tremblay, E., Hauw, J.J. & Ben-Ari, Y. (1988). Is senile dementia of the Alzheimer's type associated with hippocampal plasticity? *Brain Research*, **457**, 355–9.

Saper, C.B., German, D.C. & White, C.L. (1985). Neuronal pathology in the nucleus basalis and associated cell groups in senile dementia of the Alzheimer's type: Possible role in cell loss. *Neurology*, **35**, 1089–95.

Schellenberg, G.D., Bird, T.D., Wijsman, E.M. et al. (1992). Genetic linkage evidence for a familial Alzheimer's disease locus on chromosome 14. *Science*, **258**, 668–71.

Scoville, W.B. & Milner, B. (1957). Loss of recent memory and bilateral hippocampal lesions. *Journal of Neurology, Neurosurgery and Psychiatry*, **20**, 11–21.

Selkoe, D.J. (1993). Physiological production of the b-amyloid protein and the mechanism of Alzheimer's disease. *Trends in Neurosciences*, **16**, 403–09.

Slater, N.T., Stelzer, A. & Galvan, M. (1985). Kindling-like stimulus patterns induce epileptiform discharges in the guinea pig *in vitro* hippocampus. *Neuroscience Letters*, **60**, 25–31.

Squire, L.R. & Zola-Morgan, S. (1991). The medial temporal-lobe memory system. *Science*, **253**, 1380–6.

Swartzwelder, H.S., Lewis, D.V., Anderson, W.W. & Wilson, W.A. (1987). Seizure-like events in brain slices: suppression by interictal activity. *Brain Research*, **410**, 362–6.

Traub, R.D., Colling, S.B. & Jefferys, J.G. (1995). Enhanced NMDA conductance can account for epileptiform activity induced by low Mg^{2+} in the rat hippocampal slice. *Journal of Physiology*, **489**, 127–40.

Traub, R.D. & Jefferys, J.G. (1994a). Simulations of epileptiform activity in the hippocampal CA3 region *in vitro*. *Hippocampus*, **4**, 281–5.

Traub, R.D. & Jefferys, J.G. (1994b). Are there unifying principles underlying the generation of epileptic afterdischarges in vitro? *Progress in Brain Research*, **102**, 383–94.

Traub, R.D., Jefferys, J.G. & Whittington, M.A. (1994). Enhanced NMDA conductance can account for epileptiform activity induced by low Mg^{2+} in the rat hippocampal slice. *Journal of Physiology*, **478**, 379–93.

Traub, R.D. & Miles, R. (1991). *Neural Networks of the Hippocampus*. Cambridge: Cambridge University Press.

Traub, R.D., Miles, R. & Wong, R.K.S. (1989). Model of the origin of rhythmic population oscillations in the hippocampal slice. *Science*, **243**, 1319–25.

Traub, R.D., Wong, R.K.S., Miles, R. & Michelson, H. (1991). A model of a CA3 hippocampal pyramidal neuron incorporating voltage-clamp data on intrinsic conductances. *Journal of Neurophysiology*, **66**, 635–50.

Troster, A.I., Jacobs, D., Butters, N., Cullum, C.M. & Salmon, D.P. (1989). Differentiating Alzheimer's disease from Huntington's disease with the Wechsler Memory Scale – Revised. *Clinics in Geriatric Medicine*, **5**, 611–32.

Turner, R.W., Baimbridge, K.G. & Miller, J.J. (1982). Calcium-induced long-term potentiation in the hippocampus. *Neuroscience*, **7**, 1411–16.

Wallenstein, G.V. & Hasselmo, M.E. (1997). Functional transitions between epileptiform-like activity and associative memory in hippocampal region CA3. *Brain Research Bulletin*, **43**, 485–93.

Whitehouse, P.J., Price, D.L., Struble, R.G., Clark, A.W., Coyle, J.T. & DeLong, M.R. (1982). Alzheimer's disease and senile dementia: Loss of neurons in the basal forebrain. *Science*, **215**, 1237–9.

Wigstrom, H. & Gustafsson, B. (1986). Postsynaptic control of hippocampal long-term potentiation. *Journal of Physiology*, **81**, 228–36.

Wigstrom, H., Gustafsson, B., Huang, Y.-Y. & Abraham, W.C. (1986). Hippocampal long-term potentiation is induced by pairing single afferent volleys with intracellularly injected depolarizing current pulses. *Acta Physiologica Scandinavica*, **126**, 317–19.

Wilson, R.S., Kaszniak, A.W. & Fox, J.H. (1981). Remote memory in senile dementia. *Cortex*, **17**, 41–8.

Wilson, M.A. & McNaughton, B.L. (1994). Reactivation of hippocampal ensemble memories during sleep. *Science*, **265**, 676–9.

Zador, A., Koch, C. & Brown, T.H. (1990). Biophysical model of a Hebbian synapse. *Proceedings of the National Academy of Sciences*, **87**, 6718–22.

Epilogue

The patient in the machine: challenges for neurocomputing

DAVID V. FORREST

This volume has provided many examples of how connectionist models may allow clinicians to replace vague and nonquantitative approaches to psychopathology with a more sophisticated and quantitative paradigm. Nevertheless, several challenges remain for clinicians and researchers interested in consolidating the intersection between connectionism and psychiatry. In this closing contribution, a number of these challenges are discussed.

The challenge of education

The first challenge for neural network modelers is to become included in the mainstream of general psychiatry. It may be argued that neural networks look more mathematical than they are on a practical level. Nevertheless, neural networks may involve more mathematics than many psychiatrists are willing to countenance. At least some preparation is required for comprehension.

However, there is reason to be optimistic that the challenge of education will be met. When the author first presented a grand rounds on neural networks in 1990, he found few psychiatric residents had any computer preparation. Since then, the wave of children who have grown up with computers has reached our residencies, and most are now willing to consider these logicomathematical structures. The author is confident that in the future a working knowledge of neurocomputation will be pushed earlier and earlier in general education, partly because its applications will be everywhere.

We can help by translating neural network models into verbal structures and by beginning to speak during our clinical rounds in the metaphors of neurocomputing. As discussed below, these metaphors are most compatible with a dynamic psychiatry that is cognitively informed. And as their currency grows, computers offer metaphors for many processes of thought. The author recently heard himself arguing against self-analysis because individually we do not have enough computational power to comprehend the totality of our minds, since so much of them must be devoted to unconscious machinery and subattentional processing, and we need a buffer in the person of the psychiatrist into whom to dump data and free ourselves up for larger self-consideration.

The penetrance of neural networks into other aspects of everyday life, such as speech and writing recognition and indoor climate control, may make them a household word, whether or not most people know how they work. Similar wide-ranging terminological examples are thermostats, elevator automata, cybernetics, cruise control, smart appliances, and web browsers.

The challenge of biological verisimilitude

Several authors have commented that neural networks are not capable of very much on their own, or are limited as an explanatory mechanism for the self-emergence of mind. One complaint has been that neural networks rely on extraneous rule-based instructions, and in particular the back-propagation of errors, which has no exact biological correlate.

Criteria of what is biologically verisimilar not only help build better models of the brain, they also, at this stage of neurocomputation, help build better, brainier computers. But, to turn the problem around, computational successes that seem nonbiological may suggest that we look more closely at them for parallels in the brain. For example, the departure from pure neural nets in the form of hybrids with rule-based features is typical of Grossberg's complex biomodeling of perceptual and adaptive learning biofunctions. But is this not a feature of many brains in animals? An inborn genetically determined programming often initiates the birdsong, in natural neural nets, of species-specific behavior, such as birdsong, which hierarchically represented in the avian forebrian (Yu and Margolish, 1996).

The neuroscientific understanding of neural function is anything but a stationary target for modelers. As Sejnowski (1997) summarizes, new work has shown that the dendrites of pyramidal neurons in the neocortex and hippocampus have fast sodium and high-threshold calcium currents that make for highly nonlinear synaptic integration in their dendritic trees. Other studies suggest such back-propagating action potentials do influence the strength of dendritic synapses in both the neocortex and the hippocampus, regulating LTP, LTD, and the coupling between synapses and the spike-initiating zone near the cell body, findings which Sejnowski says would have pleased Hebb.

Another aspect of brains overlooked in requiring neural nets to be totally self-organizing and self-sustaining is the programmatic nature of environmental input. Data that input via sensory apparatuses are not solely raw data lacking any organization; rather, they are often specifically coded and user-friendly signals for the individual from other members of its species. These signals and much of the species' habitat are genetically prewired expectancies, starting from the expectancy of the shadow patterns of a single overhead solar light source. In a sense, part of the elusive homunculus is outside the brain, contributing and reaffirming rule-based knowledge. Dennett (1996) has proposed differentiating levels of brains in the animal kingdom according to the use of this coding: Darwinian creatures are simply hardwired; Skinnerian creatures have wired-in reinforcers that favor smart moves, i.e., actions better for the creature than alternative actions; Popperian creatures employ preselection among possible moves, and insight rather than chance; and Gregorian creatures (named for Richard Gregory, the British psychologist), the top of the line, are 'informed by the designed portions of the outer environment' (p. 99), importing 'mind tools' (p. 100) from the cultural environment.

One interesting class of neural phenomena for modeling that also has correlates in the nonbiological sphere might be termed readiness activity. An example is the dedicated 'chattering' pyramidal cells that contribute to synchrony in the visual cortex (Gray and McCormick, 1996). A good number of psychiatric functions could conceivably be related to problems with such readiness activity, including signal anxiety, paranoid perceptive tendencies, phobic conditioning, schizophrenic attention problems, registration problems in delirium, kindling, and priming. Similarly, unconscious (or 'unaware') perception has recently attracted new credibility. Greenwald, Draine and Abrams (1996) have investigated subliminal semantic activation of very short (100 ms) duration by means of priming procedures. A related challenge would be modeling the demand function of brain. Just et al. (1996) demonstrated by functional MRI (fMRI) that brain activity increases with the linguistic complexity of visually presented sentences. Now that 'thinking harder' can be imaged, further work could elucidate the activation basis for emotional work.

The shackles of our new traditions

Modelers, unless they are creating a prototype, hark back to the source they are imitating, and neurocomputational researchers try to emulate brains as more and more is known about them. But artificial life and artificial minds have been launched in their own right, and are developing at an astonishing rate. A survey on the world economy in *The Economist* (1996) notes the 'vertiginous decline in the price of computer-processing power, which has fallen by an average of around 30% a year in real terms over the past couple of decades' (p. 8); '70% of the computer industry's revenues come from products that did not exist two years ago' (p. 10).

It is entirely possible that artificial minds will evolve faster than the 'explosion' in neuroscientific knowledge. The result may be that the evolution of artificial life will branch off from models based on biological minds. Indeed, what is being done in this, the first generation of simulation of mind and its pathology, may be important in determining the models used by future generations. Current models could perhaps be as determinative as earbones from gill arches. The very techniques we use, of error minimization by back-propagation, cyclic updating, and so forth, may achieve such currency that they will be comparable to life's choice of a carbon over a silicon basis, unless we strive to free our computers from traditions that can become as excluding of alternatives as evolution in the biosphere has been. The most difficult creative challenge is to think beyond our traditions.

Closeness to what we do and lack of a perspective threaten to blind us to other possibilities. Even the fact that the students of artificial mind, perhaps less than students of mind generally, are often the students of pathological biological mind, should give us pause. To be sure, many aspects of normal and supernormal function in communication, recognition, locomotion, etc. have attracted neurocomputational research and development. But the emulation of higher and more unifying cortical function tends to be in pursuit of models of derangement. These models include aspects of error and delusion, degrees of signal misapprehension, information or stimulus overload, disorders of drive parameters, bias of the response, etc. Although these are generalizable features of the networks, in our particular usages of them we may overly commandeer them for psychopathological models.

Again and again, the seminal models cited by modelers have been those of Hoffman and Cohen and Servan-Schreiber, whose particular choices for models, though highly heuristic, may by their very strength create traditions that overly influence the development of future models.

Challenges from nonbiology

There are also nonbiological neural networks that are of interest. Let us take, for example, pyramidal neural networks, as described by Bischof (1995). Here, the term pyramidal in the title does not refer to the imitation of an anatomical, bioneural component such as a pyramidal cell, as does, for example, the term cerebellar neural network (Burgin, 1992), which denotes a computational structure that imitates, by a profusion of input-level neurons, the proximal arborization of Purkinje cells to provide for the modeling of coordinated motion control. 'Pyramidal' here refers to image pyramids in computer vision, a technique of reshaping the tractability (number of steps) of visual search through approximating and optimizing the resources devoted to visual processing, dividing and conquering the task by converting global features to local ones and finding regions of interest for guided analysis at low cost in low-resolution images, ignoring irrelevant details. 'An image pyramid tries to combine the advantages of high and low resolution. An image pyramid is a collection of images of a single scene at exponentially decreasing resolutions. The bottom level of the pyramid is the original image. In the simplest case, each successive level of the pyramid is obtained from the previous level by a filtering operation followed by a sampling operator' (Burgin, 1992, p. 20). This involves the localization of visual fields, noting that objects and events are not arbitrarily spread out spatiotemporally, a bioneural feature. Indeed, image pyramids have been noted to be similar to the human visual system by Rosenfeld (see Chapter 1) and others cited in this book. Related to the concept of scale space, each pyramidal cell (except the base level) has a set of children at the input level below, a set of neighbors at the same level, some of whom do not survive stochastic decimation, and a set of parents at the level above. Cell and level in image pyramids correspond to unit and layer in neural networks. The contents of the cell, which may be pixels, edges, grey levels, numbers, or symbolic values, correspond to the activation of units. The bottom-up reduction corresponds to the activation function familiar in neural networks. In sum, the effects of pyramids are impressive, and while they do not particularly derive from the neurology of vision, they may yet help us to understand some of the logical steps necessary for the independent adaptability of human vision and visual attention.

Should the psychiatric modeler eschew all such architectures that do not slavishly follow a bioprototype? Or can we learn from and be stimulated by the seemingly nonphysiological? For one thing, it is not always immediately clear what is a nonbiological mechanism. How, for example, does a pyramidal vision system compare with the neural wiring of an insect's faceted eye? If a given system is getting the job done, perhaps there is some logical, if not anatomic, throwoff. Some version of the artificial vision system may ultimately be implantable in a human nervous system.

We have already seen that some of the least biologically likely materials in the world of physical chemistry, namely metals in the process of annealing, and spin glasses, which are metallic alloys approaching ferromagnetism – frozen paramagnets attempting to line up their molecular poles and become magnets – have deeply impacted the philosophy of mind as it has been expressed in neural networks. Thus, models of minor impurities have been used to discuss jumpstarting the otherwise homogeneous and therefore unstartable elements in a brain's neural net (Forrest, 1996).

Interest in the nonbiological, at the very least, provides a check against parochialism in modeling. We may have the consolation of modeling life elsewhere in the universe, if not the future of life in the universe. We have no idea how diverse life is on other planets, and, in the end, it may not matter. Human–machine hybrids are probable in the not-too-distant future, and our only constraint for that evolution is the limits of mathematical logic.

The challenge of surmountability

Any too facile assumption that the structure of hardware or wetware is function will founder on the demonstrated potentiality that, with sufficient complexity or speed, a thinking apparatus or a brain can surmount its basic structure and, within limits, simulate an entirely different structure as an enclosed mega-object in its software programming. The best example is right before our eyes: the very neural networks we have all been playing with, all of which are simulations on serial digital computers of parallel and netlike processes.

Brains, too, are so complex they also may have similar tricks up their sleeves. For example, we can think like a serial computer. Many of our more obsessive patients try to do this as an emotion-avoiding technique of thought. Information modulation may occur at so many sites of the neuron (dendrites as well as synapses) that a broad range of computational processes is possible. Our brains' functions are so highly dependent on our cultural and educational programming that we may be oblivious to other ways of using them. A simple example is the almost unlimited potential of our minds for rote memorization of series of digits (80 or more) when this is encouraged, and the peculiar way in which the brain accomplishes this by associational chunking. Mathematical and musical memory and thinking may also seem to mimic the serial computer.

The challenge of evolution

It is clear that the evolutionary process is overwhelmingly and exponentially conditioned by its starting points, however ultimately distant from them. To overcome the weight of our own traditions, evolutionary networks could be given the task of searching for things reminiscent of our minds through a much wider domain of possible neurocomputational models for appropriation as artificial brain timber. The fact that the brain is our most evolved organ and that evolution is stamped all over its oddly burgeoning shape should remind us that evolution is intrinsic to all biology. Our brains can be more fully understood as evolving from previous adaptations toward new adaptations to changing selection pressures. In some way, perhaps using genetic algorithms, evolution should be built into our models of brain and psychopathology.

The challenge of normality

The parochialism of modeling pathology leads to aspirations of modeling normality, or the body's attempts to return itself to the homeostatic balance of health. Certainly, pathology is a whole lot simpler than normality, when normality is defined as all the processes that must function to maintain homeostasis and lead the person back to homeostasis from the derangement of disease and disorders. Elsewhere (Forrest, 1994) homologies have been suggested between neuropathologies and robotic mechanopathologies in motoric action systems. Perhaps, in building neural network models, we tend too much to look in the light of obvious deviations for our solutions rather than in the dark where homeostatic processes silently work their restorations.

The search for monkey wrenches is like the search for silver bullets: it rarely pays off a jackpot, easy wins are serendipitous and unanticipated, and it is less a heuristic for full understanding than an edifice of science. A simple thought experiment, relevant to Park's contribution to this volume (see Chapter 4), is to ask what the complete computational modeling of a psychopharmacologic agent would amount to. A program for chlorpromazine or fluoxetine might be very long, incorporating a great deal not yet known, and one might keep finding objections that certain contexts and contingencies of response to its use had been omitted.

From the static to the kinematic to the dynamic

Another consideration in modeling life processes of any kind is the desirability of a progression in our models toward dynamic animation. All that is alive changes, transforms, moves, grows, and is in dynamic conflict and disequilibrium. Our outstar and avalanche neural networks are kinematic in that they are based on formulas that employ lots of 't's for time units and run like an animated movie that allows for a serial output, for example simply to spell out a sequence like the alphabet. This is done by having the travel time between the neurodes be a unit of time and a decay function be two units, so there is an overlap and a stored sequential process (Forrest, 1996, p. 65; see also Chapter 6).

Inherent in the models of the Parallel Distributed Processing (PDP) group (McClelland and Rumelhart, 1988) is an interactive competition that could be a starting point for a model of dynamic conflict: the weighting of attributes in the sorting of many-featured percepts. But a truer model of the dynamic will emerge when the computational entity must enact its conceptualizations against opposing demands, preferably embodied in an ambulatory robot. Old-time science fiction provided us with stationary computers that began to smoke and spark when confronted with irresolvable conflicts of a purely logical nature fed to them by some wily human hero. Or it provided robots that became lost in endless repetitive indecision about a logicomathematical paradox such as Epimenides about the Cretans being liars, Russell's class of all the classes that are not members of themselves, or Zeno's that motion is impossible. This would be comparable to a purely cognitive explanation of content dilemmas in obsessive–compulsive disorder. One way out would be to adduce a reality check function, as Hestenes has discussed (see Chapter 6). In Ludik and Stein's model (see Chapter 9), the modeling of an OCD defect in negative priming, equivalent to impaired cognitive inhibition (increasing the cycle number), is along this line, as is decreasing the gain of the context module. The incorporation of a temporal component makes the model more kinematically lifelike.

Implicit in this multiple neurotransmitter model is the idea, which psychiatry understands better than cognitive psychology, that minds employ drives to override the inevitable mathematical paradoxes of existence and to live practically in the world, which OCD patients find difficult. The modeling of the increased impulsiveness of OCD patients portrays an OCD pathological solution in place of normal emotional thought. The dynamic viewpoint adds to this the realization that once the drives are necessarily brought into play to avoid cognitive paralysis, we are in a dynamic playground of conflicting drives struggling for resolutions which are (to use a Freudian term) always compromise formations. The performance of a computational entity under these conditions will add a poignancy, as in the learned helplessness animal models. Beyond cerebral conflict there is the clash of wants, needs, and drives.

Our new logical beasties, to be properly driven, must have something to lose by erroneous choice. A device even as simple as the recharging of their batteries, if they must struggle for this replenishment against obstacles, prohibitions, time limits or conflicting demands, would be a start. They should be capable of pleasure and pain, unpleasure and relief. And they might also have an affiliative longing, or even a desire, like Commander Data of the television series Star Trek: The Next Generation, to become more human. One of the more intriguing predictions (by Professor Masohiro Mori of the Tokyo Institute of Technology, quoted in Reichardt, 1978) about the eventual development of near-human equivalence in androids is that when they become very close to human resemblance, and not until then, they will engender feelings of creepiness in humans. Brilliant as the modeling of psychopathology is, the reader will probably agree that none of it is creepy yet!

The challenge of complexity and decipherment

Deciphering the decisions of neural networks in the sense of retracing how they arrive at a particular result or decision has always been problematic because of their distributed nature and the very unpredictability and unrepeatability that we value as biologic. Neural networks may decide by a variety of feature criteria and, like humans, by patterns of absences of features. Understanding them is like understanding a person: one has to 'interview' or test them by submitting known test data sets and observing outcomes, or subjecting them to differing conditions and settings. Fully reading them would be like reassembling shredded documents. In Chapter 4, Park discusses nonintuitive results and raises critical issues about the abstractness of neural networks and their degree of falsifiability, which may increase as they are made more explicit.

As the complexity of neural network models increases, the limits of human ability to comprehend may be left in the dust. It is true human processing has not been tested in this way, and our capacity, like our storage for rote memory, may be much greater than we realize, but eventually there will be limits of multiple system interaction that will be beyond us, and better handled by other neural networks. Indeed, this very complexity should be the trump card for neural networks to convert the unpersuaded and unwooed: their use in the thought process of comprehending the fully modeled thought process. Like all computer systems, the totality of the neural system is greater than the system's ability to self-report, or to identify with as a self-concept. In other words, in neural modeling, we have met the adversary and it is not us, or not entirely us.

The challenge of mathematical limits

It is sobering to consider that the complete modeling of a human being, even in the prospect of exponential growth in computational capacity, will not be soon. A physicist (Krauss, 1995, pp. 76–8) has estimated the information encoded in the human body, specifying the conditions of each of our 10^{28} atoms, as 10^{28} kilobytes. All the information in all the books ever written would take 10^{12} kilobytes – 16 orders of magnitude less. Stacked 10-gigabyte hard disks storing one human would reach a third of the way to the center of the galaxy. At the fastest digital transfer rate of 100 megabytes per second, it would take 2000 times the present age of the universe of 10 billion years to write the data of a human pattern to tape. Krauss (1995, p. 78) estimates that at the current progress of computers' improvement in storage and speed by a factor of 100 each decade, the task of recording a human will not be possible for another 210 years. Or should I say *only* 210 years?

The challenge of the quantum level

The concept of multiple scales in the understanding of mind has been pushed to the quantum level in a collection of papers edited by Pribram and King (1995). Beginning with Searle's listing of features of consciousness, including subjectivity, unity, intentionality, attention, Gestalt, familiarity, mood, and situatedness, the opening papers contend that the comprehensive, unified and instantaneous properties of consciousness and memory do not seem, to a number of our best scientific thinkers, to be accounted for by our neurotransmitter theories alone.

In the model of consciousness proposed by Stuart Hameroff and Roger Penrose (1995), there is an 'orchestrated reduction of quantum coherence' in brain microtubules. Cytoskeletal microtubules are hollow cylinders, 25 nm in diameter and of varying length, comprised of 13 longitudinal protofilaments, each of which is a series of subunit proteins known as tubulins. These microtubules mediate the delicate quantum effects proposed to exist within the 'wild, wet and noisy' brain. How this occurs is that subunits of microtubules undergo coherent conformational excitations when energy is supplied by the surrounding 'heat bath.' The metaphor that comes to mind is the moving border of lights on old-fashioned movie marquees. The stationary bulbs can be either on or off, and, when coherent, the emergent pattern of stripes seems to move. This takes on the aspects of a quantum computer, and can self-collapse, a quality suitable for consciousness.

Hameroff and Penrose continue (King and Pribram, 1995, p. 253): 'by considering only classical computing and local neighbor interactions, microtubule automata fail to address the problematic features of consciousness for which quantum theory holds promise.' What consciousness is, is still stranger. When the degree of mass–energy difference leads to sufficient separation of space–time geometry, the system must choose and decay (reduce, collapse) to a single universe state, thus preventing 'multiple universes' (e.g., Wheeler, 1957). In this way, a transient superposition of slightly differing space–time geometries persists until an abrupt quantum to classical reduction occurs and one or the other is chosen.

Quantum coherence in microtubules is theoretically prevented by anesthesia, slowed in dreaming, and speeded up in altered states and heightened experience. In quantum physics, such states are called Bose–Einstein condensates (BEC), which were proposed in 1924 and have received much attention lately, being named 1995 Molecule of the Year by Science (Bloom, 1995; Culotta, 1995). The suggestion is that BEC are responsible for the rapid, holistic, global properties of thought, consciousness, and subjectivity. Amoroso and Martin (King and Pribram, 1995, pp. 351–77) bring from California the thought that 'reality as it were surfs on a standing wave of spacetime' (p. 365). They present a list of 21 'mentons' (p. 354), or quanta possibly related to mind, of which the ions we are used to considering are only one class. The quantum level has been breached, and the computational modeling of mental phenomena must eventually enter it. What remains as a further challenge is to decide what is the relevant scale for each psychopathology, although there may be perturbations on several levels.

The challenge of the narrative

In their approach to delusional thinking in Chapter 8, Vinogradov, Poole and Willis-Shore discuss Hoffmann and McGlashan's (1993) linking of reduced synaptic density and excessive axonal pruning in schizophrenia to a loss of control of narrative memory. In Chapter 10, Lloyd concludes from his neural net simulation of Freud's case of Lucy R. that psychopathology is a narrative, not simple cause and effect but a scientifically demonstrable network of events leading to a complex outcome. Narrative is no simple stringing together in a sequence. Roemer (1995), for example, has discussed the concepts of fate, deriving from Greek sources, and individual freedom in narratives from ancient drama to television, arguing against the deconstructivist idea that our deeds, perceptions, and experience are structured by culture. The contradictions and conflicts that Roemer finds arising from the problems of narrative challenge our concepts with their complexity and passions. Ultimately, our models need to account for the brain as a storymaking mechanism.

The challenge of intersubjectivity

Individual psychodynamic approaches to the theory of mind are currently undergoing a refocusing in psychoanalytic circles. The interpersonal model first proposed by Sullivan (1953) is considered more explanatory of the psychotherapeutic process, especially when interacting mental processes are construed in full intrapersonal psychodynamic richness. Lloyd's 'Lucynet' for Freud's Lucy R. (see Chapter 10) is not intersubjective, but there would seem to be no obstacle to incorporating the subjective experiences of the others in her story, if they were known. Neural nets could potentially simulate dyadic couple dynamics, and family or small group dynamics, especially if they focused on affective and transference phenomena.

When the author was engaged in training international psychiatric residents, he decided to present videotapes of patients for an exercise in calibrating affect perception and description. An intrapsychic model would have required extended soliloquies of the patients, speaking into a video camera, and the author elected to employ 3–5-minute samples of videotapes with psychiatrists. It is interesting that when these were scored from 0–4+ points for the six basic objects – joy, fear, anger, shame, guilt, and sadness – and the results averaged, groups of only 20 upward would agree with other groups within a few tenths of a point, whether the groups were of a particular nationality (e.g., Indian) or region in the United States where the author had gone to give the exercise as a grand rounds at various psychiatry departments. The point is that inter-personal processes can have a certain quantitative purity, and all science does not have to stop at the boundary of the cerebral membranes. When brain and mind are considered as information, the flow between brains may be considered similarly to chip allocation, porting, and display problems in computation.

Humans are social animals, and our well-being is frequently linked to the well-being of small identificatory groups with whom we have a relation of heterostasis (Forrest, 1997), a homeostatic process relying upon others. The eventual social limits of neural modeling, from dyadic relationships to anthropology, are yet to be explored. Larger-scale human interaction science, like predicting the weather, could employ the mathematics of chaos and assemble results from multiple model runs (Kerr, 1996), and will eventually be advanced by the further development of computer power.

The teleology of artificial mind

Much of this book has focused on modeling as it relates to practical clinical issues. This concluding section addresses some of the more speculative issues currently being raised about computational science. Like Moravec (1988), Tipler (1994) calculates that the next stage of intelligent life is information-processing machines. Taking issue with the ideas of Freeman Dyson (1979), Tipler (1994) argues: 'using the standard physics measure of complexity, it is possible for an infinite amount of complexity to be produced, and hence an infinite amount of subjective time, between now and the collapse of the universe.' This is because 'the total energy diverges to infinity, so there is plenty for everybody.' The physics for this assertion is provided.

Eventually, conscious intelligence will sweep the spatial universe. Our current bodies implemented in matter (p. 242) could not survive the final singularity's extreme heat, but a computer simulation could. Tipler argues that 'the drive for total knowledge' (p. 219) and for the re-creation of all past lives is inevitable in the eschaton (last times); we humans shall be emulated in the unlimited capacity of the computers of the far future. The best way to immortalize any past human's quantum state (at the moment of death) is to generate all 10 to the 10th to the 70th possible humans, who will be brought to life with their children and familiar environment (p. 224). Of course, people will be emulated who never lived.

One of the obsessive delights of Tipler's book is his use of the power of double exponents to determine and put a number on the farthest limits of human possibility. We learn that if we have 10 000 genes, it is possible for them to code 10 to the 10th to the 6th power genetically distinct human beings. We could resurrect all humans merely by simulating the finite number of possible life forms that could be coded by DNA. The human brain can store about 2^{17} informational bits, and there would be 2 to the 10th to the 17th possible human memories.

The lens of physics allows Tipler to say fresh things about some of the most difficult problems of theology. It does not require a great deal of imagination to realize that, even short of ultimate teleology, the philosophical bases of psychiatry as a science of mind are even now beginning to be affected by projections of computer potentiality, and the present book on neural network simulations of psychopathology is one example. Tipler's book is good natured and leaves one with a feeling between exhilaration and hope. Viewed from the future – a future of human-engendered artificial intelligence – the predictions of the universal expansion of mind may become classics beside early attempts, like the present volume, to computerize the intimate psychiatric agonies of the human spirit.

References

Bischof, H. (1995). *Pyramidal Neural Networks*. Hillsdale, NJ: Lawrence Erlbaum.

Bloom, F.E. (1995). Molecule of the Year 1995. *Science*, **270**, 1901.

Burgin, G. (1992). Using cerebellar arithmetic computers. *AI Expert*, **June**, 32–41.

Culotta, E. (1995). A new form of matter unveiled. *Science*, **270**, 1902–03.

Dennett, D.C. (1996). *Kinds of Minds: Towards an Understanding of Consciousness*. London: Weidenfeld & Nicolson.

Dyson, F. (1979). Time without end: physics and biology in an open universe. *Reviews of Modern Physics*, **51**, 447–60.

The Economist. Survey of world economy: The hitchhiker's guide to cybernomics. Insert, Sept. 28, 46 pp.

Forrest, D.V. (1994). Mind, brain and machine: action and creation. *Journal of the American Academy of Psychoanalysis*, **22**(1), 29–56.

Forrest, D.V. (1996). Artificial mind: the promise of neural networks. *Journal of the Indian Psychoanalytical Society*, **49**, 45–72.

Forrest, D.V. (1997). Psychotherapy of patients with neuropsychiatric disorders. In *American Psychiatric Press Textbook of Neuropsychiatry*, 3rd edition, ed. R.E. Hales & S.C. Yudofsky, pp. 983–1017. Washington, DC: American Psychiatric Press.

Gray, C.M. & McCormick, D.A. (1996). Chattering cells: Superficial pyramidal neurons contributing to the generation of synchronous oscillations in the visual cortex. *Science*, **274**, 109–13.

Greenwald, A.G., Draine, S.C. & Abrams, R.L. (1996). Three cognitive markers of unconscious semantic activation. *Science*, **273**, 1699–707.

Hameroff, S. & Penrose, R. (1995). Orchestrated reduction of quantum coherence in brain microtubules: a model for consciousness. In *Scale in Conscious Experience: is the Brain too important to be left to Specialists to Study?*, ed. J. King & K.H. Pribram, pp. 271–4. Hillsdale, NJ: Lawrence Erlbaum.

Hoffman, R.E. & McGlashan, T.H. (1993). Parallel distributed processing and the emergence of schizophrenic symptoms. *Schizophrenia Bulletin*, **19**(1), 119–40.

Just, M.A., Carpenter, P.A., Keller, T.A., Eddy, W.F. & Thulborn, K.R. (1996). Brain activation modulated by sentence comprehension. *Science*, **274**, 114–16.

Kerr, R.A. (1996). Weather forecasting: Budgets stall but forecasts jump forward. *Science*, **273**, 1658–9.

King, J. & Pribram, K.H., eds. (1995). *Scale in Conscious Experience: is the Brain too important to be left to Specialists to Study?* Hillsdale, NJ: Lawrence Erlbaum.

Krauss, L.M. (1995). *The Physics of Star Trek*. New York: Basic Books.

McClelland, J.L. & Rumelhart, D.E. (1988). *Explorations in Parallel Distributed Processing: a Handbook of Models, Programs and Exercises*. Cambridge, MA: MIT Press.

Moravec, H. (1988). *Mind Children: The Future of Robot and Human Intelligence*. Cambridge, MA: Harvard University Press.

Reichardt, J. (1978). *Robots: Fact, Fiction and Prediction*. Harmondsworth: Penguin.

Roemer, M. (1995). *Telling Stories: Postmodernism and the Invalidation of Traditional Narrative*. Lanham, MD: Rowman and Littlefield.

Sejnowski, T.J. (1997). The year of the dendrite. *Science*, **275**, 178–9.

Sullivan, H.S. (1953). *The Interpersonal Theory of Psychiatry*. New York: WW Norton.

Tipler, F.J. (1994). *The Physics of Immortality*. New York: Anchor/Doubleday.

Wheeler, J.A. (1957). Assessment of Everett's 'relative state' formulation of quantum theory. *Reviews of Modern Physics*, **29**, 463–5.

Yu, A.C. & Margolish, D. (1996). Temporal hierarchical control of singing in birds. *Science*, **273**, 1871–5.

Index

Note: **bold** page numbers indicate illustrations